Translational Multimodality Optical Imaging

Artech House Series
Bioinformatics & Biomedical Imaging

Series Editors
Stephen T. C. Wong, The Methodist Hospital and Weill Cornell Medical College
Guang-Zhong Yang, Imperial College

Advances in Diagnostic and Therapeutic Ultrasound Imaging, Jasjit S. Suri, Chirinjeev Kathuria, Ruey-Feng Chang, Filippo Molinari, and Aaron Fenster, editors

Biological Database Modeling, Jake Chen and Amandeep S. Sidhu, editors

Biomedical Informatics in Translational Research, Hai Hu, Michael Liebman, and Richard Mural

Genome Sequencing Technology and Algorithms, Sun Kim, Haixu Tang, and Elaine R. Mardis, editors

Life Science Automation Fundamentals and Applications, Mingjun Zhang, Bradley Nelson, and Robin Felder, editors

Microscopic Image Analysis for Life Science Applications, Jens Rittscher, Stephen T. C. Wong, and Raghu Machiraju, editors

Next Generation Artificial Vision Systems: Reverse Engineering the Human Visual System, Maria Petrou and Anil Bharath, editors

Systems Bioinformatics: An Engineering Case-Based Approach, Gil Alterovitz and Marco F. Ramoni, editors

Text Mining for Biology and Biomedicine, Sophia Ananiadou and John McNaught, editors

Translational Multimodality Optical Imaging, Fred S. Azar and Xavier Intes, editors

Translational Multimodality Optical Imaging

Fred S. Azar
Xavier Intes
Editors

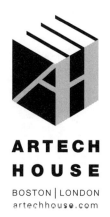

ARTECH
HOUSE

BOSTON | LONDON
artechhouse.com

Library of Congress Cataloging-in-Publication Data
A catalog record for this book is available from the U.S. Library of Congress.

British Library Cataloguing in Publication Data
A catalogue record for this book is available from the British Library.

ISBN-13: 978-1-59693-307-1

Cover design by Yekaterina Ratner

© 2008 ARTECH HOUSE, INC.
685 Canton Street
Norwood, MA 02062

All rights reserved. Printed and bound in the United States of America. No part of this book may be reproduced or utilized in any form or by any means, electronic or mechanical, including photocopying, recording, or by any information storage and retrieval system, without permission in writing from the publisher.

All terms mentioned in this book that are known to be trademarks or service marks have been appropriately capitalized. Artech House cannot attest to the accuracy of this information. Use of a term in this book should not be regarded as affecting the validity of any trademark or service mark.

10 9 8 7 6 5 4 3 2 1

DISCLAIMER OF WARRANTY

The technical descriptions, procedures, and computer programs in this book have been developed with the greatest of care and they have been useful to the author in a broad range of applications; however, they are provided as is, without warranty of any kind. Artech House, Inc. and the author and editors of the book titled *Translational Multimodality Optical Imaging* make no warranties, expressed or implied, that the equations, programs, and procedures in this book or its associated software are free of error, or are consistent with any particular standard of merchantability, or will meet your requirements for any particular application. They should not be relied upon for solving a problem whose incorrect solution could result in injury to a person or loss of property. Any use of the programs or procedures in such a manner is at the user's own risk. The editors, author, and publisher disclaim all liability for direct, incidental, or consequent damages resulting from use of the programs or procedures in this book or the associated software.

Contents

Foreword   xv
Preface   xvii

CHAPTER 1
Introduction to Clinical Optical Imaging   1

1.1 Introduction   1
1.2 Tissue Optics   2
    1.2.1 Scattering   2
    1.2.2 Raman Scattering   3
    1.2.3 Absorption   3
    1.2.4 Fluorescence   4
1.3 Light Propagation   6
    1.3.1 Fundamentals   6
    1.3.2 Forward Model   7
1.4 Multimodality Imaging   9
    1.4.1 A Brief History of Clinical Multimodality Imaging   9
    1.4.2 Multimodality Optical Imaging   10
1.5 Conclusions   13
    References   13

CHAPTER 2
In Vivo Microscopy   19

2.1 Introduction   19
2.2 Confocal Microscopy   20
2.3 Endoscope-Compatible Systems   20
2.4 MKT Cellvizio-GI   23
2.5 Dual-Axes Confocal Microscope   25
2.6 Molecular Imaging   27
    References   30

CHAPTER 3
Endoscopy   33

3.1 Introduction   33
3.2 Point-Probe Spectroscopy Techniques   33
    3.2.1 Scattering Spectroscopy   34
    3.2.2 Fluorescence Spectroscopy   36
    3.2.3 Raman Spectroscopy   38

		3.2.4	Multimodality Spectroscopy	38
3.3	Wide-Field Imaging			39
		3.3.1	Fluorescence Imaging	39
		3.3.2	Molecular Imaging	41
		3.3.3	Chromoendoscopy	42
		3.3.4	Narrowband Imaging	43
		3.3.5	Multimodality Wide-Field Imaging	43
3.4	Cross-Sectional Imaging			44
		3.4.1	Endoscopic Optical Coherence Tomography	44
		3.4.2	Ultrahigh-Resolution OCT (UHROCT)	45
		3.4.3	Three-Dimensional OCT	46
		3.4.4	Multimodality Imaging with OCT	47
3.5	Summary			51
	Acknowledgments			51
	References			51

CHAPTER 4
Diffuse Optical Techniques: Instrumentation — 59

4.1 Introduction: Deterministic "Diffuse" Detection of Probabilistic Photon Propagation — 59
4.2 Methods of Differentiating the Origin of Diffuse Photons — 60
    4.2.1 The Source-Encoding Requirement in DOT — 61
    4.2.2 Methods of Source Encoding and Detector Decoding for Diffuse Optical Tomography — 62
4.3 Techniques of Decoupling the Absorption and Scattering Contributions to the Photon Remission — 65
    4.3.1 Time-Domain Detection — 66
    4.3.2 Frequency-Domain Detection — 68
    4.3.3 Continuous-Wave Detection — 70
4.4 Principles of Determining the Heterogeneity of Optical Properties — 70
    4.4.1 Tomographic Image Reconstruction and Prior Utilization — 70
    4.4.2 Diffuse Optical Tomography Imaging in the Context of Multimodality Imaging — 73
4.5 Novel Approaches in Instrumentation of Diffuse Optical Tomography: Source Spectral Encoding — 76
    4.5.1 Discrete Spectral Encoding by Use of Multiple Laser Diodes — 76
    4.5.2 Imaging Examples of Spectral-Encoding Rapid NIR Tomography — 78
    4.5.3 Spread Spectral Encoding by Use of Single Wideband Light Source — 80
    4.5.4 Light Sources for Spread Spectral Encoding — 81
    4.5.5 Characteristics of Spread Spectral Encoding — 82
    4.5.6 Hemodynamic Imaging by Spread-Spectral-Encoding NIR Tomography — 84
4.6 Novel Approaches in Instrumentation of Diffuse Optical Tomography: Transrectal Applicator — 85
    4.6.1 Transrectal Applicator for Transverse DOT Imaging — 86
    4.6.2 Transrectal Applicator for Sagittal DOT Imaging — 88

4.7	Potential Directions of Instrumentation for Diffuse Optical Measurements	93
4.8	Conclusions	94
	Acknowledgments	94
	References	94

CHAPTER 5
Multimodal Diffuse Optical Tomography: Theory — 101

5.1	Introduction	101
5.2	Diffuse Optical Tomography	102
	5.2.1 The Forward Problem and Linearization	103
	5.2.2 Inverse Problem	106
5.3	Multimodality Reconstruction: Review of Previous Work	108
5.4	Multimodality Priors and Regularization	111
	5.4.1 Structural Priors	111
	5.4.2 Regularization Using Mutual Information	113
5.5	Conclusions	119
	Acknowledgments	119
	References	120

CHAPTER 6
Diffuse Optical Spectroscopy with Magnetic Resonance Imaging — 125

6.1	Introduction	125
6.2	Anatomical Imaging	126
6.3	Combining Hemodynamic Measures of MRI and Optical Imaging	128
6.4	MRI-Guided Optical Imaging Reconstruction Techniques	131
6.5	Other MR-Derived Contrast and Optical Imaging	133
6.6	Hardware Challenges to Merging Optical and MRI	134
6.7	Optical/MR Contrast Agents	135
6.8	Outlook for MR-Optical Imaging	136
	References	136

CHAPTER 7
Software Platforms for Integration of Diffuse Optical Imaging and Other Modalities — 141

7.1	Introduction	141
	7.1.1 A Platform for Diffuse Optical Tomography	141
	7.1.2 A Platform for Diffuse Optical Spectroscopy	142
7.2	Imaging Platform Technologies	143
	7.2.1 Multimodal Imaging Workflow for DOT Applications	143
	7.2.2 3D-DOT/3D-MRI Image-Registration Algorithm	144
	7.2.3 Breast MRI Image Segmentation	151
	7.2.4 Image-Based Guidance Workflow and System for DOS Applications	152
7.3	Computing the Accuracy of a Guidance and Tracking System	153
	7.3.1 Global Accuracy of the System	153
	7.3.2 Motion Tracking	154

7.4	Application to Nonconcurrent MRI and DOT Data of Human Subjects	155
7.5	Conclusion	157
	Acknowledgments	158
	References	158
	Selected Bibliography	162

CHAPTER 8
Diffuse Optical Spectroscopy in Breast Cancer: Coregistration with MRI and Predicting Response to Neoadjuvant Chemotherapy — 163

8.1	Introduction	163
8.2	Coregistration with MRI	164
	8.2.1 Materials and Methods	164
	8.2.2 Results	167
	8.2.3 Discussion	175
8.3	Monitoring and Predicting Response to Breast Cancer Neoadjuvant Chemotherapy	176
	8.3.1 Materials and Methods	176
	8.3.2 Results	177
	8.3.3 Discussion	180
8.4	Summary and Conclusions	181
	Acknowledgments	182
	References	182

CHAPTER 9
Optical Imaging and X-Ray Imaging — 185

9.1	Introduction	185
	9.1.1 Current Clinical Approach to Breast Cancer Screening and Diagnosis	185
	9.1.2 The Importance of Fusing Function and Structural Information	186
	9.1.3 Recent Advances in DOT for Imaging Breast Cancer	187
9.2	Instrumentation and Methods	188
	9.2.1 Tomographic Optical Breast-Imaging System and Tomosynthesis	188
	9.2.2 3D Forward Modeling and Nonlinear Image Reconstruction	190
	9.2.3 Simultaneous Image Reconstruction with Calibration Coefficient Estimation	190
	9.2.4 Utilizing Spectral Prior and Best Linear Unbiased Estimator	191
	9.2.5 Utilizing Spatial Prior from Tomosynthesis Image	192
9.3	Clinical Trial of TOBI/DBT Imaging System	192
	9.3.1 Image Reconstruction of Healthy Breasts	193
	9.3.2 Imaging Breasts with Tumors or Benign Lesions	193
	9.3.3 Region-of-Interest Analysis	194
9.4	Dynamic Imaging of Breast Under Mechanical Compression	194
	9.4.1 Experiment Setup	194
	9.4.2 Tissue Dynamic from Healthy Subjects	195

	9.4.3 Contact Pressure Map Under Compression	197
9.5	Conclusions	198
	References	199

CHAPTER 10
Diffuse Optical Imaging and PET Imaging — 205

10.1	Introduction	205
10.2	Positron Emission Tomography (PET)	207
	10.2.1 PET Fundamentals	207
	10.2.2 PET Image Reconstruction	208
	10.2.3 PET Instrumentation	209
10.3	Diffuse Optical Imaging (DOI)	210
	10.3.1 DOI Instrumentation	210
	10.3.2 DOI Image Reconstruction	211
10.4	Fluorescence Diffuse Optical Imaging (FDOI)	212
10.5	Clinical Observations	214
	10.5.1 Whole-Body PET and DOI	214
	10.5.2 Breast-Only PET and DOI	216
	10.5.3 ICG Fluorescence	216
10.6	Summary	219
	Acknowledgments	220
	References	220

CHAPTER 11
Photodynamic Therapy — 225

11.1	Introduction	225
11.2	Basics of PDT	227
11.3	Superficial Applications	230
11.4	PDT in Body Cavities	231
11.5	PDT for Solid Tumors	233
11.6	Delivery and Monitoring of PDT	235
11.7	The Future of PDT and Imaging	236
	Acknowledgments	236
	References	236

CHAPTER 12
Optical Phantoms for Multimodality Imaging — 241

12.1	Introduction	241
12.2	Absorption and Scatter Phantom Composition	242
12.3	Typical Tissue Phantoms for Multimodal and Optical Imaging	245
	12.3.1 Hydrogel-Based Phantoms	245
	12.3.2 Polyester Resin and RTV Silicone Phantoms	249
	12.3.3 Aqueous Suspension Phantoms	251
12.4	Conclusions	253
	Acknowledgments	254
	References	254

CHAPTER 13

Intraoperative Near-Infrared Fluorescent Imaging Exogenous Fluorescence Contrast Agents — 259

13.1 Introduction — 259
13.2 Unmet Medical Needs Addressed by Intraoperative NIR Fluorescence Imaging — 259
  13.2.1 Improving Long-Term Efficacy of Primary Treatment — 260
  13.2.2 Reducing the Rate of Complications — 261
13.3 Imaging Considerations — 262
  13.3.1 Contrast Media — 262
  13.3.2 Tissue Penetration Depth — 263
  13.3.3 Autofluorescence — 265
  13.3.4 Optical Design Considerations — 265
  13.3.5 Excitation — 267
  13.3.6 Collection Optics and Emission Filtering — 267
  13.3.7 Detectors — 268
13.4 Future Outlook — 268
References — 269

CHAPTER 14

Clinical Studies in Optical Imaging: An Industry Perspective — 275

14.1 Introduction — 275
14.2 Breast Cancer — 276
14.3 Optical Breast-Imaging Technology — 277
14.4 Development Process — 277
  14.4.1 Product Definition — 278
  14.4.2 Clinical Indication — 279
  14.4.3 Target Markets — 280
  14.4.4 Regulatory Risk Classification — 282
  14.4.5 General Device Description — 282
  14.4.6 Design Control — 285
14.5 Clinical Trials and Results — 286
  14.5.1 Clinical Plan — 286
  14.5.2 Pilot Studies — 286
  14.5.3 Tissue-Characterization Trials — 287
14.6 Conclusions — 294
Acknowledgments — 294
References — 295

CHAPTER 15

Regulation and Regulatory Science for Optical Imaging — 299

15.1 Introduction — 299
15.2 Fundamental Concepts in Medical Device Regulation — 300
  15.2.1 Premarket and Postmarket — 301
  15.2.2 Safety — 301
  15.2.3 Effectiveness — 301
  15.2.4 Risk Evaluation — 301

		15.2.5	Labeling	302
		15.2.6	Standards	302
	15.3	Medical Device Regulation Throughout the World		302
		15.3.1	International Harmonization of Medical Device Regulation	303
	15.4	FDA Background		304
		15.4.1	FDA Mission	304
		15.4.2	FDA History and Authorizing Legislation	304
		15.4.3	Organizational Structure of the FDA	305
	15.5	Overview of FDA Regulations		305
		15.5.1	Classification	307
		15.5.2	Early Premarket Interactions	310
		15.5.3	Premarket Submissions	311
		15.5.4	Postmarket Issues	312
		15.5.5	Combination Products and Contrast Agents	313
		15.5.6	Regulatory Submission Aids	313
		15.5.7	Good Practices	314
	15.6	Regulatory Science: Optical Safety Hazards		315
		15.6.1	Photochemical Damage	316
		15.6.2	Photosensitivity	318
		15.6.3	Photothermal Effects	318
		15.6.4	Photomechanical Damage	320
	15.7	Conclusions		322
		Acknowledgments		322
		References		322

CHAPTER 16

Emerging Optical Imaging Technologies: Contrast Agents — 327

16.1	Introduction		327
16.2	Optical Probes		328
	16.2.1	Fluorophores as Contrast Agents for Optical Imaging	328
	16.2.2	Fluorophore Conjugates for Targeting and Activation	330
	16.2.3	Fluorescent Nanoparticles	331
16.3	Multimodality Probes for Optical Imaging		332
	16.3.1	Probes for Optical Imaging and MRI	332
	16.3.2	Probes for Optical Imaging and SPECT/PET	335
	16.3.3	Probes for Optical Imaging and Therapy	336
16.4	Summary and Conclusions		337
	References		337

CHAPTER 17

Emerging Optical Imaging Techniques: Fluorescence Molecular Tomography and Beyond — 343

17.1	Introduction		343
17.2	From Planar Imaging to Tomography		344
	17.2.1	Prerequisites	344
	17.2.2	Bioluminescence and Fluorescence Imaging	345
	17.2.3	Data-Collection Modes	345

17.3	Fluorescence Molecular Tomography	347
	17.3.1 Hardware Development	347
	17.3.2 Image Reconstruction	349
	17.3.3 Intrinsic Resolution Limits	350
17.4	FMT-Derived Imaging Modalities	351
	17.4.1 Noncontact FMT	351
	17.4.2 Fluorescent Protein Tomography	351
	17.4.3 Mesoscopic Fluorescence Tomography	353
	17.4.4 Further Developments	354
17.5	Photoacoustic Tomography	355
	17.5.1 Photoacoustic Theory	356
	17.5.2 Combined FMT-PAT Imaging	357
17.6	Summary	357
	References	359

CHAPTER 18
From Benchtop to Boardroom: Staying Market Focused — 363

18.1	Identify the Market	363
18.2	Technology Alone Has Little Value	364
18.3	Find a Business Mentor	365
18.4	Tell a Story Using the Right Terms	365
18.5	Focus Is the Key	366
18.6	Build Value	367
18.7	Conclusions	367
	References	368

About the Editors	369
List of Contributors	371
Index	375

Foreword

The novel field of NIR spectroscopy and imaging began with the work of Glenn Millikan, who applied photoelectric methods to the kinetics of the reaction of oxygen and myoglobin, superceding the hemoglobin studies of Hartridge and Roughton. The 1935 ear oxymeter of Karl Matthes, the father of oximetry, was the first clinical quantitative application of optics to tissues. Applications such as Millikan's aviation ear oxymeter during World War II with lightweight and practical instrumentation followed shortly thereafter, establishing optical spectrophotometry as an invaluable functional monitoring tool. Since then, pulse oximeters have become a staple clinical tool in numerous areas such as emergency medicine, anesthesia, postoperative recovery, endoscopy, dentistry and oral surgery, sleep apnea, neonatology, and others.

Along parallel lines, in the late 1920s, Cutler generated "shadowgrams" of human breast cancer without regard to tissue scattering. Even if the concept fell into desuetude for a while due to patient discomfort associated with skin overheating and low sensitivity specificity due to scattering blurring, this concept presaged much of the current work. With the advent of new optical sources and detectors, the field of optical mammography regained strength and led to multispectral transillumination systems in the 1980s, though the clinical evaluation of dual-wavelength systems demonstrated a marginal contribution over mammography and an undesirable number of false positives due to the lack of quantitative light propagation models.

The field soon attracted the attention of physicists following the demonstration of absorption separation and scattering in studies by Patterson and Yodh, using time and phase resolution of photon propagation in tissues. The development of new software for quantification has been an intense field of research with tremendous success in the past two decades. However, such studies underlined some of the inherent weaknesses of optical imaging and led to the consideration of complementing optical techniques with information derived from other imaging modalities.

Following the pioneer work at University of Pennsylvania, the fusion of the optical technique with well-established clinical modalities blossomed. The flexibility of optical techniques, their relative low costs, and the unique set of information provided enable software and/or hardware fusion. The potential of multimodality optical imaging has been widely demonstrated for optical mammography and, to a lesser extent, with brain functional imaging. This active area of research and development is growing rapidly with an exceptionally bright future in sight.

Academic achievements were not unnoticed by the industrial community. Giants such as GE, Phillips, and Siemens formed in-house teams to evaluate the potential of optical techniques in the 1990s. With numerous small and mid-size companies striving to develop optical-based clinical systems, this industrial impetus has grown steadily in the last decade. Developing optical products for clinical use is a challenging task regulated by ISO 13485 and the FDA. For instance, in 1991, the U.S. Food and Drug Administration (FDA) Obstetrics and Gynecology Devices Panel recommended that breast transilluminators be classified as Class III devices and that premarket approval (PMA) would be required to allow the distribution and use of transilluminators in the United States. In 1994, the FDA classified breast illuminators as Class III devices, thus mandating that a PMA be submitted and approved prior to commercial distribution of this device.

As history teaches us, the effort to establish optical techniques as clinical modalities is a long and treacherous path. The stringent regulatory constraints and specific technical challenges associated with optical techniques make the transition from bench to clinical product arduous.

This is the first book to provide an expert and timely comprehensive overview of the present and future outlook of clinical multimodality optical imaging from the academic to the industrial perspective. Written by pioneers in the field, it will become a useful reference to clinicians, nonclinicians, researchers, scientists, educators, and students alike.

Britton Chance
Eldridge Reeves Johnson
University Professor Emeritus of
Biophysics, Physical Chemistry,
and Radiological Physics
Philadelphia, Pennsylvania
September 2008

Preface

Translational Research

In 2002, the NIH began a process of charting a road map for medical research in the twenty-first century [1] in order to identify gaps and opportunities in biomedical research. A key initiative that came out of this review was an effort to strengthen translational research.

Translational research is pushing a fundamental change in the way that science has operated for decades, bridging the gaps that separate basic scientists and clinical researchers. To improve human health, scientific discoveries must be translated into practical applications. Such discoveries typically begin at "the bench" with basic research, in which scientists study disease at a molecular or cellular level, and then progress to the clinical level, or the patient's "bedside." Translational research has the potential to significantly improve clinical trials and to transform fundamental discoveries from the lab, clinic, or population into specific products or interventions ready for human testing [2].

Translational research faces three major challenges. The first challenge is to ensure that the most promising and important discoveries are identified and moved forward into development. The second challenge is to ensure that these discoveries advance through the multidisciplinary, goal-oriented development process as efficiently as possible. The third challenge is to ensure a smooth and timely transition between early translational research and late-stage human trials, product commercialization, and dissemination among communities [2]. The position of translational research in the medical devices evolution cycle is depicted in Figure P.1.

Optical Imaging

Optical imaging technologies, which exploit the physics of optical propagation in tissue, may add many important advantages to the imaging options currently available to physicians and researchers. Optical methods may offer low-cost imaging systems based on robust physical principles. They are fast and nonionizing and have the capacity of offering excellent signal-to-noise capabilities. The time resolution of the biophysical processes monitored span the range from femto-seconds to multiday longitudinal studies, and spatial resolutions span from subcellular, micro- to mesostructural anatomy up to organ level features. Optical imaging and spectroscopy technologies may provide dynamic molecular, structural, and functional imaging with the potential to expand clinical opportunities for screening, early disease

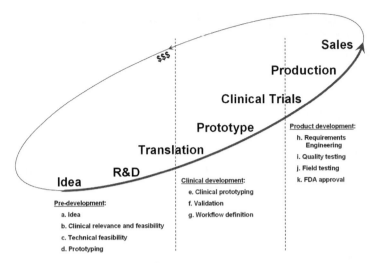

Figure P.1 Medical devices evolution cycle.

detection, diagnosis, image-guided intervention, safer therapy, and monitoring of therapeutic response. Furthermore, optical imaging technologies are unobtrusive enough that they may be efficiently combined with established imaging modalities, and yield significant decreases in patient morbidity (examples of combinations are optical/MRI and optical/ultrasound). These unique sets of features position optical techniques as one of the most promising new clinical modalities with a major impact on clinical research, clinical care, and drug development.

A Case Example of Translational Optical Imaging: The Network for Translational Research in Optical Imaging

The NCI-funded Network for Translational Research: Optical Imaging (NTROI) [3, 4] was started in 2002 and lasted five years to support four multisite teams, including broad national and international representation from academia, NIH intramural, and device and drug industry investigators. The broad goals of the NTROI, as defined by the steering committee, were to develop validated optical platforms that address oncology clinical needs, to develop IT solutions for standardizing data collection and analysis across different platforms, to formulate the role of optical imaging for drug discovery, response, and localized delivery, and finally, to plan the building of standardized prototypes for multisite clinical trials.

The network recognized the need for standards in development and cross-validation of new academic optical modalities. The NTROI worked to establish pathology standards for assessing the predictability of novel optical technologies and created informatics solutions to standardize both data collection and analysis across different imaging platforms, with the help of the industrial partners. Figure P.2 describes the broad goals of the industry to facilitate translation to the clinic.

In the end, the tight and structured collaboration of academic and industry partners has enabled optical imaging research prototypes to be significantly improved and ready for clinical trials by decreasing diagnostic uncertainty (improving reliabil-

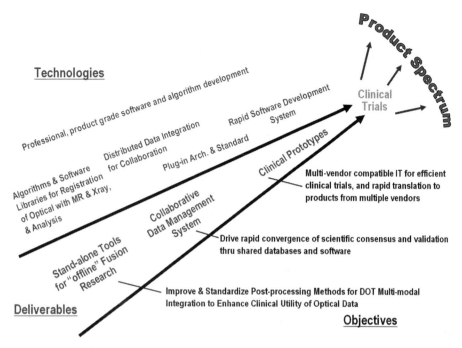

Figure P.2 Broad objectives of the industry to facilitate translation to the clinic.

ity, repeatability of measurements over time, minimizing operator error), validating the imaging technologies, comparing/combining the optical imaging technologies with orthogonal imaging approaches (e.g., MRI), and personalizing the workflows to benefit the patient. The lessons learned from this exceptional academic endeavor underlined the necessity to provide a comprehensive overview of the different facets of the clinical translation of optical techniques.

Aim and Scope of This Book

The aim and scope of this book are to provide a different strong and established source of information to introduce nonoptical imaging experts to this technology and its clinical applications; to review and share recent developments in new optical multimodal imaging techniques; to highlight development of novel computational methods; to demonstrate the clinical potential of optical imaging; and to provide the key steps necessary to translate this technology into successful clinical products. Multimodality optical imaging is evolving at a fast pace. The contributors to this book are renowned scientists and industry leaders who set the trend in this field.

This book is divided into chapters spanning all aspects of the technology and its translation. Thus, different chapters address a wide range of technical, clinical, and regulatory materials. This book provides the necessary technical information to successfully understand/develop a clinical optical imaging platform within acceptable regulatory practices. Highly technical chapters rely on current developments as demonstrative examples. Thus, a general understanding of biomedical imaging is required, but no specific technical expertise is necessary.

This is the first book providing a comprehensive overview of the clinical applications of multimodality optical imaging, related technological development, and translational steps towards wide clinical acceptance. It will provide the reader with a full picture of the development and applications of multimodality optical imaging platforms from bench to bedside, from an academic, regulatory, and industrial standpoint.

Chapters in the book are clustered by technical content. Due to the interdisciplinary aspect of the subject, readers will have different background and interests. The chapters cover all aspects of multimodality optical imaging in clinical settings. Readers may navigate easily through the book to find information relevant to their interests.

We have included a CD-ROM with the book. This CD-ROM contains full-color versions of all figures in the book, which further illustrate the topics discussed herein. Additionally, we have provided three freely installable software platforms for development of advanced imaging applications:

- *XIP (eXtensible Imaging Platform)*: XIP is an open-source environment for rapidly developing medical imaging applications from a set of modular software elements. This platform makes it easy to access specific postprocessing applications at multiple sites; it supports the DICOM standard and is fully compatible with the ITK (www.itk.org) and VTK (www.vtk.org) open-source libraries. XIP has the capability of simplifying workflows and speeding data processing and analysis. XIP is an initiative of the Cancer Bioinformatics Grid (caBIG) program created by the National Cancer Institute to facilitate the sharing of IT infrastructure, data, and applications.
- TOAST *(Time-resolved Optical Absorption and Scattering Tomography)*: TOAST is a software toolbox for the simulation of light transport in highly scattering media (the forward model) and the reconstruction of the spatial distribution of absorption and scattering coefficients from time-resolved transillumination measurements at the boundary (the inverse model). TOAST is under active development at University College London, Department of Computer Science and the Centre for Medical Image Computing (CMIC).
- NIRFAST (Near Infrared Frequency domain optical Absorption and Scatter Tomography): NIRFAST is an open source FEM-based software package designed for modeling near infrared frequency domain light transport in tissue. NIRFAST solves for the frequency domain diffusion approximation, for 2D or 3D problems. It also solves for the image reconstruction to provide simultaneous solution of optical properties using log amplitude and phase data. NIRFAST was developed and is maintained by the Near Infrared Imaging Group, Thayer School of Engineering at Dartmouth College, and by the School of Physics at the University of Exeter.

Overall, we expect this book will help the reader obtain a better understanding of:

- The main concepts and physical phenomena involved in optical imaging, as well as the detailed theory behind diffuse optical imaging;

- The major applications of optical imaging in the clinical world and what translation means in this context;
- The techniques used to combine optical imaging techniques with the established modalities (MRI, X-ray, PET, and so forth);
- The instrumentation required and involved in building a diffuse optical imaging device;
- How clinical trials are set up for an optical imaging device;
- How to build a test phantom for optical imaging;
- The business and regulatory aspects of the technology;
- The future of optical imaging and contrast agent technologies.

We believe this work will be useful to a wide array of readers, including researchers, clinicians, educators, students, and potential investors in the technology. We hope you will enjoy reading the book as much as all contributors and we were delighted to write it.

Acknowledgments

We both would like to thank our spouses, parents, and relatives for their inspiration and loving support. We editors gratefully thank the many friends and colleagues who made this work possible. It is also with great pleasure that we acknowledge the contributions of all 42 contributors to the 18 chapters of this book. Lastly, we would like to mention the positive influence and inspiration of the father of the field, who helped shape our views of biomedical optics: Britton Chance.

References

[1] Zerhouni, E. "Medicine. The NIH Roadmap." *Science*, 2003, 302:63–72.
[2] Report of the Translational Research Working Group of the National Cancer Advisory Board, *Transforming Translation—Harnessing Discovery for Patient and Public Benefit*, Executive Summary, http://www.cancer.gov/aboutnci/trwg/executive-summary.pdf.
[3] Cancer Imaging Program. *Network for Translational Research: Optical Imaging (NTROI)*, http://imaging.cancer.gov/programsandresources/specializedinitiatives/ntroi.
[4] Network for Translational Research: Optical Imaging, Request for Applications (RFA), http://grants.nih.gov/grants/guide/rfa-files/rfa-ca-03-002.html.

Fred S. Azar
Siemens Corporate Research Inc.
Princeton, New Jersey

Xavier Intes
Rensselaer Polytechnic Institute
Troy, New York
Editors
September 2008

CHAPTER 1
Introduction to Clinical Optical Imaging

Xavier Intes and Fred S. Azar

1.1 Introduction

The diagnostic and healing properties of light have been known to mankind for thousands of years. Sunlight alone or in combination with topical unguents was successfully employed to treat many diseases in ancient Egypt, India, and China [1]. A common practice among the Greeks and Romans was treatment by sunlight, known as heliotherapy, which Herodotus is supposed to have introduced [2]. However, only recently has light become a significant modern medical tool. Thanks to technological breakthroughs such as the laser [3], biomedical applications based on optical devices have flourished and are changing medicine as we know it [4, 5]. These applications provide tools to detect, image, monitor, and cure diseases from single molecules to large organs.

Optical sensing techniques for medical applications have been receiving increased attention in the last decade [6]. Clinical systems such as the pulse oxymeter have already found a unique place in the medical environment [7, 8]. New fundamental research developments and technological advances promise the widespread acceptance of many more optical monitoring and diagnostic systems. The specific light-tissue interaction from the ultraviolet to the infrared spectral regions reveals fundamental properties of biological tissues such as structure, physiology, and molecular function. In turn, these fundamental properties enable noninvasive tracking with low-power sources of specific biochemical events of interest to the medical community.

Light examination of tissue is already well established as a modality in medicine, especially optical surface imaging as commonly practiced in endoscopy or ophthalmology. These areas are still actively investigated as new approaches emerge, bringing more in-depth monitoring of epithelial tissue [9–12]. Moreover, some intrinsic compounds, such as nicotinamide adenine dinucleotide (NADH) or flavins fluorescence imaging, are reemerging as new modalities [13], providing additional discrimination between healthy and diseased tissues [14–16].

However, light propagation in biological samples is highly dependent on the wavelength selected. The most favorable spectral window in terms of depth penetration is situated in the near-infrared (NIR) range (wavelengths between $\lambda \in [600–1,000]$ nm). Thus, NIR techniques are the optical techniques of choice to image large organs. In this spectral range, biological tissues exhibit relatively weak absorption [17], allowing imaging through several centimeters of a sample. Outside this spectral window, the strong absorption of hemoglobin and water, respectively, for lower and higher wavelengths restricts the optical examination to shallow interrogation.

Not intended to provide a complete survey of optical imaging, this chapter aims primarily to provide the reader with basic tools necessary to understand the principles of optical biomedical applications as well as the underlying medical and physical background.

1.2 Tissue Optics

The spectral range of the electromagnetic spectrum employed in optical clinical applications spans the near infrared (NIR) to the ultraviolet (UV). This spectral range encompasses wavelengths from 100 nm to 1 μm: UV-C from 100 to 280 nm, UV-B from 280 to 315 nm, UV-A from 315 to 400 nm, the visible spectra from 400 to 760 nm, and a portion of the I-A band from 760 to 1,400 nm. The interaction of electromagnetic waves at these wavelengths with matter is dependent on specific physical phenomena that provide the unique wealth of information attainable with light (see Color Plate 1).

Overall, four photophysical processes are the basis of biomedical optics: elastic scattering, Raman scattering, absorption, and fluorescence. These photophysical processes are the fundamental properties of the tissues providing diagnostic contrast functions and necessary to cast the theoretical model describing light propagation. We provide below a brief description of these four light-tissue interactions.

1.2.1 Scattering

One of the fundamental quantities describing the propagation of light is the index of refraction. It is defined for a material as the ratio of the speed of light in vacuum to the speed of light in that material. When a light wave propagating in a material with a given index encounters a boundary with a second material with a different index, the path of light is redirected. Thus, the index of refraction of biological tissue plays a crucial role in biophotonics.

Biological tissues comprise many different molecules that are bound into a vast variety of small and large molecules. Cells are composed of this large variety of molecules. All these cell components exhibit different indices of refraction, which are spectrally dependent. Table 1.1 provides a list of approximate values for the optical refractive index of different cellular components. At a microscopic scale, the sharp transitions of the index of refraction at the cellular and subcellular level induce a change in the direction of the light propagation. The overall effect of these light redirections occurring at different scales is termed *scattering* and partially characterizes the propagating medium.

Light scattering is a wavelength-dependent phenomenon conveying significant information about microscopic and tissue structure. In particular, scattering depends on the sizes, indices of refraction, and structures of the denser subcellular components. Experimental evidence demonstrates that nuclear size [28], cell mem-

1.2 Tissue Optics

Table 1.1 Index of Refraction Values of Cell Components Taken from Previously Published Data

Cell Component	Index of Refraction	Reference
Water	1.33	
Extracellular fluid	1.35–1.38	[18, 19]
Cytoplasm	1.35–1.37	[20–23]
Nucleus	1.38–1.47	[18, 24]
Mitochondria	1.38–1.42	[18, 25]
Lipid	1.48	[18]
Protein	1.50	[20]
Melanin	1.7	[26]
Dried protein	1.58	[27]

branes [18], and mitochondria [29] are the major contributors to scattering in vivo. The cell nuclei (5 to 10 μm) are appreciably larger than the probing optical wavelength (0.01 to 1 μm). They predominantly scatter light in the forward direction, and there is also appreciable scattering in the backward direction (Mie scattering). Mitochondria are oblong scatterers with a 1 to 4 μm length and a 0.2 to 0.5 μm diameter and are responsible for scattering at larger angles (Rayleigh scattering). Contrasts in the size, density, distribution, and refraction index of these organelles generate optical signatures that may be disease specific [30].

1.2.2 Raman Scattering

In the 1920s, Sir Chandrasekhara Venkata Raman noticed that light incident on a variety of surfaces is sometimes scattered with wavelengths different from that of the incident light [31]. Conversely to scattering, which is an elastic, energy-conservative phenomenon, in Raman scattering the incident light is scattered inelastically. This is the result of an energy transition from the scattering molecule to a virtual state and its return to a higher or lower vibrational state with the emission of a photon of different energy. The efficiency of Raman scattering is weak, and typically only 1 out of 10^5 photons will be inelastically scattered. The energy transition can sometimes involve a real state, leading to a considerable enhancement in the scattering process. This specific case is termed *resonance Raman scattering*.

Raman signals are rich in spectral features, which in many cases are associated with the vibration of a particular chemical bond in a molecule. Most biological molecules exhibit specific spectral Raman "fingerprints." Thus, Raman scattering allows the quantitative evaluation of tissue composition (see Section 3.2.3) [32, 33].

1.2.3 Absorption

As light interacts with biological tissue, some of the incident energy is transformed. Especially, some atoms or molecules have the property to absorb the excitation energy and transform it into heat or light of different color (fluorescence). The probability of a specific molecular species extracting energy from the incident light is ruled by quantum mechanics. The absorption of energy could involve electronic transitions, vibrational transitions, and rotational transitions.

Light absorption in tissue originates from many different analytes. The main relevant chromophores are oxy- and deoxyhemoglobin, melanin, water, lipids, porphyrins, NADH, flavins, and other structural components [17]. These chromophores exhibit spectrally dependent absorbing properties providing specific optical signatures that are used to discriminate them and quantify their concentration in vivo. For instance, optical investigations of the blood properties have been an active research field since the nineteenth century [34]. These investigations led to the seminal works of Millikan [35] and Drabkin and Austin [36] in the 1930s, studies that furthered contemporary tissue oximetry.

The strong spectral dependence of tissue chromophores is of key importance in biophotonics and correlates with light penetration depth. The overall absorption of the tissue restricts light penetration. The most favorable spectral window in terms of depth penetration is situated in the near-infrared (NIR) range ($\lambda \in [600-1{,}000]$ nm). In this specific spectral window, the so-called therapeutic window, blood and water are minimally absorbing, thereby allowing successful examination of centimeters-thick samples. Figure 1.1 provides an example of the spectrally absorbing properties of the main tissue chromophores.

1.2.4 Fluorescence

Fluorescence is an absorption-mediated phenomenon related to an electronic transition from the excited state to the ground state of a molecule. In some cases, this

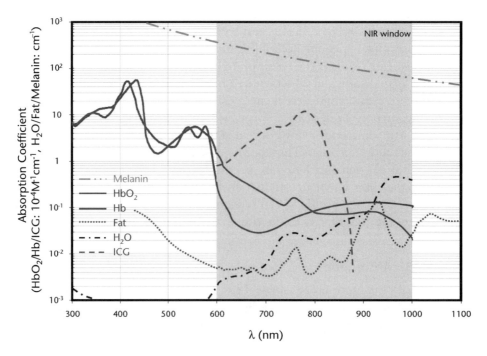

Figure 1.1 Absorption coefficient spectra for the main tissue absorbers.

Table 1.2 Maximum Excitation and Emission Wavelengths of the Primary Endogenous Fluorophores

Fluorophore	Wavelength of Maximum Fluorescence Excitation (nm)	Wavelength of Maximum Fluorescence Emission (nm)
Tryptophan	280	350
Collagen	330	390
Elastin	350	420
NADH	340	450
FAD	450	515
Porphyrins	405	635

relaxation may generate a photon of lower energy. Such photon generation will be specific to a molecular species and can be characterized by two intrinsic molecular parameters: the quantum yield and the lifetime.

The quantum yield is defined as the ratio of the number of fluorescent photons emitted to the number of photons emitted. The lifetime is defined as the average amount of time the molecule spends in the excited state following absorption of photons. Both parameters are dependent (however weakly) on environmental factors such as temperature, solvent, pH, and the like [37].

Biological tissues are constituted of many molecules with fluorescence properties [38]. Such molecules are generally referred to as endogenous fluorophores conversely to exogenous chromophores, which are externally administered compounds. The primary molecules accounting for endogenous fluorescence (i.e., autofluorescence) are proteins, collagen, elastin, a reduced form of NADH, various flavins, and porphyrins. The emission spectra of these molecules are mainly confined within 300 to 600 nm. Intrinsic fluorescence of proteins occurs at 280 to 350 nm, requires an excitation of between 250 and 280 nm, and is linked to the aromatic amino acids tryptophan, tyrosin, and phenylalaline (with predominance of tryptophan) [37]. Collagen and elastin fluoresce broadly between 400 and 600 nm (maxima around 400, 430, and 460 nm), with an excitation occurring from 300 to 400 nm. NADH fluorescence peaks around 460 nm, whereas fluorescence of the oxidized form (NAD+) peaks at 435 nm. Flavins monocleotide (FMN) and dinucleotide (FAD) fluoresce within the 500 to 600 nm window [39]. The resulting autofluorescence spectra of tissues are thus typically very broad. Table 1.2 presents a summary of the main spectral characteristics of the endogenous fluorophores of interest.

Many fluorescent compounds have been synthesized with appropriate spectral features for optical applications. The interest in such dyes is based on relatively high quantum yields and favorable spectral behavior, as compared to the endogenous markers. The first dye of interest was synthesized in 1871 by Adolf von Baeyer and is still the most dominant fluorophore for clinical uses: fluorescein. Characterized by a relatively high absorptivity (also known as extinction coefficient) and high quantum yield, the dye exhibits a fluorescence peak around 520 nm. Since its advent, many exogenous markers have been developed to overcome the limitation of fluorescein. In particular, numerous cyanine dyes have been synthesized with excellent fluorescent properties [40]. An in-depth review of the current status of optical contrast agents, especially with multimodality emphasis, is provided in Chapter 16. The use of functional exogenous contrast agents is expected to play an increased role in the translational effort of optical-based medical techniques and to contribute to establishing molecular imaging as a clinical practice.

1.3 Light Propagation

In this section we present a brief overview of several approaches employed to model light propagation in tissue. We restrict ourselves to the commonly used approaches that are applicable to in vivo cases. A more complete review of theoretical approaches for modeling light scattering and propagation is available in [4, 5].

1.3.1 Fundamentals

Tissues are complex heterogeneous assemblies of different components altering light propagation. Such complexity generally forbids the use of classical Maxwell's wave propagation theory due to inextricable computational difficulties. Thus, simpler approaches must be devised to describe light propagation in tissue.

First, scattering and absorption processes are simply described by the notion of cross section. With such an approach, scatterers and absorbers within tissues are considered to be localized particles characterized by a cross section (respectively, σ_s and σ_a in m^{-2}). Both cross sections are defined as the ratio of the power scattered/absorbed to the incident power. In the case of scattering, this parameter is dependent on the polarization and the direction of the incident beam [4]. If a medium contains a uniform distribution of identical scatterers (absorbers), then it is characterized by a scattering (absorbing) coefficient (m^{-1}):

$$\mu_{s(a)} = \rho \sigma_{s(a)} \tag{1.1}$$

where ρ (m^{-3}) is the number density of scatterer (absorbers). These coefficients represent the inverse of the average distance a photon travels before being scattered (absorbed). As light propagates more deeply in the sample, it will experience increased scattering and absorbing interactions. With each scattering interaction, the coherent information of the incident light (phase and polarization) is degraded until it is completely lost. Thus, the light-propagation regimes are generally divided into three components: the nonscattered light, the single scattering regime in which the wave nature of light can still be harnessed, and finally the multiple scattering regime in which we consider only the average propagating energy. To illustrate the three components of light, consider a short pulse of light propagating through tissue (see Figure 1.2) [41].

First, light emerging from the tissue surface is composed of photons traveling in straight lines or reflected from an object. These coherent photons are referred to as the ballistic photons. These photons are very sensitive to the internal structure of the sample. However, they can be efficiently detected only across short distances. Ballistic photons are used in coherent high-resolution imaging systems such as ultrafast

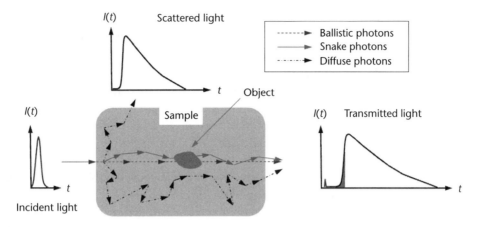

Figure 1.2 Propagation of a laser pulse through a turbid medium. (*After:* [41].)

time gating [42] and optical coherence tomography [43] (see Chapters 2 and 3) to produce diffraction-limited images.

Second, light emerging from the tissue surface is composed of photons that have undergone few scattering events, all of which are in the forward or near-forward direction (snake photons). Consequently, they retain some degree of coherence (phase and polarization), hence, to some extent, the image-bearing characteristics. They are also used in coherent high-resolution imaging systems and become predominant over ballistic photons as the photon path length increases (thicker sample or scattering-dominant regimes).

Third, light emerging from the tissue is composed of the remaining multiple-scattering photons. They are incoherent photons that will experience random paths in the sample and are called diffuse photons. They carry information on the variations in tissue; however, this information is blurred by the random walk process. Unlike ballistic and snake photons, they can be detected efficiently through several centimeters of tissue. Coupled with an appropriate light-propagation model, they can noninvasively provide unique functional quantities of the tissue sampled but with low resolution. To achieve high-resolution imaging with such photons, multimodality techniques are necessary to alleviate the loss of spatial information due to scattering (see Chapter 5).

1.3.2 Forward Model

Beyond the potential to provide high-resolution images based on coherent or spatially coherent photons, optical techniques strive to render quantitative 2D or 3D maps of the tissue optical properties and/or their associated functional/molecular/structural parameters [44]. This is a classical subsurface imaging problem that relies on a quantitative light-propagation model (forward model). Such models can be summarily divided in two categories: Monte Carlo simulations and the deterministic methods—the radiation transport equation (RTE) and its approximation, the diffusion equation) [45].

1.3.2.1 Monte Carlo

The Monte Carlo (MC) method is considered the gold standard to simulate light propagation through tissues. The MC method uses a numerical approach to calculate the light energy fluence rate at any location in the tissue. This model follows one photon at a time and calculates the probability of scattering or absorption of this photon [46]. At each interaction point, the scattering direction, absorption, and distance to the next interaction point are modeled as random variables on the basis of the optical properties of the tissue. This process is repeated for a certain predetermined number of photons.

The Monte Carlo technique is easy to implement, flexible, proven to be accurate over a large span of optical properties (or conversely over a large spectral range) as well as for small finite interrogated volumes [47, 48], and able to model coherent photons [49]. Since it is a statistical method, large packets of photons need to be simulated to obtain simulation results with good signal-to-noise ratio. This translates into large computing power requirements to achieve acceptable simulations within hours, even with parallel computing implementations [50]. Due to this drawback, the Monte Carlo method for simulating light propagation is used as a validating tool for other forward models or to estimate the bulk optical properties of tissues [51, 52].

1.3.2.2 Radiation Transport Equation

The radiation transport equation (RTE) allows modeling light in a relatively more computationally efficient framework than MC methods. The RTE is an integro-differential equation describing the energy flow per unit normal area, per unit solid angle, per unit time. It can be derived via conservation of energy [53]. Briefly, the RTE states that a beam of light loses energy through divergence and extinction (including both absorption and scattering away from the beam) and gains energy from light sources in the medium and scattering directed toward the beam [54]. Coherence and nonlinearity are neglected. Polarization is also generally neglected, even though it can be considered in some cases [55]. Optical properties such as the refractive index n, the absorption coefficient μ_a, the scattering coefficient μ_s, and the scattering anisotropy g are taken as time invariant but may vary spatially [56, 57].

Analytical solutions to the RTE are difficult to derive, and generally the equation is solved numerically with finite-element or finite-difference solvers. The RTE offers the same advantages as the MC method—it is flexible and proven to be accurate over a large span of optical properties as well as for small, interrogated finite volumes—but it too is more complex to implement. The RTE has been successfully employed as the forward model to perform optical tomography [58, 59]. However, it is generally used only when certain conditions are met: small source-detector separations [60, 61], tissue with low-absorbing/scattering regions (e.g., cerebrospinal fluid, synovial fluid in joints) [62, 63]. In other cases, approximations to the RTE are introduced to provide more computationally efficient methods.

1.3.2.3 Diffusion Equation

Numerous implementations of optical techniques for clinical scenarios capitalize on the relative transparency of tissue in the NIR window [44]. In this spectral range, the majority of tissues exhibit scattering-dominant transport characteristics (high-albedo). For such a scattering-dominant regime, the light propagation can be accurately modeled by an approximation to the RTE: the diffusion equation.

In the RTE, six different independent variables define the optical radiance at any spatiotemporal point. In the scattering-dominant regime, the radiance becomes nearly isotropic, thus enabling a reduction in the number of independent variables (after making the appropriate assumptions). The resulting differential equation, the diffusion equation, can be solved analytically for specific geometries. These analytical solutions that have the form of Green's function are extremely computationally efficient [64]. In the case of arbitrary geometries, the diffusion equation can be solved numerically [65], or a more sophisticated analytical model of the boundary conditions is required [66, 67].

Even though the diffusion equation is less accurate than MC methods or the RTE, it is the most commonly used forward model in optical tomography. It has been employed successfully to provide 3D functional maps of activities in brain [68, 69], breast [70–72], and muscle [73, 74] tissue.

1.4 Multimodality Imaging

1.4.1 A Brief History of Clinical Multimodality Imaging

Historically, medical imaging devices were developed independently to image either the structure or functional state of tissues. Different imaging techniques were devised based on different spectral regions of the electromagnetic spectrum [magnetic resonance imaging (MRI); visible and near-infrared light; X-rays, gamma rays, and single photon emission computed tomography (SPECT); annihilation photons and positron emission tomography (PET)] or on high-frequency sound waves (ultrasound) [75]. However, it was recognized that none of these stand-alone modalities provided a complete picture of the structure and function of tissue. Figure 1.3 proposes a spectrum of established anatomical and functional imaging modalities in oncology [76]. Only recently, cross-fertilization between imaging modalities has become a major research area [77].

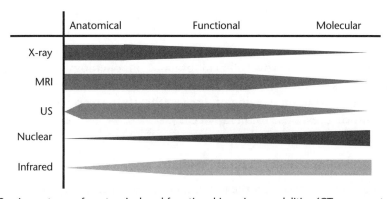

Figure 1.3 A spectrum of anatomical and functional imaging modalities (CT = computed tomography, MRI = magnetic resonance imaging, SPECT = single photon emission computed tomography, PET = positron emission tomography).

CT and MRI dominate the structural imaging modalities. CT was introduced in the early 1970s, initially for brain imaging and later for whole-body imaging [78, 79]. MRI was introduced to the clinical world in the 1980s and was well received as it does not require ionizing radiation [80]. Both imaging techniques are routinely employed for imaging the human anatomy in exquisite detail; however, in diagnosing and staging disease or monitoring response to therapy, they provide a partial picture. They lack the ability to track functional or metabolic changes that can occur in the absence of corresponding anatomical correlates. Clinicians rely on nuclear medicine techniques to reveal such functional or metabolic information. These techniques, initiated in the late 1940s, are based on radioactive tracers. The first human tomographic images with positron-emitting isotopes were presented in 1972 [81]. Single photon emission tomography (SPECT) results followed very shortly thereafter, establishing nuclear techniques as valuable clinical tools [82, 83].

Until the development of image fusion algorithms in the late 1980s to register images from stand-alone clinical systems [84], the acquisition and interpretation of anatomical and functional data were performed in different departments (radiology and nuclear medicine). Since then, physicians have recognized the usefulness of combining anatomical and functional images, and image fusion using software techniques has evolved considerably [85, 86] from its first inceptions. Commercial software is available to perform PET/CT, SPECT/CT, PET/MR, and PET/CT/MRI fusion for a wide variety of diagnostic clinical scenarios [87, 88], longitudinal studies, and treatment planning [89, 90]. Besides these successes, software fusion is not yet well adapted for certain body parts, such as lung [91] or pelvis imaging [92], or indications such as recurrent colorectal cancer [93]. Figure 1.4 shows an example of clinical software fusion abilities [94]. Alternatively, coregistration studies acquired on combined systems are simpler and more convenient, and they alleviate some of the common problems encountered with software-based fusion.

Clinicians are rapidly adopting multimodality imaging systems. For instance, between 2001 and 2006, sales of PET-only scanners decreased to zero to be replaced by PET/CT, as recorded by the Nuclear Equipment Manufacturers Association (NEMA) [77] (see Figure 1.5). The attempts to integrate two imaging modalities in one stand-alone system can be tracked to the late 1980s [95]. Since then, commercial multimodality systems have been available to perform PET/CT (Biograph Truepoint, Siemens Medical Solutions; Discovery, GE Healthcare; Gemini, Philips) and SPECT/CT (Symbia T, Siemens Medical Solutions; Hawkeye, GE Healthcare; Precedence, Philips Medical Solutions). Recently, combined clinical MRI/PET scanners have been also developed with success for preclinical applications [96–98]. These systems improve clinical practice in oncology compared to stand-alone modalities. Clinical literature illustrates the benefit of these multimodality platforms in the diagnosis and staging of disease [99, 100], treatment planning [90, 101], and monitoring response to therapy [102].

1.4.2 Multimodality Optical Imaging

Optical techniques offer the potential to contribute greatly to the expansion of clinical multimodality techniques. Their ability to image structural, functional, and molecular information at different spatial and temporal scales makes them very

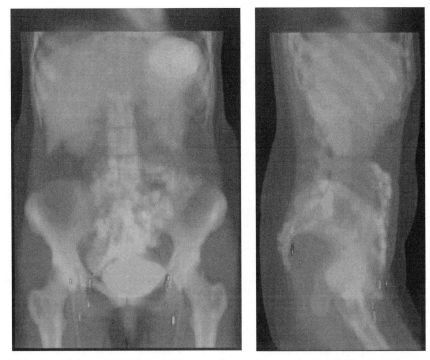

Figure 1.4 Coregistered MR, PET/CT data from the same patient with highlighted MR-segmented lymph nodes. Most patients with cancer are currently staged using PET/CT. While this strategy provides adequate primary-tumor and distant-metastases information, there is a need for better nodal staging. Lymphotrophic nanoparticle-enhanced MRI can overcome this handicap for nodal staging by accurately identifying subtle areas of nodal metastases. The mutually fused images allow for accurate staging and provide a time-saving approach for planning patient therapy [94].

attractive. In this case, the multimodality approach can be understood as the combination of multiple optical techniques in one instrument and/or the fusion of an optical technique with another well-established clinical modality, such as CT, MRI, or PET.

All-optical multimodality (or multidimensional) techniques benefit from the unique contrast mechanisms of stand-alone optical techniques. Complementary information about the biochemical, architectural, and morphological state of tissue is obtained through combination of different optical techniques and provides unprecedented diagnostic potential. For instance, Georgakoudi et al. found that by combining the fluorescence, reflectance, and light-scattering spectroscopies, superior separation between dysplastic and nondysplastic epithelium was achieved [103]. Fluorescence spectroscopy monitors the biochemical information, reflectance spectroscopy quantifies the bulk morphology of the tissue, and light-scattering spectroscopy provides the nuclei-population information. Such techniques are mainly associated with endoscopic imaging techniques (mucosa imaging) or minimally invasive techniques since at least one technique relies on coherent photons. An in-depth review of the different all-optical multimodality techniques is provided in Chapters 2 and 3.

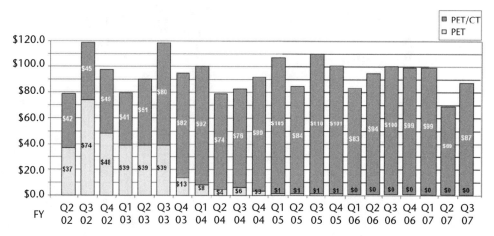

Figure 1.5 Shipments of PET and PET/CT scanners for the U.S. market as recorded by the Nuclear Equipment Manufacturers Association (NEMA) for the period from January 2002 to October 2007. Note that the figures (in millions of dollars) reflect the total revenue for all shipments from which the selling price and individual unit type cannot be determined. Shipments of PET-only scanners declined during this period to zero from January 2006 onwards. The overall market for PET or PET/CT remained fairly constant throughout this period, although since January 2007, with the reduction in reimbursement due to the introduction of the Deficit Reduction Act, sales declined somewhat. (*From:* [77]. © 2008 IOP. Reprinted with permission.)

Another active area of research is the combination of optical techniques with other clinical modalities. Similarly to other fusion approaches, software fusion and hardware fusion are actively pursued. Software fusion is generally preferred for handheld optical devices when the primary care physician would ideally examine the patient (see Chapter 7) or when an optimal optical imaging platform design is to be retained. Such software fusion faces the same challenges as other nonconcurrent fusion such as CT-PET. Chapter 7 provides a review of the challenges and technical implementation of software fusion. Software fusion provides greater flexibility than physically integrated multimodality systems, thereby removing the requirements of the "other" imaging modality, for example, restrictions on metallic instrumentation for MRI, hard breast compression for X-ray mammography, limited optode combinations for ultrasound (as well as MRI and X-ray), and time constraints. It is therefore desirable to develop quantitative and systematic methods for data fusion that utilize the high-quality data and versatility of the stand-alone imaging systems.

Hardware fusion follows the same development path of MR/PET fusion [104]. Light can be efficiently delivered to tissue and detected from tissue using light guides. Such flexibility allows efficient integration of optical techniques with clinical platforms such a CT (see Chapter 9) and MRI (see Chapter 6 and 8). The concurrent acquisition of data is then feasible, leading to minimized errors in registration and reduced bias in anatomically assisted optical imaging (see Chapter 5). In this case, accurate anatomical templates allow alleviation of some of the intrinsic weaknesses of thick-tissue optical imaging. Chapter 5 provides a concise description of the methods and benefits that employ accurate anatomical maps obtained from other imaging modalities for use with optical imaging.

1.5 Conclusions

Advances in clinical imaging are being made through the combination of imaging techniques and multimodal imaging platforms, such as PET/CT, PET/MRI, and MRI/US. More recently, optical imaging methods have been used in multimodal imaging platforms such as MRI/DOT, PET/DOT, MRI/DOS (diffuse optical spectroscopy), X-ray/DOT, US/DOS, and other combinations using optical methods as a complementary imaging modality. Each imaging technique relies on different physical tissue interaction principles and, in some cases, on the use of different molecular probes. As a result, multimodal imaging methods may provide a unique combined set of structural, functional, molecular, and/or metabolic information. The complexities of integrating different methods are offset by the potential for increased performance in both sensitivity and specificity (by reducing false-positive and false-negative results) in screening, diagnosis, staging, treatment monitoring, or image-guided intervention. There is a critical need today to translate research and optical systems development and to produce robust and cost-effective medical products. The National Cancer Institute Translational Research Working Group (TRWG) defines translational research in the following way [105]: "Translational research transforms scientific discoveries arising from laboratory, clinical, or population studies into clinical applications to reduce cancer incidence, morbidity, and mortality." Translational optical imaging relies on the synthesis of knowledge from many fields, including fundamental optical science, medicine, chemical and biomedical engineering, and medical imaging and device technology. The combination of diagnostic imaging with molecular characterization of disease is leading to practical techniques that will impact or modify clinical practice and commercial products.

References

[1] Ackroyd, R., C. Kelty, N. Brown, and M. Reed, "The history of photodetection and photodynamic therapy," *Photochem. Photobiol.* 74(5) (2001): 656–669.

[2] Daniell, M. D., and J. S. Hill, "A history of photodynamic therapy," *ANZ J. Surgery* 61(5) (1991): 340–348.

[3] Bertolotti, M., *Masers and lasers: A historical approach*, Bristol, UK: Adam Hilger, 1983.

[4] Vo-Dinh, T., *Biomedical photonics handbook*, Boca Raton, FL: CRC Press, 2003.

[5] Tuchin, V., *Handbook of optical biomedical diagnostics*, Washington, DC: SPIE Press, 2002.

[6] Kincade, K., "Optical diagnostics continue migration from bench top to bedside," *Laser Focus World* (January 2004): 130–134.

[7] Vora, V. A., and S. H. Ahmedzai, "Pulse oximetry in supportive and palliative care," *Support. Care Canc.* 12 (2004): 758–761.

[8] Sola, A., L. Chow, and M. Rogido, "Pulse oximetry in neonatal care in 2005: A comprehensive state of the art review," *Annales de Pediatra* 62(3) (2005): 266–281.

[9] Farkas, D., and D. Becker, "Application of spectral imaging: Detection and analysis of human melanoma and its precursor," *Pigm. Cell Res.* 14 (2001): 2–8.

[10] Zonios, G., J. Bykowski, and N. Kollias, "Skin melanin, hemoglobin, and light scattering properties can be quantitatively assessed in vivo using diffuse reflectance spectroscopy," *J. Invest. Dermatol.* 117 (2001): 1452–1457.

[11] Bono, A., et al., "The ABCD system of melanoma detection: A spectrophotometric analysis of the asymmetry, border, color, and dimension," *Cancer* 85 (1999): 72–77.

[12] Popp, A., M. Valentine, P. Kaplan, and D. Weitz, "Microscopic origin of light scattering in tissue," *Appl. Opt.* 42 (2003): 2871–2880.

[13] Wagnieres, G., W. Star, and B. Wilson, "In vivo fluorescence spectroscopy and imaging for oncological applications," *Photochem. Photobiol.* 68 (1998): 603–632.

[14] Ramanujam, N., et al., "Cervical cancer detection using a multivariate statistical algorithm based on laser-induced fluorescence spectra at multiple wavelength," *Photochem. Photobiol.* 64 (1996): 720–735.

[15] Stepp, H., R. Sroka, and R. Baumgartner, "Fluorescence endoscopy of gastrointestinal diseases: Basic principles, techniques, and clinical experience," *Endoscopy* 30 (1998): 379–386.

[16] Moesta, K. T., et al., "Protoporphyrin IX occurs naturally in colorectal cancers and their metastases," *Canc. Res.* 61 (2001): 991–999.

[17] Cheong, W., S. Prahl, and A. Welch, "A review of the optical properties of biological tissues," *IEEE J. Quant. Electron.* 26 (1990): 2166–2185.

[18] Beuthan, J., O. Minet, J. Helfman, and G. Muller, "The spatial variation of the refractive index in biological cells," *Phys. Med. Biol.* 41 (1996): 369–382.

[19] Beauvoit, B., T. Kitai, and B. Chance, "Contribution of the mitochondrial compartment to the optical properties of rat liver: A theoretical and practical approach," *Biophys. J.* 67 (1994): 2501–2510.

[20] Kohl, M., and M. Cope, "Influence of glucose concentration on light scattering in tissue," *Opt. Lett.* 17 (1994): 2170–2172.

[21] Brunsting, A., and P. Mullaney, "Differential light scattering from spherical mammalian cells," *Biophys. J.* 14 (1974): 439–453.

[22] Lanni, F., A. Waggoner, and D. Taylor, "Internal reflection fluorescence microscopy," *J. Cell Biol.* 100 (1985): 1091.

[23] Bereiter-Han, J., C. Fox, and B. Thorell, "Quantitative reflection contrast microscopy of living cells," *J. Cell Biol.* 82 (1979): 767–779.

[24] Sloot, P. M., A. G. Hoekstra, and C. G. Figdor, "Osmotic response of lymphocytes measured by means of forward light-scattering-theoretical considerations," *Cytometry* 9 (1988): 636–641.

[25] Liu, H., B. Beauvoit, M. Kimura, and B. Chance, "Dependence of tissue optical properties on solute-induced changes in refractive index and osmolarity," *J. Biomed. Opt.* 1 (1996): 200–211.

[26] Vitkin, I., J. Woolsey, B. Wilson, and R. Anderson, "Optical and thermal characterization of natural (sepia officinalis) melanin," *Photochem. Photobiol.* 59 (1994): 455–462.

[27] Barer, R., and S. Joseph, "Refractometry of living cells," *Quart. J. Microscopic. Sci.* 95 (1954): 399–423.

[28] Backman, V., R. Gurjar, K. Badizadegan, I. Itzkan, R. R. Dasari, L. T. Perelman, and M. S. Feld, "Polarized light scattering spectroscopy for quantitative measurement of epithelial structures in situ," *IEEE J. Sel. Top. Quant. Electron.* 5 (1999): 1019–1026.

[29] Beauvoit, B., S. M. Evans, T. W. Jenkins, E. E. Miller, and B. Chance, "Correlation between the light scattering and the mitochondrial content of normal tissues and transplantable rodent tumors," *Analyt. Biochem.* 226 (1995): 167–174.

[30] Backman, V., et al., "Detection of pre-invasive cancer cells," *Nature* 406 (2000): 35–36.

1.5 Conclusions

[31] Raman, C. V., and K. S. Krishnan, "A new type of secondary radiation," *Nature* 121 (1928): 501–502.

[32] Rinia, H. A., M. Bonn, E. M. Vartiainen, C. B. Schaffer, and M. Müller, "Spectroscopic analysis of the oxygenation state of hemoglobin using coherent anti–Stokes Raman scattering," *J. Biomed. Opt.* 11(5) (2006): 050502.

[33] Römer, T. J., et al., "Intravascular ultrasound combined with Raman spectroscopy to localize and quantify cholesterol and calcium salts in atherosclerotic coronary arteries," *Arterioscl. Thromb. Vasc. Biol.* 20(2) (2000): pp. 478–483.

[34] Hoppe-Sleyer, F., "Ueber das verhakte des blutfarbstoffes im spectrum des sonnenlichtes," *Arch. Pathol. Anat. Physiol. Klin. Med.* 23 (1862): 446.

[35] Millikan, G. A., "Photometric methods of measuring the velocity of rapid reactions. III. A portable micro-apparatus applicable to an extended range of reactions," *Proc. Royal Soc. A* 155 (1936): 277–292.

[36] Drabkin, D. L., and H. Austin, "Spectrophometric studies. I. Spectrophotometric constants for common hemoglobin derivatives in human, dog and rabbit blood," *J. Biolog. Chem.* 98 (1932): 719–733.

[37] Lackowicz, J. R., *Principles of fluorescence spectroscopy*, New York: Kluwer Academic/Plenum Publishers, 1999.

[38] Mycek, M.-A., and B. W. Pogue, *Handbook of biomedical fluorescence*, Boca Raton, FL: CRC Press, 2003.

[39] Schneckenburger, H., R. Steiner, W. Strauss, K. Stock, and R. Sailer, "Fluorescence technologies in biomedical diagnostics," ch. 15 in V. V. Tuchin (ed.), *Optical biomedical diagnostics*, Bellingham, WA: SPIE Press, 2002.

[40] Zheng, G., Y. Chen, X. Intes, B. Chance, and J. Glickson, "Contrast-enhanced NIR optical imaging for subsurface cancer detection," *J. Porphyrin Phthalocyanines* 8 (2004): 1106–1118.

[41] Gayen, S. K., and R. R. Alfano, "Emerging biomedical imaging techniques," *Opt. Photon. News* 7(3) (1996): 17–22.

[42] Farsiu, S., J. Christofferson, B. Eriksson, P. Milanfar, B. Friedlander, A. Shakouri, and R. Nowak, "Statistical detection and imaging of objects hidden in turbid media using ballistic photons," *Appl. Opt.* 46(23) (2007): 5805–5822.

[43] Huang, D., et al., "Optical coherence tomography," *Science* 254(5035) (1991): 1178–1181.

[44] Intes, X., and B. Chance, "Non-PET functional imaging techniques optical," *Radiolog. Clin. N. Am.* 43(1) (2005): 221–234.

[45] Arridge, S. R., and J. C. Hebden, "Optical imaging in medicine II: Modeling and reconstruction," *Phys. Med. Biol.* 42 (1997): 841–854.

[46] Keijzer, M., S. L. Jacques, S. A. Prahl, and A. J. Welch, "Light distributions in artery tissue: Monte Carlo simulations for finite-diameter laser beams," *Lasers Med. Surg.* 9 (1989): 148–154.

[47] Cheong, W-F., S. A. Prahl, and A. J. Welch, "A review of the optical properties of biological tissues," *IEEE J. Quant. Electron.* 26 (1990): 2166–2185.

[48] Okada, E., M. Schweiger, S. R. Arridge, M. Firbank, and D. T. Delpy, "Experimental validation of Monte Carlo and finite-element methods for the estimation of the optical path length in inhomogeneous tissue," *Appl. Opt.* 35(19) (1996): 3362–3371.

[49] Moon, S., D. Kim, and E. Sim, "Monte Carlo study of coherent diffuse photon transport in a homogeneous turbid medium: A degree-of-coherence based approach," *Appl. Opt.* 47(3) (2008): 336–345.

[50] Kirkby, D. R., and D. T. Delpy, "Parallel operation of Monte Carlo simulations on a diverse network of computers," *Phys. Med. Biol.* 42 (1997): 1203–1208.

[51] Bevilacqua, F., D. Piguet, P. Marquet, J. D. Gross, B. J. Tromberg, and C. Depeursinge, "In vivo local determination of tissue optical properties: Applications to human brain," *Appl. Opt.* 38(22) (1999): 4939–4950.

[52] Hayakawa, C. K., J. Spanier, F. Bevilacqua, A. K. Dunn, J. S. You, B. J. Tromberg, and V. Venugopalan, "Perturbation Monte Carlo methods to solve inverse photon migration problems in heterogeneous tissues," *Opt. Lett.* 26(17) (2001): 1335–1137.

[53] Chandrasekhar, S., *Radiative transfer*, New York: Dover, 1960.

[54] Ishimaru, A., *Wave propagation and scattering in random media*, New York: IEEE Press, 1997.

[55] Mishchenko, M. I., "Vector radiative transfer equation for arbitrarily shaped and arbitrarily oriented particles: A microphysical derivation from statistical electromagnetics," *Appl. Opt.* 41(33) (2002): 7114–7134.

[56] Klose, A. D., and A. H. Hielscher, "Iterative reconstruction scheme for optical tomography based on the equation of radiative transfer," *Med. Phys.* 26(8) (1999): 1698–1707.

[57] Arridge, S. R., et al., "Reconstruction of subdomain boundaries of piecewise constant coefficients of the radiative transfer equation from optical tomography data," *Inverse Problems* 22 (2006): 2175–2196.

[58] Aronson, R., R. L. Barbour, J. Lubowsky, and H. Graber, "Application of transport theory to infra-red medical imaging," *Mod. Mathemat. Methods Transport Theory* (1991): 64–67.

[59] Abdoulaev, G. S., and A. H. Hielscher, "Three-dimensional optical tomography with the equation of radiative transfer," *J. Elec. Imag.* 12(4) (2003): 594–601.

[60] Dunn, A., and D. A. Boas, "Transport-based image reconstruction in turbid media with small source-detector separations," *Opt. Lett.* 25(24) (2000): 1777–1779.

[61] Ren, K., G. Bal, and A. H. Hielscher, "Transport- and diffusion-based optical tomography in small domains: A comparative study," *Appl. Opt.* 46(27) (2007): 6669–6679.

[62] Firbank, M., S. R. Arridge, M. Schweiger, and D. T. Delpy, "An investigation of light transport through scattering bodies with non-scattering regions," *Phys. Med. Biol.* 41 (1998): 767–783.

[63] Scheel, A. K., et al., "First clinical evaluation of sagittal laser optical tomography for detection of synovitis in arthritic finger joints," *Ann. Rheumat. Dis.* 64 (2005): 239–245.

[64] O'Leary, M. A., D. A. Boas, B. Chance, and A. G. Yodh, "Experimental images of heterogeneous turbid media by frequency-domain diffusing-photon tomography," *Opt. Lett.* 20 (1995): 426–428.

[65] Arridge, S. R., "Topical review: Optical tomography in medical imaging," *Inverse Problems* 15 (1999): R41–R93.

[66] Ripoll, J., V. Ntziachristos, R. Carminati, and M. Nieto-Vesperinas, "Kirchhoff approximation for diffusive waves," *Phys. Rev. E* 64 (2001): 051917-8.

[67] Ripoll, J., S. R. Arridge, H. Dehghani, and M. Nieto-Vesperinas, "Boundary conditions for light propagation in diffusive media with non-scattering regions," *J. Opt. Soc. Am. A.* 17 (2000): 1671–1681.

[68] Hebden, J., et al., "Three-dimensional optical tomography of the premature infant brain," *Phys. Med. Biol.* 47 (2002): 4155–4166.

[69] Chen, Y., D. Tailor, X. Intes, and B. Chance, "Correlation between near-infrared spectroscopy (NIRS) and magnetic resonance imaging (MRI) on rat brain oxygenation modulation," *Phys. Med. Biol.* 48 (2003): 417–427.

[70] Leff, D. R., et al., "Diffuse optical imaging of the healthy and diseased breast: A systematic review," *Breast Canc. Res. Treat.* 108(1) (2008): 9–22.

[71] Intes, X., et al., "Time-domain optical mammography SoftScan: Initial results," *Acad. Radiol.* 12 (2005): 934–947.

[72] Intes, X., J. Ripoll, Y. Chen, S. Nioka, A. Yodh, and B. Chance, "In vivo continuous-wave optical breast imaging enhanced with indocyanine green," *Med. Phys.* 30 (2003): 1039–1047.

[73] Hamaoka, T., K. K. McCully, V. Quaresima, K. Yamamoto, and B. Chance, "Near-infrared spectroscopy/imaging for monitoring muscle oxygenation and oxidative metabolism in healthy and diseased humans," *J. Biomed. Opt.* 12(6) (2007) 1–16.

[74] Lin, Y., G. Lech, S. Nioka, X. Intes, and B. Chance, "Noninvasive, low-noise, fast imaging of blood volume and deoxygenation changes in muscles using light-emitting diode continuous-wave imager," *Rev. Sci. Instr.* 73 (2002): 3065–3074.

[75] Bushberg, J. T., J. A. Seibert, E. M. Leidhodlt, and J. M. Boone, *The essential physics of medical imaging*, Philadelphia: Lippincott Williams and Wilkins, 2002.

[76] Laking, G. R., P. M. Price, and M. J. Sculpher, "Assessment of the technology for functional imaging in cancer," *Eur. J. Cancer* 38 (2002): 2194–2199.

[77] Townsend, D. W., "Multimodality imaging of structure and function," *Phys. Med. Biol.* 53 (2008): R1–R39.

[78] Hounsfield, G. N., "Computerised transverse axial scanning (tomography): Part 1. Description of system," *Br. J. Radiol.* 46 (1973): 1016–1022.

[79] Ambrose, J., "Computerized transverse axial scanning (tomography): Part 2. Clinical application," *Br. J. Radiol.* 46 (1973): 1023–1047.

[80] Mattson, J., and M. Simon, *The pioneers of NMR and magnetic resonance in medicine: The story of MRI*, Jericho, NY: Dean Books Co., 1996.

[81] Chesler, D. A., "Positron tomography and three-dimensional reconstruction techniques," *Proc. Symp. Tomog. Imag. Nucl. Med.*, New York: Society of Nuclear Medicine, 1972, 176–183.

[82] Jaszczak, R. J., and R. E. Coleman, "Single photon emission computed tomography (SPECT). Part I: Principles and instrumentation," *Invest. Radiol.* 20(9) (1985): 897–910.

[83] Coleman, R. E., R. A. Blinder, and R. J. Jaszczak, "Single photon emission computed tomography (SPECT). Part II: Clinical applications," *Invest. Radiol.* 21(1) (1986): 1–11.

[84] Levin, D. N., C. A. Pelizzari, G. T. Chen, C. T. Chen, and M. D. Cooper, "Retrospective geometric correlation of MR, CT and PET images," *Radiology* 169 (1988): 817–236.

[85] Hawkes, D. J., D. L. Hill, L. Hallpike, and D. L. Bailey, *Coregistration of structural and functional images, positron emission tomography: Basic science and clinical practice*, New York: Springer-Verlag, 2004, 181–198.

[86] Slomka, P. J., "Software approach to merging molecular with anatomic information," *J. Nucl. Med.* 45 (2004): 36S–45S.

[87] Duarte, G. M., et al., "Fusion of magnetic resonance and scintimammography images for breast cancer evaluation: A pilot study," *Ann. Surg. Oncol.* 14(10) (2007): 2903–2910.

[88] Jin, J. Y., S. Ryu, K. Faber, T. Mikkelsen, Q. Chen, S. Li, and B. Movsas, "2D/3D image fusion for accurate target localization and evaluation of a mask-based stereotactic system in fractionated stereotactic radiotherapy of cranial lesions," *Med. Phys.* 33(12) (2006): 4557–4566.

[89] Cai, J., et al., "CT and PET lung image registration and fusion in radiotherapy treatment planning using the chamfer-matching method," *Int. J. Radiat. Oncol.*Biol.*Phys.* 43(4) (1999): 883–891.

[90] Gregoire, V., K. Haustermas, X. Geets, S. Roels, and M. Lonneux, "PET-based treatment planning in radiotherapy: A new standard?" *J. Nucl. Med.* 48 (2007): 68S–77S.

[91] Wahl, R. L., L. E. Quint, R. D. Cieslak, A. M. Aisen, R. A. Koeppe, and C. R. Meyer, "Anatometabolic tumor imaging: Fusion of FDG PET with CT or MRI to localize foci of increased activity," *J. Nucl. Med.* 34 (1993): 1190–1197.

[92] Hamilton, R. J., M. J. Blend, C. A. Pelizzari, B. D. Milliken, and S. Vijayakumar, "Using vascular structure for CT-SPECT registration in the pelvis," *J. Nucl. Med.* 40 (1999): 347–351.

[93] Kim, J. H., et al., "Comparison between 18F-FDG Pet, in-line PET/CT, and software fusion for restaging of recurrent colorectal cancer," *J. Nucl. Med.* 46 (2005): 587–595.

[94] Azar, F. V., B. de Roquemaurel, A. Khamene, R. T. Seethamraju, R. Weissleder, and M. G. Harisinghani, "Feasibility of MRI-PET-CT mutual image co-registration for cancer staging and therapeutic planning," *Novel Imaging for Clinical Studies, Joint Molecular Imaging Conference,* Providence, RI, September 2007.

[95] Hasegawa, B., E. L. Gingold, S. M. Reilly, S. C. Liew, and C. E. Cann, "Description of simultaneous emission-transmission CT system," *Proc. SPIE* 1231, 1990, 50–60.

[96] Buchanan, M., P. K. Marsden, C. H. Mielke, and P. B. Garlick, "A system to obtain radiotracer uptake data simultaneously with NMR spectra in a high field magnet," *IEEE Trans. Nucl. Sci.* 43(3) (1996): 2044–2048.

[97] Catana, C., et al., "Simultaneous in vivo positron emission tomography and magnetic resonance imaging," *PNAS* 105(10) (2008): 3705–3710.

[98] Judenhofer, M. S., et al., "Simultaneous PET-MRI: A new approach for functional and morphological imaging," *Nat. Med.*, 2008, doi:10.1038/nm1700.

[99] Czernin, J., M. Allen-Auerbahc, and H. Schelberg, "Improvements in cancer staging with PET/CT: Literature-based evidence as of September 2006," *J. Nucl. Med.* 48 (2007): 78S–88S.

[100] Roach, P. J., G. P. Schembri, I. A. Ho Shon, E. A. Bailey, and D. L. Bailey, "SPECT/CT imaging using a spiral CT scanner for anatomical localization: Impact on diagnosis accuracy and reporter confidence in clinical practice," *Nucl. Med. Communic.* 27 (2006): 977–987.

[101] Yap, J. T., D. W. Townsend, and N. C. Hall, *PET-CT in IMRT planning, intensity modulated radiation therapy: A clinical perspective,* Amsterdam, NH: Elsevier, 2004, 115–130.

[102] Weber, W. A., and R. Figlin, "Monitoring cancer treatment with PET/CT: Does it make a difference?" *J. Nucl. Med.* 48 (2007): 36S–44S.

[103] Georgakoudi, I., et al., "Fluorescence, reflectance, and light-scattering spectroscopy for evaluating dysplasia in patients with Barrett's esophagus," *Gastroenterology* 120(7) (2001): 1620–1629.

[104] Christensen, N. L., B. E. Hammer, B. G. Heil, and K. Fetterly, "Positron emission tomography within a magnetic field using photomultiplier tubes and light guides," *Phys. Med. Biol.* 40 (1995): 691–697.

[105] TRWG report, http://www.cancer.gov/aboutnci/trwg/order-final-report, June 2007.

CHAPTER 2
In Vivo Microscopy

Thomas D. Wang

2.1 Introduction

Histological interpretation of diseased tissue is currently being performed by taking the specimen to the microscope to look for microarchitectural differences in tissue. Processing artifact, sampling error, and interpretive variability can limit this process. Instead, a greater understanding of the disease process may be attained by taking the microscope to the tissue, where pathology can be assessed on viable tissue. Confocal microscopes provide a clear image of tissue using the technique of optical sectioning. Tabletop versions are common laboratory instruments used to perform fluorescence microscopy and immunohistochemistry in excised specimens of tissue. Significant progress has been made recently in scaling down the instrument dimensions for endoscope compatibility, thus providing an unprecedented opportunity to assess viable tissue in real time. These techniques are now being developed for use in the clinic to help with endoscopic surveillance of cancer by guiding tissue biopsy, reducing the risks of screening (i.e., bleeding, infection, and perforation), and lowering the costs associated with tissue pathology. Furthermore, these instruments can be combined with affinity probes to assess the molecular expression pattern of cells and tissues in vivo, providing an exciting opportunity to explore new frontiers in biological investigation.

Recent advances in the availability of flexible optical fibers, quality of microoptics, and performance of high-speed scanners [1–5] have allowed for the miniaturization of confocal microscopes for clinical use. These instruments have a size compatible with medical endoscopes and the speed to image in vivo without motion artifact in dynamically active tissue, such as that of the gastrointestinal tract [6–10]. A plethora of confocal microscope instruments in various stages of development collect either backscattered light to provide details about tissue microarchitecture or fluorescence images to reveal properties of mucosal function [11–13]. The key performance parameters of these prototypes are determined by the microoptical design and the scanning mechanism, which also determine the trade-offs allowed for reduction of instrument size. Refractive optical approaches for focusing the beam include the use of gradient index (GRIN) lenses and polydimethylsiloxane (PDMS) objectives, while nonrefractive designs include the use of parabolic surfaces. Scanning can be performed by either mechanically translating the fiber or objective lens or by steering the beam. The former approach is simpler but slower than the latter and ultimately determines the frame rate, which needs to be at least about 5 Hz to overcome in vivo motion artifact. A promising direction is the development of high-speed scanners with microelectromechanical systems (MEMS) technology to perform beam scanning [14, 15].

2.2 Confocal Microscopy

Confocal microscopy is an imaging method that provides high-resolution images from tissue using the technique of optical sectioning where a pinhole is placed between the objective lens and the detector to allow collection only of the light that originates from within a tiny volume below the tissue surface. Light from all other origins does not have the correct path to enter the pinhole and thus becomes "spatially filtered." This approach can provide clear images that reveal fine details about cells and subcellular structures [1]. Recently, this technique has been adapted for in vivo imaging by using an optical fiber rather than a pinhole. Most confocal microscopes use a single-axis design, as shown in Color Plate 2(a), where the pinhole and objective are located along the main optical axis. A high-numerical-aperture (NA) objective is used to achieve subcellular resolution and efficient light collection. The same objective is used for both the illumination and collection of light. The working distance is often limited, given the geometry of the high-NA objective; thus, the scanning mechanism (mirror) is placed on the pinhole side of the objective (preobjective position). Furthermore, a large amount of the light that is scattered by the tissue present between the objective and focal volume (dashed lines) is collected, reducing the dynamic range of detection.

The dual-axes architecture, shown in Color Plate 2(b), is an alternate optical design that employs two fibers and low-NA objectives [16, 17]. The illumination and collection of light are performed separately, and the region of overlap between the two beams (focal volume) achieves subcellular resolution. The low-NA objectives create a long working distance so that the scan mirror can be placed on the tissue side of the lens (postobjective position). Very little of the light that is scattered by tissue along the illumination path is collected (dashed lines), resulting in a high dynamic range [18]. Consequently, optical sections can be collected in both vertical (V) and horizontal (H) planes with dual axes, as compared to horizontal planes only with a single-axis configuration.

2.3 Endoscope-Compatible Systems

Two endoscope-compatible confocal microscopy systems are commercially available for clinical use and are shown in Figure 2.1. The EC-3870K (Pentax Precision Instruments, Tokyo, Japan) integrates a confocal microscope (Optiscan Pty. Ltd., Victoria, Australia) into the distal tip of the endoscope, as shown in Figure 2.1(a), resulting in an overall endoscope diameter of 12.8 mm [19, 20], and the dimension of the confocal microscope alone is approximately 5 mm. Two light guides illuminate the mucosa for generating the conventional white-light images that are imaged onto the charge-coupled device (CCD) detector by the objective. The instrument

2.3 Endoscope-Compatible Systems

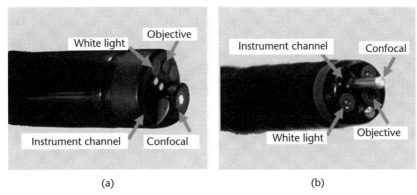

Figure 2.1 Clinical confocal imaging system. (a) The Pentax EC-3870K integrates a confocal microscope (Optiscan Pty. Ltd., Victoria, Australia) into the distal tip of the endoscope. Two white-light guides provide illumination for the wide-area imaging by the objective onto a CCD detector, and the instrument channel is used to obtain tissue biopsies. (b) The Cellvizio-GI (Mauna Kea Technologies, Paris, France) consists of a miniprobe that passes through the instrument channel of a standard medical endoscope and moves independently of the endoscope so that the white-light image can be used to guide confocal placement.

channel has a standard diameter of 2.8 mm and can be used to obtain pinch biopsies of the mucosa. With the confocal window placed into contact with the tissue for confocal image collection, the white-light image becomes unavailable to guide confocal placement. Alternatively, the Cellvizio-GI (Mauna Kea Technologies, Paris, France) is a miniprobe that passes through the instrument channel of most standard medical endoscopes [Figure 2.1(b) shows the Olympus CFQ-180 colonoscope with a diameter of 11 mm]. In this approach, the confocal moves independently of the endoscope so that placement onto the tissue can be guided by the white-light image [21, 22]. The miniprobe is retracted from the instrument channel in order to collect standard pinch biopsies of tissue.

The EC-3870K incorporates an Optiscan confocal microscope, a single-axis [Figure 2.1(a)] optical configuration that uses one single-mode fiber aligned with a GRIN objective with an NA ≈ 0.6 to focus the beam into the tissue. Scanning of the distal tip of the optical fiber is performed mechanically by coupling the fiber to a tuning fork and vibrating at resonance, as shown in Figure 2.2(a). Axial scanning is performed with a nitinol actuator that can translate the focal volume over a distance of 0 to 250 μm below the tissue surface. Excitation is provide at 488 nm (peak absorption of fluorescein) by a semiconductor laser, and a transverse and axial resolution of 0.7 and 7 μm, respectively, has been achieved. The images are collected at a frame rate of either 0.8 or 1.6 Hz to achieve a field of view of either 1,024 × 1,024 or 1,024 × 512 pixels, respectively. Figure 2.2(b) summarizes the performance parameters of this instrument.

This instrument has been demonstrated in the gastrointestinal tract for a number of clinical applications. In the colon, patients scheduled for routine screening colonoscopy were recruited and prepared with 4L of golytely. Confocal images were collected following intravenous administration of fluorescein sodium (5 to 10

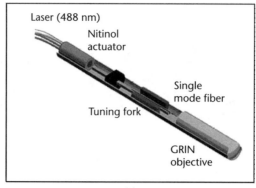

(a)

Parameter		EC3870K
Working distance (μm)	0–250	0–250
Trans. res. (μm)	0.7	0.7
Axial res. (μm)	7	7
Field of view (pixels^2)	1024 × 1024	1024 × 512
Diameter* (mm)	12.8	12.8
Frame rate (Hz)	0.8	1.6

(b)

Figure 2.2 Optiscan confocal imaging system. (a) Scanning of a single-mode optical fiber is performed by a tuning fork in resonance, and z-scanning is provided by a nitinol actuator that is activated in the hand piece. (b) Performance of this confocal microscope includes a transverse and axial resolution of 0.7 and 7 μm, respectively, at a frame rate of 0.8 and 1.6 Hz. The diameter represents that for the overall endoscope; the confocal microscope itself is approximately 5 mm.

mL at 10% solution). When a suspicious region of mucosa was found on white light, the distal tip of the endoscope was placed in gentle contact with the mucosa, and the position of the confocal plane was adjusted to achieve the best image. More than 70% of the images were found to be satisfactory in quality. The others were affected by motion artifacts. The images collected with 1,024 × 1,024 pixels typically contained 6 to 12 crypts in the field of view.

Color Plate 3 shows in vivo confocal images collected with the Pentax EC-3870K. An image of normal colonic mucosa in Color Plate 3(a) reveals mucin-containing goblet cells and the columnar epithelial cells, scale bar 80 μm. With intravenous administration, fluorescein becomes distributed throughout the entire mucosa within seconds, providing contrast to highlight the epithelium and the connective tissue and microvasculature within the intervening lamina propria. Fluorescein also enhances the microstructures within the villi in the terminal ileum, as shown in Color Plate 3(b). Significant distortion of the microarchitecture can be seen in the images of intraepithelial neoplasia and colonic adenocarcinoma, shown in Color Plate 3(c, d), respectively. The corresponding histology for each image obtained from pinch biopsy is shown in Color Plate 3(e–h), respectively.

2.4 MKT Cellvizio-GI

The Cellvizio-GI uses a significantly different design in the same single-axis [Color Plate 2(a)] optical configuration. A bundle of multimode optical fibers (~30,000), rather than one single mode, is aligned to a GRIN objective with an NA ≈ 0.6 to focus the beam into the tissue. The core of each individual fiber acts as the collection pinholes for rejecting out-of-focus light to perform optical sectioning. Scanning is performed at the proximal end of the bundle in the instrument control unit with a 4 kHz oscillating mirror for horizontal lines and a 12 Hz galvo mirror for frames. Because transverse scanning is not performed at the distal tip, these miniprobes have much smaller diameters of 1.5 to 1.8 mm. No axial scanning is performed; thus, separate miniprobes with different working distances are needed to section at different depths. Excitation is provided at 488 nm, and at this wavelength, the transverse and axial resolution ranges from 2.5 to 5 and 15 to 20 μm, respectively. Images are collected at a frame rate of 12 Hz with a field of view of either 600 × 500 or 240 × 200 μm. Figure 2.3(b) summarizes the performance parameters of this instrument.

The use of beam scanning in this system enables the fast frame rate (12 Hz) and allows for mucosal function to be evaluated and quantified [23]. Transient ($t < 5$s) and steady-state ($t > 5$s) images of normal colonic mucosa, hyperplasia, tubular

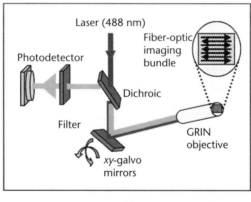

(a)

Parameter	S	HD
Working distance (μm)	0	50
Trans. res. (μm)	5	2.5
Axial res. (μm)	15	20
Field of view (μm^2)	600 × 500	240 × 200
Diameter* (mm)	1.5	1.8
Frame rate (Hz)	12	12

(b)

Figure 2.3 Cellvizio-GI confocal imaging system. (a) Scanning of the fiber-optic imaging bundle is performed by *xy*-galvo mirrors located in the instrument control unit to perform horizontal cross-sectional imaging. (b) Optical imaging parameters of two confocal miniprobes available for clinical use are shown.

adenoma, and villous adenoma have been collected in vivo following topical administration of fluorescein onto colonic mucosa. Mucosal function was quantified by measuring the steady-state fluorescence contrast ratio defined by a ratio of the mean intensity from the lamina propria to that of a crypt using an average of three sites from each region with an area of $35 \times 35\ \mu m^2$, sufficient to span several cells and to account for image variability. Images that displayed discrete glands with centrally located lumens and well-defined space between the glands (lamina propria) were included in the analysis. A pinch biopsy was obtained from all sites imaged and processed for routine histology.

The steady-state images, along with the corresponding histology (H&E), are shown in Figure 2.4, scale bar 20 μm. For normal mucosa, shown in Figure 2.4(a), individual colonocytes (c) can be seen surrounding the lumen (l) of the crypt, and the apical and basolateral epithelial cell membranes can be clearly distinguished. Contrast enhances the lamina propria (lp) between the glands. The crypts are circular in shape, are approximately uniform in size, and have oval lumens. For hyperplasia, shown in Figure 2.4(b), proliferative colonocytes (c) line an irregularly shaped lumen (l) that displays inward buckling in a serrated or saw-toothed appearance. The crypts are circular in shape but significantly larger in size than those of normal mucosa. Contrast can be seen in the lamina propria (lp) beyond the border of the gland. For the tubular adenoma, shown in Figure 2.4(c), distorted colonocytes (c) surround an elongated lumen (l), and the crypts appear eccentric in shape and are slightly larger in size than those of normal mucosa. Contrast appears to accumulate along the basolateral border of the epithelial cells rather than the apical surface. Moreover, the fluorescence intensity in the lamina propria (lp) appears reduced. For the villous adenoma, shown in Figure 2.4(d), enlarged colonocytes (c) surround a significantly elongated lumen (l).

Contrast accumulates within the colonocytes in a punctuate fashion with multiple filling defects. The adenomatous mucosa exhibits a papillary appearance, with elliptical mucosal profiles that are significantly larger in size than those of normal mucosa. Moreover, the fluorescence intensity in the lamina propria (lp) of these pap-

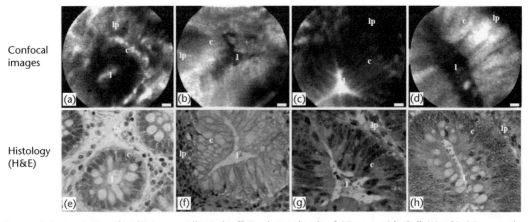

Figure 2.4 In vivo confocal images collected, affected at a depth of 50 μm, with Cellvizio-GI: (a) normal colonic mucosa, (b) hyperplasia, (c) tubular adenoma, and (d) villous adenoma following topical administration of fluorescein. Corresponding histology is shown in (e–h); scale bar = 20 μm.

illary profiles is significantly reduced. A greater lamina propria:crypt fluorescence-contrast-ratio value was found for normal than for lesional mucosa. On average, the fluorescence contrast ratios (mean ± std. dev.) for normal, hyperplasia, tubular adenoma, and villous adenoma are 1.29 ± 0.24 (range 0.85 to 1.74), 0.92 ± 0.10 (range 0.69 to 1.08), 0.60 ± 0.10 (range 0.43 to 0.81), and 0.41 ± 0.03 (range 0.38 to 0.44), respectively. The difference in the mean contrast ratio is statistically significant for normal versus lesional mucosa (including hyperplasia, tubular adenoma, and villous adenoma), $p < 0.001$; hyperplasia versus adenoma (including tubular and villous), $p < 0.001$; and tubular versus villous adenoma, $p < 0.001$.

The key features of the Cellvizio-GI system have recently been adapted for use in the lung. This system is called the F400/S, and the fluorescence collected by the fiber bundle is divided for imaging (80%) and spectroscopy (20%) by a beam splitter. A 1.4 mm diameter miniprobe (BronchoFlex) has similar imaging parameters to that of the S instrument and is passed through the instrument channel of a bronchoscope. The miniprobe is placed in contact with the bronchial epithelium and can collect both the autofluorescence spectra (530 to 750 nm) and confocal image from the same location. This system was used to study autofluorescence from the bronchial mucosa and found the origin to be from the elastin component of the basement membrane zone [22].

2.5 Dual-Axes Confocal Microscope

A miniature, endoscope-compatible (5 mm diameter) confocal microscope has been developed with the dual-axes architecture [shown in Figure 2.5(a)]. This instrument passes easily through the 6 mm diameter instrument channel of a therapeutic endoscope. The design of the scanhead is based on the simple optics principle of focusing two parallel beams on a common point in the tissue with a parabolic surface (mirror), as shown in Figure 2.5(a) [24]. This approach provides for tremendous flexibility in the choice of wavelengths used because no refractive optics are required. This avoids defocusing of the region of overlap between the two beams from chromatic aberrations and allows for future development of multispectral imaging. Scanning of the beam is performed with use of a high-speed MEMS mirror mounted on a chip that contains the control and power wires. A parabolic mirror with NA ≈ 0.12 focuses the beam into the tissue at either 488 or 785 nm to achieve a transverse and axial resolution of approximately 1 and 2 μm or approximately 2 and 4 μm, respectively, as shown in Figure 2.5(b). The images can be collected at a frame rate of 5 Hz to obtain a field of view of approximately $400 \times 800\ \mu m^2$. These dimensions are much larger than those achieved with the single-axis configuration because postobjective scanning is used. The performance of this instrument will be clinically demonstrated in the near future.

The MEMS mirror performs high-speed scanning while maintaining a fixed intersection of the two beams below the tissue surface [25]. The geometry of this scanner is barbell in shape and has an active mirror surface of $600 \times 650\ \mu m^2$ each connected by a 300 μm wide strut. Actuation is performed with use of vertical combdrives. Fabrication of the scanner involves four deep-reactive-ion-etching (DRIE) steps to self-align the comb fingers in the device layers by transferring mask

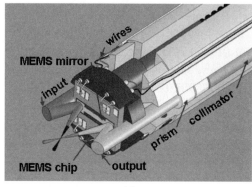

(a)

Parameter	488 nm	785 nm
Working distance (μm)	0–250	0–500
Trans. res. (μm)	1	2
Axial res. (μm)	2	4
Field of view (μm^2)	400 × 800	400 × 800
Diameter* (mm)	5	5
Frame rate (Hz)	5	5

(b)

Figure 2.5 Dual-axes confocal imaging system. (a) The dual-axes architecture uses two fibers (input/output) for separate illumination and collection of light, using the region of overlap between the two beams (focal volume) to achieve subcellular resolution. The scanhead design focuses two parallel beams on a common point in the tissue with a parabolic mirror, and scanning of the beam is performed with use of a high-speed MEMS mirror. (b) A parabolic mirror with NA ≈ 0.12 focuses the beam into the tissue at 488 (785) nm to achieve a transverse and axial resolution of approximately 1 and 2 μm (~2 and 4 μm), respectively. The images can be collected at a frame rate of 5 Hz to obtain a field of view of 400 × 800 μm^2 using postobjective scanning.

features sequentially from upper to lower layers and to remove the backside of the substrate behind the mirror, releasing the gimbal for rotation. The mirror surfaces were coated with aluminum using a blanket evaporation technique to achieve greater than 90% reflectivity at visible wavelengths. The maximum dc optical scan angles are ±3.3° on the inner axis and ±1.0° on the outer axis, and the corresponding resonance frequencies are 3.54 and 1.1 kHz. Images can be acquired at rates of up to 30 frames/s with a maximum field of view of 800 × 400 μm^2, but the process is often run more slowly to improve signal collection.

Fluorescence is detected with a photomultiplier tube (Hamamatsu, H7422-50) whose gain is modulated to achieve amplification of the fluorescence signal from the deeper regions of tissue and digitized with 8 bits (Data Translation, DT3152) [26]. A long-pass filter (Semrock, LP02-785RU-25) is used to reject the excitation light. Figure 2.5(a) shows an ex vivo demonstration of vertical cross-sectional imaging. A freshly excised specimen of colonic mucosa was soaked for 1 minute in a near-infrared dye (LI-COR Biosciences, IRDye 800CW) at a concentration of 0.1 mg/mL (90 μM) with 5% DMSO to facilitate dye penetration into the tissue. Figure 2.6(a)

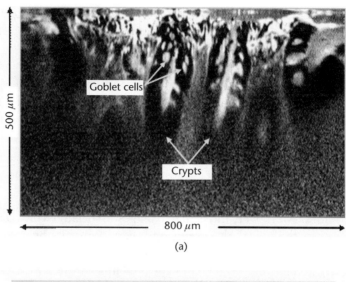

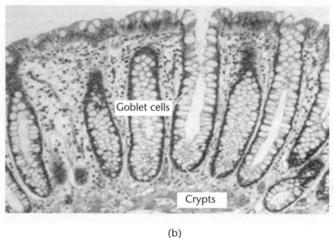

Figure 2.6 Vertical cross-sectional image of colonic mucosa: (a) collected with dual-axes confocal microscope on excised mucosa stained with IRDye 800CW and revealing individual goblet cells within vertical crypts, and (b) corresponding histology.

shows a vertical cross-sectional image with a tissue-penetration depth of 500 μm and a horizontal field of view of 800 μm. Individual goblet cells can be seen within a vertical view of several crypts, and the corresponding histology is shown in Figure 2.6(b) for purposes of comparison. Table 2.1 compares the key imaging parameters used for in vivo confocal imaging among the Pentax EC-3870, MKT Cellvizio, and dual-axes microendoscopes.

2.6 Molecular Imaging

Because of its sensitivity to fluorescence, confocal microscopy has potential for great impact in clinical medicine as a tool for performing molecular imaging. Transformed cells and tissues express molecular changes well in advance of architectural

Table 2.1 Comparison of Key Imaging Parameters Used for In Vivo Confocal Imaging Among the Pentax EC-3870, MKT Cellvizio, and Dual-Axes Microendoscopes

Parameters	Pentax EC-3870	MKT Cellvizio	Dual Axes
Excitation	Fixed at 488 nm	Variable (488–660 nm)	Variable (488–785 nm)
Resolution	Very good (<10 μm)	Good (15–20 μm)	Very good (<10 μm)
Size	Good (5 mm)	Excellent (1–2 mm)	Good (5 mm)
Field of view	Good (<400 μm)	Fair (<200 μm)	Excellent (400–800 μm)
Frame rate	Slow (0.8–1.6 Hz)	Very fast (12 Hz)	Fast (5 Hz)
z-scanning	Good (0–250 μm)	Fair (fixed—0, 50,100 μm)	Excellent (0–500 μm)

deformities. Moreover, molecular changes associated with genetic instability precede histopathological alterations and may ultimately be a more useful parameter for diagnostic evaluation. Molecular probes that bind to targets of disease can be topically administered safely and conveniently through medical endoscopes. These probes can be labeled with fluorescent dyes and used to guide tissue biopsy, assess for submucosal invasion, and monitor response to therapy. There has been a great deal of research in developing the use of molecular probes to target neoplasia in preclinical (small-animal) models. For example, monoclonal antibodies have been investigated for tumor detection and drug delivery because of their high specificity [27, 28]; however, delivery challenges, immunogenicity, and the cost of reagent development have limited their use in vivo [29]. The molecular targets for detection have included proteolytic enzymes [30], matrix metalloproteinases [31], endothelial-specific markers [32], and apoptosis reporters [33, 34]. Recently, a number of near-infrared fluorescent-labeled probes have been developed to detect neoplasia and have potential to image with deep tissue penetration [35].

Peptides have tremendous potential for use as molecular probes because of their high clonal diversity, small size, compatibility with fluorescence labels, and minimal immunogenicity, and they are well suited for clinical use because of their rapid binding kinetics, deep tissue penetration, and lack of toxicity. Methods of targeted detection of cancer with peptides have been demonstrated in the ex vivo setting [36, 37]. A recent study has demonstrated the use of fluorescent-labeled peptides to target dysplastic colonocytes in vivo with confocal microscopy [38]. When premalignant colonic mucosa, such as the adenoma shown in Color Plate 4(a), was identified on white-light endoscopy, the Cellvizio-GI miniprobe was passed through the instrument channel and placed in contact with the lesion. The in vivo confocal image shown in Color Plate 4(b) reveals preferential binding of the FITC-labeled target peptide to transformed colonocytes within a dysplastic crypt. Color Plate 4(c) shows preferential binding to the dysplastic crypt in comparison to the adjacent normal crypt. Color Plate 4(d) shows a hyperplastic polyp (no malignant potential), the confocal image in Color Plate 4(e) reveals absence of binding by the target peptide due to the lack of fluorescence. Furthermore, no peptide binding to the adjacent normal mucosa is seen either, as Color Plate 4(f) shows (scale bar 20 μm).

Images were quantitatively evaluated that met the following criteria: (1) minimum motion artifact; (2) lack of stool, debris, or excess mucus obscuring the image; and (3) the presence of crypt morphology. The mean fluorescence intensity associated with peptide binding was calculated using the average of three independent regions (size $25 \times 25\ \mu m^2$) within a dysplastic and adjacent normal crypt from five consecutive images. The target-to-background ratio was calculated from the ratio of the mean fluorescence intensities from regions of dysplastic and adjacent normal mucosa. A mean target-to-background ratio of 4.7 ± 0.5 was calculated for the target peptide from a total of $n = 57$ adenomas. The detection criterion for each site was compared to a threshold intensity, designated positive if greater (negative if less), that was varied over the range of fluorescence intensities measured (0 to 80), as displayed in Figure 2.7. Figure 2.7(a) shows the sensitivity, specificity, positive predictive value (PPV), and negative predictive value (NPV) for this technique as a function of the target-to-background ratio. In Figure 2.7(b), the ROC curve shows the optimal trade-off in performance for the detection of dysplasia. An optimum

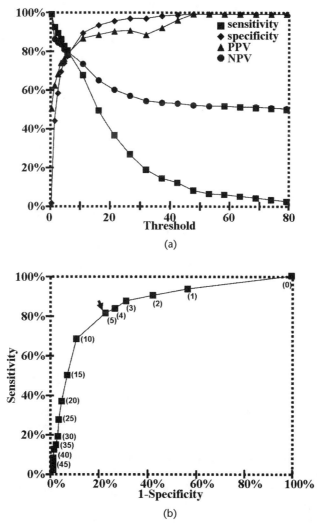

Figure 2.7 Performance for peptide binding on confocal microscopy. (a) The sensitivity, specificity, PPV, and NPV for targeted detection of colonic dysplasia is shown as a function of the target-to-background ratio. (b) ROC curve shows optimal sensitivity and specificity of 81% and 78% achieved at threshold of five (arrow).

sensitivity of 81% and specificity of 78% were achieved at a threshold of five (arrow). This result is very promising, as the use of multiple probes that bind to independent targets can achieve very high detection accuracy. No toxicity associated with peptide administration was observed in any of the patients.

In summary, confocal microscopy is a well-known method for creating high-resolution images in unprocessed tissue using the technique of optical sectioning that has recently been demonstrated in vivo, resulting from significant advances in the miniaturization of optics and scanning mechanisms. Imaging instruments based on optical fibers are now being used in the clinic via medical endoscopes. Various designs are being developed that have advantages in resolution (Optiscan), size (MKT), and tissue penetration (dual axes). In general, microscopes that perform distal scanning require a larger form factor (~5 mm) than those that scan proximally (~2 mm), and beam scanning techniques achieve a faster frame rate than mechanical scanning methods, which is necessary to reduce in vivo motion artifact and to collect functional images. Commercially available systems use the single-axis design where the fiber and objective lie along the main optical axis and collect images in the horizontal cross sections. In vivo images have been collected using excitation at 488 nm and either intravenous or topical fluorescein for contrast. Images with subcellular resolution of mucosal microanatomy have been demonstrated that exhibit striking resemblance to the corresponding histology. The dual-axes architecture minimizes the effects of tissue scattering with off-axis light collection and results in an improvement in dynamic range, allowing for the collection of vertical cross sections (preferred pathologist's view). This configuration is being scaled down in dimension for in vivo use with high-speed MEMS scanning mirrors. Finally, confocal microscopy has been used to validate in vivo binding of fluorescent-labeled probes to molecular targets and is promising as a tool to guide tissue biopsy, assess response to therapy, and monitor disease recurrence. This integrated imaging methodology can assess the presence of subtle molecular changes in cells and tissues expressed well prior to gross morphological changes in the disease process.

References

[1] Pawley, J. B., ed., *Handbook of biological confocal microscopy*, 3rd ed., New York: Springer-Verlag, 2006.

[2] Yelin, D., Rizvi, I., White, W. M., Motz, J. T., Hasan, T., Bouma, B. E., and Tearney, G. J. "Three-dimensional miniature endoscopy," *Nature* 443 (2006): 765.

[3] Rouse, A. R., Kano, A., Udovich, J. A., Kroto, S. M., and Gmitro, A. F. "Design and demonstration of a miniature catheter for a confocal microendoscope," *Appl. Opt.* 43 (2004): 5763–5771.

[4] Laemmel, E., Genet, M., Le Goualher, G., Perchant, A., Le Gargasson, J. F., and Vicaut, E. "Fibered confocal fluorescence microscopy (Cell-viZio) facilitates extended imaging in the field of microcirculation: A comparison with intravital microscopy," *J. Vasc. Res.* 41 (2004): 400–411.

[5] Kiesslich, R., Burg, J., Vieth, M., Gnaendiger, J., Enders, M., Delaney, P., Polglase, A., McLaren, W., Janell, D., Thomas, S., Nafe, B., Galle, P. R., and Neurath, M. F. "Confocal laser endoscopy for diagnosing intraepithelial neoplasias and colorectal cancer in vivo," *Gastroenterology* 127 (2004): 706–713.

[6] Thiberville, L., Moreno-Swirc, S., Vercauteren, T., Peltier, E., Cave, C., Bourg Heckly, G. "In vivo imaging of the bronchial wall microstructure using fibered confocal fluorescence microscopy," *Am. J. Respir. Crit. Care Med.* 175 (2007): 22–31.

[7] Kitabatake, S., Niwa, Y., Miyahara, R., Ohashi, A., Matsuura, T., Iguchi, Y., Shimoyama, Y., Nagasaka, T., Maeda, O., Ando, T., Ohmiya, N., Itoh, A., Hirooka, Y., and Goto, H. "Confocal endomicroscopy for the diagnosis of gastric cancer in vivo," *Endoscopy* 38 (2006): 1110–1114.

[8] Kiesslich, R., Goetz, M., Burg, J., Stolte, M., Siegel, E., Maeurer, M. J., Thomas, S., Strand, D., Galle, P. R., and Neurath, M. F. "Diagnosing helicobacter pylori in vivo by confocal laser endoscopy," *Gastroenterology* 128 (2005): 2119–2123.

[9] Meining, A., Bajbouj, M., and Schmid, R. M. "Confocal fluorescence microscopy for detection of gastric angiodysplasia," *Endoscopy* 39 (2007): S1:E145.

[10] Meining, A., Schwendy, S., Becker, V., Schmid, R. M., and Prinz, C. "In vivo histopathology of lymphocytic colitis," *Gastrointest. Endosc.* 66 (2007): 398–399.

[11] Sabharwal, Y. S., Rouse, A. R., Donaldson, L., Hopkins, M. F., and Gmitro, A. F. "Slit-scanning confocal microendoscope for high-resolution in vivo imaging," *Appl. Opt.* 38 (1999): 7133–7144.

[12] Liang, C., Sung, K., Richards-Kortum, R., and Descour, M. R. "Design of a high-numerical-aperture miniature microscope objective for an endoscopic fiber confocal reflectance microscope," *Appl. Opt.* 41 (2002): 4603–4610.

[13] Delaney, P. M., Harris, M. R., and King, R. G. "Fiber-optic laser scanning confocal microscope suitable for fluorescence imaging," *Appl. Opt.* 94(33) (1994): 573–577.

[14] Dickensheets, D. L., and Kino, G. S. "A micromachined scanning confocal optical microscope," *Opt. Lett.* 21 (1996): 764–766.

[15] Piyawattanametha, W., Barretto, R. P. J., Ko, T. H., Flusberg, B. A., Cocker, E. D., Ra, H., Lee, D., Solgaard, O., and Schnitzer, M. J. "Fast-scanning two-photon fluorescence imaging based on a microelectromechanical systems two-dimensional scanning mirror," *Opt. Lett.* 31(13) (2006): 2018–2020.

[16] Wang, T. D., Mandella, M. J., Contag, C. H., and Kino, G. S. "Dual axes confocal microscope for high resolution in vivo imaging," *Opt. Lett.* 28 (2003): 414–416.

[17] Wang, T. D., Contag, C. H., Mandella, M. J., Chan, N. Y., and Kino, G. S. "Dual axes confocal microscope with post-objective scanning and low coherence heterodyne detection," *Opt. Lett.* 28 (2003): 1915–1917.

[18] Wong, L. K., Mandella, M. J., Kino, G. S., and Wang, T. D. "Improved rejection of multiply scattered photons in confocal microscopy using dual-axes architecture," *Opt. Lett.* 32 (2007): 1674–1676.

[19] Kiesslich, R., Burg, J., Vieth, M., Gnaendiger, J., Enders, M., Delaney, P., Polglase, A., McLaren, W., Janell, D., Thomas, S., Nafe, B., Galle, P. R., and Neurath, M. F. "Confocal laser endoscopy for diagnosing intraepithelial neoplasias and colorectal cancer in vivo," *Gastroenterology* 127 (2004): 706–713.

[20] Kiesslich, R., Gossner, L., Goetz, M., Dahlmann, A., Vieth, M., Stolte, M., Hoffman, A., Jung, M., Nafe, B., Galle, P. R., and Neurath, M. F. "In vivo histology of Barrett's esophagus and associated neoplasia by confocal laser endomicroscopy," *Clin. Gastroenterol. Hepatol.* 4 (2006): 979–987.

[21] Meining, A., Saur, D., Bajbouj, M., Becker, V., Peltier, E., Höfler, H., von Weyhern, C. H., Schmid, R. M., and Prinz, C. "In vivo histopathology for detection of gastrointestinal neoplasia with a portable, confocal miniprobe: An examiner blinded analysis," *Clin. Gastroenterol. Hepatol.* 5 (2007): 1261–1267.

[22] Thiberville, L., Moreno-Swirc, S., Vercauteren, T., Peltier, E., Cave, C., and Bourg Heckly, G. "In vivo imaging of the bronchial wall microstructure using fibered confocal fluorescence microscopy," *Am. J. Respir. Crit. Care Med.* 175 (2007): 22–31.

[23] Wang, T. D., Friedland, S., Sahbaie, P., Soetikno, R., Hsiung, P., Liu, J. T. C., Crawford, J. M., and Contag, C. "Functional imaging of colonic mucosa with a fibered confocal microscope for real time in vivo pathology," *Clin. Gastroent. Hepatol.* 5 (2007): 1300–1305.

[24] Liu, J. T. C., Mandella, M. J., Ra, H., Lee, D., Kino, G. S., Solgaard, O., Piyawattanametha, W., Contag, C. H., and Wang, T. D. "Miniature near-infrared dual-axes confocal microscope utilizing a two-dimensional microelectromechanical systems scanner," *Opt. Lett.* 32 (2007): 256–258.

[25] Ra, H., Piyawattanametha, W., Taguchi, Y., Lee, D., Mandella, M. J., and Solgaard, O. "Two-dimensional MEMS scanner for dual-axes confocal microscopy," *J. Microelectromech. Syst.* 16(4) (2007): 969–976.

[26] Liu, J. T. C., Mandella, M. J., Crawford, J. M., Contag, C. H., Wang, T. D., and Kino, G. S. "Effective rejection of scattered light enables deep optical sectioning in turbid media with low-NA optics in a dual-axes confocal architecture," *J. Biomed. Opt.*, 13(03) (2008).

[27] Orlova, A., Magnusson, M., Eriksson, T. L., Nilsson, M., Larsson, B., Hoiden-Guthenberg, I., Widstrom, C., Carlsson, J., Tolmachev, V., Stahl, S., and Nilsson, F. Y. "Tumor imaging using a picomolar affinity HER2 binding affibody molecule," *Canc. Res.* 66 (2006): 4339–4348.

[28] Keller, R., Winde, G., Terpe, H. J., Foerster, E. C., and Domschke, W. "Fluorescence endoscopy using a fluorescein-labeled monoclonal antibody against carcinoembryonic antigen in patients with colorectal carcinoma and adenoma," *Endoscopy* 34 (2002): 801–807.

[29] Goldsmith, S. J. "Receptor imaging: Competitive or complementary to antibody imaging?" *Semin. Nucl. Med.* 27 (1997): 85–93.

[30] Tung, C. H., Mahmood, U., Bredow, S., and Weissleder, R. "In vivo imaging of proteolytic enzyme activity using a novel molecular reporter," *Canc. Res.* 60 (2000): 4953–4958.

[31] Bremer, C., Bredow, S., Mahmood, U., Weissleder, R., and Tung, C. H. "Optical imaging of matrix metalloproteinase-2 activity in tumors: Feasibility study in a mouse model," *Radiology* 221 (2001): 523–529.

[32] Kang, H. W., Torres, D., Wald, L., Weissleder, R., and Bogdanov, A. A., Jr. "Targeted imaging of human endothelial-specific marker in a model of adoptive cell transfer," *Lab. Invest.* 86 (2006): 599–609.

[33] Laxman, B., Hall, D. E., Bhojani, M. S., Hamstra, D. A., Chenevert, T. L., Ross, B. D., and Rehemtulla, A. "Noninvasive real-time imaging of apoptosis," *PNAS* 99 (2002): 16551–16555.

[34] Messerli, S. M., Prabhakar, S., Tang, Y., Shah, K., Cortes, M. L., Murthy, V., Weissleder, R., Breakefield, X. O., and Tung, C. H. "A novel method for imaging apoptosis using a caspase-1 near-infrared fluorescent probe," *Neoplasia* 6 (2004): 95–105.

[35] Weissleder, R., Tung, C. H., Mahmood, U., and Bogdanov, A., Jr. "In vivo imaging of tumors with protease-activated near-infrared fluorescent probes," *Nat. Biotechnol.* 17 (1999): 375–378.

[36] Kelly, K., Alencar, H., Funovics, M., Mahmood, U., and Weissleder, R. "Detection of invasive colon cancer using a novel, targeted, library-derived fluorescent peptide," *Canc. Res.* 64 (2004): 6247–6251.

[37] Shukla, G. S., and Krag, D. N. "Selection of tumor-targeting agents on freshly excised human breast tumors using a phage display library," *Oncol. Rep.* 13 (2005): 757–764.

[38] Hsiung, P., Hardy, J., Friedland, S., Soetikno, R., Du, C. B., Wu, A. P. W., Sahbaie, P., Crawford, J. M., Lowe, A., Contag, C. H., and Wang, T. D. "Detection of colonic dysplasia in vivo using a targeted fluorescent septapeptide and confocal microendoscopy," *Nat. Med.* 14 (2008): 454–458.

CHAPTER 3
Endoscopy

Yu Chen, Aaron D. Aguirre, Desmond C. Adler, Hiroshi Mashimo, and James G. Fujimoto

3.1 Introduction

Conventional endoscopic diagnosis is based on the visualization of abnormal patterns from the images generated by light reflected from the mucosal surface. Recent advances in optical technologies (such as light sources, detectors, and fiber optics) and molecular biology have improved the capability for detection, classification, and monitoring of neoplastic changes. The ultimate goal is to detect lesions at their early, premalignant, and curable stages, thereby permitting effective interventions.

When light enters tissue, it undergoes several processes, including absorption, elastic scattering, fluorescence, and Raman scattering. Many promising optical imaging and spectroscopic methods have been developed based on these different mechanisms, aiming to utilize the optical properties obtained through light-tissue interactions to provide diagnostic information in vivo and in real time. These optical methods include point-probe spectroscopy (fluorescence, light scattering, and Raman spectroscopy), wide-field imaging (fluorescence imaging, chromoendoscopy, and narrowband imaging), cross-sectional imaging (optical coherence tomography), and confocal endomicroscopy. Compared to standard endoscopy, they provide improved image resolution, contrast, tissue penetration depth, and biochemical and molecular information about the diseases. In this chapter, we will first review each modality (except confocal endomicroscopy, which is described in Chapter 2), including basic principles, technology, and clinical applications. We will also discuss the approaches for multimodality imaging and their translational potentials. In this chapter, we will focus on gastrointestinal (GI) applications as the primary example because this is one of the most developed endoscopic applications for new optical technologies.

3.2 Point-Probe Spectroscopy Techniques

Point-probe spectroscopy is designed to obtain detailed information about the wavelength-dependent optical properties of tissue at a single spatial location. A typical point-probe spectroscopy instrument consists of a fiber-optic probe, a light source, and a spectrometer as the detector. The fiber-optic probe contains both the excitation fiber to illuminate the tissue volume and the closely spaced detection fibers to collect the resulting scattered and/or fluorescence light. The separation between the illumination and detection fibers is usually on the order of millimeters, with the total diameter of the optical probe being small enough to pass through the accessory channel of a standard endoscope. The detected light is dispersed in wavelength by a spectrograph, and the spectrum is recorded and analyzed. Depending on the nature of the light-tissue interaction, there are several types of spectroscopy systems, including scattering spectroscopy, fluorescence spectroscopy, and Raman spectroscopy.

3.2.1 Scattering Spectroscopy

Pathological tissue generally exhibits significant morphological changes from normal tissue at the cellular and subcellular levels. Cellular structures and subcellular organelles that cause light scattering typically have dimensions on the order of visible to near-infrared wavelengths. When the scattering particles are similar in size to the wavelength of the incident light, the elastically scattered light (i.e., without change in wavelength) will exhibit wavelength-dependent variations related to the size and density of the particles. In addition, microvascular alterations, such as inflammation and angiogenesis, will cause changes in hemoglobin concentration and oxygenation saturation, which will in turn cause wavelength-dependent absorption features in the detected spectrum. Therefore, the resulting elastic scattering spectrum will exhibit wavelength-dependent variations relating to the underlying biological and pathological state of tissue. There are several closely related scattering spectroscopic technologies: diffuse reflectance spectroscopy (DRS) [1], elastic scattering spectroscopy (ESS) [2], and light-scattering spectroscopy (LSS) [3, 4]. For DRS, the reflected spectra are fit using a diffusion model and are expressed as a function of the absorption (μ_a) and reduced scattering (μ_s') coefficients [1]. Mie theory predictions and analytical models have also been developed to extract the scattering and absorption coefficients for ESS [5, 6]. In LSS, the multiple scattered photons modeled by DRS are subtracted from the measured spectrum to enhance the contribution from single- or few-scattered photons [3]. By fitting the Mie scattering model to the periodic fine structure component of the single- or few-scattering spectra, it is possible to detect the changes in scattering-particle size and density, which can subsequently indicate alterations in nuclear enlargement and crowding caused by neoplastic changes [4].

Scattering spectroscopy techniques have shown promising results in detecting early cancers in the GI tract in vivo. Figure 3.1(a, b) shows a schematic diagram of an ESS system and representative tissue spectra. Using ESS in the upper GI tract, Lovat et al. found 92% sensitivity and 60% specificity for detecting high-risk disease [high-grade dysplasia (HGD) or cancer] associated with Barrett's esophagus (BE), with data analyzed from 181 sites in 81 patients [7]. In the lower GI tract, Dhar et al. reported 92% sensitivity and 82% specificity for differentiating pathological tissues (including colitis, dysplasia, and cancer) from normal tissue, with ESS spectra obtained from 138 sites in 45 patients [8]. Georgakoudi et al. found 86% sensitivity and 100% specificity in classifying high-grade dysplastic (HGD) versus low-grade dysplastic (LGD) and nondysplastic Barrett's esophagus (BE) with DRS

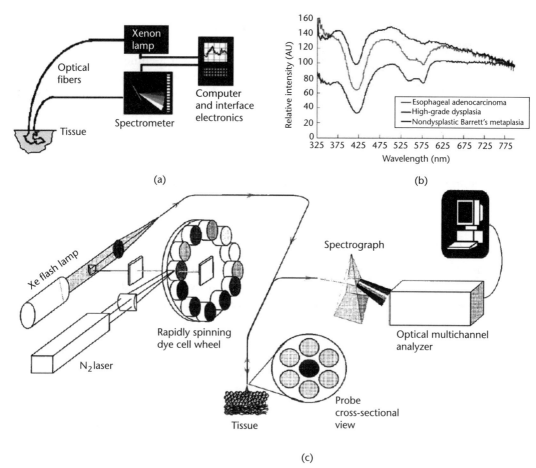

Figure 3.1 (a) Schematic diagram of elastic scattering spectroscopy (ESS) system [8]. (b) Representative spectra obtained with ESS [8]. (c) Schematic diagram of trimodal spectroscopy (TMS) system. Fluorescence measurements were performed using a fast excitation-emission matrix (EEM) instrument with a 337 nm nitrogen laser pumping 10 dye cuvettes to generate 11 different excitation wavelengths between 337 and 620 nm. Reflectance measurements were obtained using the white light (350 to 700 nm) from an Xe flash lamp (*From:* [9]. © 2001 Elsevier. Reprinted with permission.)

spectrum collected from 40 sites in 16 patients [9]. They also reported 100% sensitivity and 91% specificity in classifying HGD versus LGD and nondysplastic BE using LSS from the same patients [9]. In a retrospective study using 76 sites from 13 BE patients, Wallace et al. found that LSS detected dysplasia (either HGD or LGD) with 90% sensitivity and 90% specificity using a diagnostic threshold criteria that more than 30% of the nuclei exceed 10 μm [10].

LSS can be extended from point-probe to imaging mode by using a CCD camera and narrowband filters [11]. This allows the investigation of a wider field of view than a point sampling technique. Several new-generation light-scattering techniques have been developed recently as well. For example, azimuthal LSS (ϕ/LSS) measures the scattering spectra at different azimuthal angles (the angle between the incident light polarization and the scattering plane) $\phi = 0°$ and $90°$. For larger structures like nuclei, the scattering exhibits azimuthal asymmetry, whereas for small particles such as mitochondria, scattering is virtually independent of azimuthal angle. Therefore, this approach can isolate the scattering from nuclei from that of smaller organelles and the diffusive background [12]. Another technique, four-dimensional elastic light-scattering fingerprints (4D-ELF), enables the simultaneous measurement of the spectral (wavelength), angular (scattering angle), azimuthal (ϕ), and polarization dependence of the scattered light [13]. 4-D ELF has been demonstrated to probe the nanoscale/microscale cellular architecture in a rat model of colon carcinogenesis [14] and preneoplastic, colonic microvasculature changes in both an animal model and biopsy specimens from patients undergoing screening colonoscopy [15]. These results suggest that light-scattering spectroscopy holds promise for screening and for detecting early cancer.

3.2.2 Fluorescence Spectroscopy

Fluorescence spectroscopy uses fluorescence from either endogenous (autofluorescence) or exogenous molecules to aid in differentiating diseased mucosa from the normal tissues [16, 17]. In fluorescence spectroscopy, the tissue is illuminated with light, usually in the ultraviolet (UV) or short visible (VIS) wavelength range, thus exciting fluorescent molecules within the tissue (fluorophores). The fluorescence spectra at longer wavelengths than the excitation light are collected and analyzed [18, 19]. Endogenous fluorophores include connective tissues (collagen, elastin), cellular-metabolism-related coenzymes [reduced nicotinamide adenine dinucleotide (NADH), flavin adenine dinucleotide (FAD), and flavin mononucleotide (FMN)], and by-products of heme biosynthesis (porphyrins), among others [20]. Therefore, fluorescence spectroscopy can provide information relating to the biochemical state of the tissue.

Fluorescence spectroscopy systems generally can probe up to depths of several hundreds of microns in biological tissues. The peak wavelength and intensity of the spectra can be used to differentiate between normal versus diseased mucosa due to the changes in the concentration and distribution of metabolically related fluorophores and alterations of the tissue microstructures [16, 21, 22]. Several biochemical and morphologic factors may correlate with fluorescence changes associated with dysplastic lesions, including increased absorption of hemoglobin and loss of spectral contributions from submucosal connective tissues [23]. Abnormal thickening of epithelial tissue may cause attenuation of the excitation light, thus leading to further decreases in the fluorescence intensity. The fluorescence signal is often influenced by wavelength-dependent tissue scattering and absorption. Therefore methods have been developed to extract the intrinsic fluorescence spectroscopy (IFS) signal by measuring the fluorescence and reflectance spectra with the same light delivery/collection geometry in order to cancel these unwanted wavelength-dependent effects [24, 25].

Point-probe fluorescence spectroscopy instruments can be integrated into a fiber-optic catheter device for endoscopic applications. Previous studies have shown that fluorescence spectroscopy can increase the detection rate of high-grade dysplasia (HGD) in Barrett's esophagus [16, 21]. Using 330-nm excitation and by analyzing the fluorescence-intensity ratio at 390 and 550 nm ($I_{390\ nm}/I_{550\ nm}$),

Bourg-Heckly et al. found 86% sensitivity and 95% specificity for differentiating neoplastic tissue (HGD and intramucosal carcinoma) from normal and Barrett's mucosa in 24 patients [21]. Panjehpour et al. analyzed the fluorescence spectra from 36 patients using a differential normalized fluorescence (DNF) index technique. In DNF, the measured fluorescence spectrum is subtracted by a baseline value obtained by averaging the total-intensity-normalized spectra from the normal esophagus [16]. Based on the DNF intensity at 480 nm, the presence of HGD was detected with 90% accuracy, and the presence of nondysplastic BE mucosa was predicted with 96% accuracy [16]. Using IFS, Georgakoudi et al. found 100% sensitivity and 97% specificity in differentiating HGD from LGD and nondysplastic BE in 16 patients [9]. Mayinger et al. used the ratio of green to red fluorescence ($I_{\lambda[500-549\,nm]}/I_{\lambda[667-700\,nm]}$) and the intensity of blue excitation at 477 nm ($I_{477\,nm}$) as two parameters for tissue classification, and found 97% sensitivity and 95% specificity for diagnosis of esophageal carcinoma in 9 patients [26]. Using a similar approach, they also reported 84% sensitivity and 87% specificity for the diagnosis of gastric adenocarcinoma in 15 patients [27]. Fluorescence spectroscopy can also accurately identify dysplasia associated with adenomatous polyps in the colon [17, 28]. Using the probability distribution (bivariate normal density function) of the fluorescence intensity $I_{460\,nm}$ and the ratio of intensity $I_{680\,nm}/I_{660\,nm}$ as the diagnostic parameters, Cothren et al. found 90% sensitivity, 95% specificity, and 90% positive predictive value (PPV) for the detection of colonic dysplasia in a study with 57 patients [17]. Mayinger et al. also investigated endoscopic light-induced autofluorescence spectroscopy for the diagnosis of colorectal cancer and adenoma [29]. They found 96% sensitivity and 93% specificity for rectal cancer detection, and 98% sensitivity and 89% specificity for diagnosis of dysplastic adenomas in a study with 11 patients [29].

With the aid of exogenous contrast agents that can selectively accumulate in neoplastic tissues, it is possible to enhance the capability of fluorescence detection. One of the most widely used exogenous contrast agents is 5-aminolevulinic acid (5-ALA), which is converted intracellularly into protoporphyrin IX (PpIX). PpIX shows greater production and retention in neoplastic cells because of their increased metabolic rate and reduced ferrochelatase activity, which converts PpIX to heme [30, 31]. Therefore, the characteristic red fluorescence of PpIX is increased in neoplastic tissues [32]. Clinical studies using point fluorescence spectroscopy showed that oral administration of 5-ALA can distinguish high-grade dysplasia from nondysplastic mucosa in Barrett's esophagus [33]. By using PpIX fluorescence alone, 77% sensitivity and 71% specificity were reported in a study with 20 patients, whereas by using the fluorescence-intensity ratio $I_{635\,nm}/I_{480\,nm}$, 100% sensitivity and 100% specificity were achieved [33]. Ortner et al. investigated time-gated fluorescence spectroscopy by exploiting the long fluorescence decay time of PpIX to suppress the autofluorescence background [34]. They used nanosecond excitation pulses to illuminate the tissue and then calculated the ratio of 20 ns delayed PpIX fluorescence intensity to the immediate autofluorescence intensity. It was possible to differentiate low-grade dysplasia (LGD) from nondysplastic BE, and dysplasia was detected at a 2.8 times higher rate when compared with screening endoscopy [34]. Fluorescence spectroscopy systems can also be extended into wide-field imaging mode, which is discussed in Section 3.3.1.

3.2.3 Raman Spectroscopy

Raman spectroscopy can provide detailed biochemical information of tissue [35]. In Raman spectroscopy, a small portion of the light scattered in the tissue undergoes a transfer of energy between the photons and the molecules in a process termed *inelastic scattering*. As a result, light is reemitted at either longer or shorter wavelengths than the light that was originally incident upon the tissue. The shift in the wavelength (the Raman shift) corresponds to specific vibrational or rotational energy states of the molecular bonds of the molecules in the tissue. Each molecular species has its own set of molecular vibrations, thus resulting in a unique Raman spectrum consisting of a set of peaks or bands. Therefore, Raman spectroscopy can reveal "molecular fingerprint" information about the tissue [36]. Most biologic molecules, such as proteins, lipids, and nucleic acids, have distinct spectral characteristics. Raman spectroscopy can, therefore, be used to determine the biochemical status of tissues for the purpose of diagnosis.

However, the typical Raman signals are several orders of magnitude weaker than the tissue's autofluorescence signal; therefore, Raman signals from the tissue are often obscured by background tissue fluorescence as well as the Raman and fluorescence contamination from the optical components (such as the fiber optics) in the system. Using near-infrared (NIR) excitation can reduce the unwanted tissue autofluorescence and enable deeper penetration into tissue. Recent developments in optical technologies, including high-efficiency notch filters (to reject the incident light), high-throughput holographic spectrometers, high-sensitivity CCD detectors, and specially designed fiber-optic catheters, have facilitated the application of Raman spectroscopy for in vivo diagnostics [37–39].

NIR Raman spectroscopy has been shown to have high diagnostic accuracy for early cancer detection in the GI tract. In an ex vivo study with 44 Barrett's esophagus patients, Kendall et al. found 94% sensitivity and 93% specificity for detection of neoplasia by using a consensus pathology classification model (agreement among three pathologists) [40]. Shim et al. reported the first in vivo Raman spectra of human GI tissues measured during routine clinical endoscopy [37]. NIR Raman spectroscopy also showed significant potential for the diagnosis of lung cancer [41]. With further development, Raman spectroscopy may provide complementary information to other modalities for tissue diagnosis.

3.2.4 Multimodality Spectroscopy

Since each of the different spectroscopic methods has a unique contrast mechanism, the combination of multiple methods can provide complementary information about the biochemical, architectural, and morphologic state of tissue and the corresponding changes that occur during the neoplastic progression. Georgakoudi et al. demonstrated that superior results for differentiating dysplastic from nondysplastic epithelium can been achieved by combining fluorescence, reflectance, and light-scattering spectroscopies [9]. Figure 3.1(c) shows the schematic diagram of the combined spectroscopy system (trimodal spectroscopy). In such a multimodality approach, fluorescence spectroscopy (IFS) provides the biochemical information, reflectance spectroscopy (DRS) reveals morphologic information about the bulk tissue, and light-scattering spectroscopy (LSS) indicates the nuclei size and density information. Trimodal spectroscopy has been shown to detect HGD from LGD and nondysplastic BE with 100% sensitivity and 100% specificity from 40 sites in 16 patients [9]. The results from trimodal spectroscopy are better than those obtained using individual modalities alone (IFS: 100% sensitivity and 97% specificity; DRS: 86% sensitivity and 100% specificity; LSS: 100% sensitivity and 91% specificity) since trimodal spectroscopy combines the advantages of each modality. There is great potential to combine Raman spectroscopy. Such multimodality methods can be extended to imaging modes to enable rapid surveillance of large tissue areas.

3.3 Wide-Field Imaging

The tissue sampled in point spectroscopy systems is usually restricted to a small area comparable to the extent of conventional excisional biopsy. In contrast, wide-field techniques can image a larger surface area. Standard white-light endoscopy (WLE) uses wide-field illumination and a high-density (100,000 to 300,000 pixels) CCD camera to generate high-quality images with pixel sizes of approximately 100 μm [31]. Several methods have been developed to improve the performance of white-light endoscopy by increasing the information content of the images, thereby enhancing the diagnostic capabilities. These methods include: techniques that involve improvements in resolution by using higher density (up to 1 million pixels) CCD cameras [high-resolution endoscopy (HRE)], techniques that incorporate optical magnification (magnification endoscopy) to achieve resolution approaching the cellular level (~10 μm) [42], techniques that utilize chemical staining to enhance visualization of mucosal features (chromoendoscopy), and techniques based on the spectral characteristics of light [fluorescence imaging and narrowband imaging (NBI)]. This section will mainly focus on fluorescence imaging, chromoendoscopy, and NBI.

3.3.1 Fluorescence Imaging

Autofluorescence endoscopy can be implemented by using wide-field, blue-light excitation, fluorescence filters for wavelength selection, and CCD cameras for detection. There are several approaches to generating fluorescence images. Wang et al. used a long-pass filter (>400 nm) to select the fluorescent light and an intensified charge injection device (CID) camera to capture the fluorescence image [43]. To account for the nonuniform illumination/imaging geometry, they applied a moving average algorithm to the acquired image. The area of dysplasia was determined by the fluorescence intensity below a certain threshold. Another approach used two filters to detect the fluorescence in the green (490 to 560 nm) and red (>630 nm) wavelength ranges and two intensified CCD (ICCD) cameras to acquire the fluorescence images in the green and red channels [44, 45]. The ratio between these two channels (I_{red}/I_{green}) was used to create pseudocolor images in real time. In this laser-induced fluorescence (LIF) system, normal mucosa usually appears cyan (blue-greenish), whereas neoplastic lesions appear red, due to the higher red/green fluorescence-intensity ratio. Figure 3.2 shows the schematic diagram of the light-induced fluorescence endoscopy (LIFE) system and the representative fluorescent and

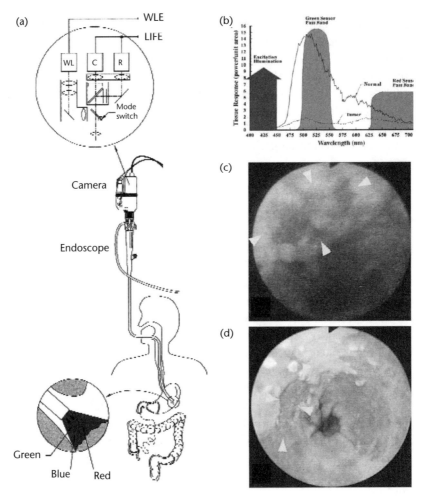

Figure 3.2 (a) Schematic diagram of the light-induced fluorescence endoscopy (LIFE) system showing the details of the special camera head with two fluorescence cameras [44], (b) spectra of normal and malignant tissue illustrating the principle of LIFE imaging [45], (c) LIFE fluorescence image, and (d) WLE image showing area of high-grade dysplasia (arrowheads) in a patient with Barrett's esophagus. (*From:* [45]. © 2001 Elsevier. Reprinted with permission.)

white-light images of the normal and dysplastic regions. To normalize the nonuniform illumination distribution and collection efficiency for each pixel, a red-near-IR diffuse reflectance image can be acquired to serve as the reference for correction (LIFR mode) [44]. In this mode, the image-acquisition components remain the same, but the illumination contains both blue light (400 to 450 nm) and red-near-IR light (>590 nm). By comparison, in the LIF mode, only blue illumination is used. Newer extensions of fluorescence endoscopy systems incorporate total autofluorescence and both green and red reflectance into the imaging algorithm. In this case, nondysplastic mucosa appears green, whereas neoplastic lesions appear blue-purple [46].

Fluorescence imaging can accurately identify dysplasia associated with adenomatous polyps in ex vivo colon specimens [43]. In an in vivo study of 30 patients, dysplasia was identified with a sensitivity of 83% [47]. Fluorescence endoscopy with LIF mode (LIFE) has been found to enhance the ability to localize small neoplastic lesions in the bronchus [48] and the GI tracts [44, 45, 49]. However, a randomized crossover study in 50 patients showed that LIFE was not superior to standard video endoscopy in detecting early neoplasia in Barrett's esophagus (sensitivity for the diagnosis of HGD/early-stage cancer in targeted biopsy were both only 62%) [50].

As in point-probe fluorescence spectroscopy, using exogenous contrast agents such as 5-ALA will enhance the detection capability in wide-field fluorescence imaging. Endlicher et al. found a sensitivity of >80% for dysplasia detection, while the specificity was only between 27% and 56% in a study of 47 patients [51]. Messmann et al. also used 5-ALA to evaluate the detection of low- and high-grade dysplasia in ulcerative colitis patients and reported a sensitivity of 87% to 100%, while the specificity was only in the range of 51% to 62% in a study of 37 patients [52]. The high false-positive rates are associated with inflamed tissue or fecal materials [32, 53].

Using the video autofluorescence imaging (AFI) system with both green and red reflectance, Kara et al. recently demonstrated that AFI detected more dysplastic and neoplastic regions in Barrett's esophagus than conventional endoscopy [46]. In a cohort of 60 patients with Barrett's esophagus, 22 patients were diagnosed with high-grade intraepithelial neoplasia (HGIN), and, among them, 7 patients were detected solely by AFI after HRE had not shown any suspicious lesions. However, the positive predictive value (PPV) from per-lesion analysis was only 49%. Further technology development and combination of other imaging modalities will improve the specificity and PPV, which will be discussed in Section 3.3.5.

3.3.2 Molecular Imaging

There have been great advances in visualizing basic molecular processes such as gene expression, enzyme activity, and disease-specific molecular interactions in vivo [54–56]. Molecular imaging promises early detection and in situ characterization of cancers [57–60]. Optical imaging in conjunction with near-infrared fluorescent imaging probes has been developed to improve early cancer detection in the colon [61, 62]. These agents either target specific biomarkers [61] or are activated by specific enzymes [62]. In the first case, Kelly et al. developed fluorescent affinity ligands derived from a phage library specific to colon cancer and demonstrated a sevenfold higher contrast than a control in orthotopic colonic tumors (HT29) using a two-channel miniaturized near-infrared fluorescent endoscopy [61]. In the later case, proteolytic enzymes were shown to play an essential role in tumor growth, including promotion of high cell turnover, invasion, and angiogenesis [63]. Cathepsin B, in particular, was shown to be up-regulated in areas of inflammation, necrosis, angiogenesis [63], focal invasion of colorectal carcinomas [64], and dysplastic adenomas [65, 66]. Marten et al. applied a fluorescent, enzyme-cleavable and activatable cathepsin B sensing probe, which is nonfluorescent at injection and locally activated after target interaction, to the APC^{min} mouse model [62]. In this study, ex vivo fluorescent imaging showed increased detection sensitivity and specificity, and the smallest lesion detected was measured to be 50 μm [62].

Miniaturized endoscope devices are under development for in vivo molecular imaging inside luminal structures. Funovics et al. developed a miniaturized 2.7 French (0.8 mm in diameter) fiber-optic sensor for the laparoscopic imaging of enzyme activity and gene expression in vivo [67]. This device includes a dichroic mirror, a bandpass filter, and two independent cameras that permit simultaneous recording of white-light and fluorescent images. Zhu et al. also demonstrated a one-dimensional, near-infrared fluorescence imaging catheter for the detection of atherosclerotic plaque in human carotid plaque specimens ex vivo [68]. Such endoscopic devices will enable intraluminal molecular imaging of the GI tract and blood vessels for early disease identification.

3.3.3 Chromoendoscopy

Chromoendoscopy utilizes chemical staining to aid the localization, characterization, or identification of various GI pathologies. Chromoendoscopy is typically used in conjunction with white-light endoscopy to enhance the ability to detect neoplastic changes in GI mucosa. Chromic agents can be divided into different categories depending on their staining mechanisms [69]. *Absorptive stains*, also referred to as vital stains, are bound, incorporated, or absorbed by cellular components. The most commonly used absorptive stains include Lugol's solution and methylene blue. Lugol's solution contains iodine and potassium iodide, which bind to glycogen in the nonkeratinized squamous epithelium to form a black or dark-brown background. The dye will not be absorbed in areas lacking glycogen, including regions of inflammation, Barrett's epithelium, dysplasia, and cancer. Methylene blue is absorbed into the cytosol of actively absorbing tissues, such as intestinal epithelium and the specialized intestinal metaplasia of Barrett's esophagus. Dysplasia and cancer are less absorptive, possibly due to relatively less cytoplasm in those cells. Methylene blue therefore helps to highlight borders of suspicious neoplastic lesions [23]. Instead of being absorbed by cellular or glandular structures, *contrast stains* are collected within mucosal surfaces such as crypts and foveolae. Indigo carmine is one of the more commonly used contrast stains. Color Plate 5(a, b) shows the endoscopic images of BE using white-light endoscopy and chromoendoscopy [70].

There is considerable interest in the use of chromoendoscopy with various dyes as an adjunct to endoscopic surveillance in Barrett's esophagus. However, due to the nonuniformity in methods, dye concentration, and classification of staining patterns, it is difficult to compare different studies. Canto et al. reported that methylene blue can significantly enhance the diagnostic yield of high-grade dysplasia or cancer when compared to conventional biopsies (12% versus 6%, $p = 0.004$) [71]. In other words, dysplasia or cancer was diagnosed significantly more in methylene-blue-directed biopsy specimens. However, other studies have reported that methylene-blue-directed biopsy is similar to conventional biopsy in detecting dysplasia in BE [72–74]. Sharma et al. showed that magnification after indigo carmine spray is useful in identifying mucosal patterns for the diagnosis of intestinal metaplasia and high-grade dysplasia [75]. In a prospective randomized crossover study with 28 patients, Kara et al. reported HRE plus indigo carmine chromoendoscopy achieved a sensitivity of 93% for the detection of HGD or early cancer [76].

Chromoendoscopy shows promising results in the detection of early cancers in the colon. Kiesslich et al. demonstrated in a prospective randomized trial with 165 patients that the use of methylene blue magnification chromoendoscopy improved the prediction of the histologic degree and extent of inflammation and allowed significantly more flat, small intraepithelial neoplasias to be diagnosed in ulcerative colitis (UC) [77]. Using a modified pit-pattern classification scheme, based on earlier work by Kudo [78], 93% sensitivity and 93% specificity for detection of neoplastic lesions were reported [77]. This work and subsequent studies confirmed a 3- to 4.75-fold increase in the diagnostic yield of chromoendoscopy-targeted biopsies over random biopsy by using either methylene blue or indigo carmine chromoendoscopy [77, 79–81]. These results suggest that chromoendoscopy-guided biopsy can be used in UC patients in lieu of the current practice of random biopsy [82].

3.3.4 Narrowband Imaging

Narrowband imaging (NBI) utilizes a set of optical filters that allow only narrow wavelength regions of blue, green, and red light to sequentially illuminate the tissue, with an increased relative contribution of blue light [83–85]. Blue light penetrates only superficially, whereas red light penetrates into deeper layers. Blue and green wavelengths are strongly absorbed by hemoglobin. Therefore, NBI enhances mucosal surface contrast and capillary patterns, thereby allowing improved visualization and diagnosis [86]. Color Plate 5(c) shows a representative NBI image of Barrett's esophagus.

NBI allows detailed inspection of the mucosal and vascular patterns with high resolution and contrast without the use of exogenous dyes. In a prospective study of 51 patients, Sharma et al. reported high sensitivity (100%), specificity (98.7%), and PPV (95.3%) for detecting irregular/distorted patterns in high-grade dysplasia [87]. In another study with 63 patients, Kara et al. used three criteria to characterize HGIN: (1) irregular/disrupted mucosal patterns, (2) irregular vascular patterns, and (3) abnormal blood vessels [88]. They showed high sensitivity (94%) and NPV (98%), with relatively lower specificity (76%) and PPV (64%). The same group also showed that HRE plus NBI yielded 83% sensitivity in detecting HGD and early cancer in BE, which is comparable to the results using HRE plus chromoendoscopy [76]. These studies have shown that NBI is promising in detecting early neoplasia.

3.3.5 Multimodality Wide-Field Imaging

An optimal approach for early cancer detection would involve a system that can first scan large areas of mucosal surface with high sensitivity to identify possible regions of neoplasia, and then follow up by close inspection to characterize the mucosal properties in detail. As mentioned previously, AFI can achieve high sensitivity in detecting dysplasia and, therefore, can be used as a technique to detect suspicious lesions. However, AFI is limited by its high false-positive rate. NBI, on the other hand, can provide magnified inspection of mucosal patterns for the detection of dysplasia. Therefore, the combination of AFI and NBI can provide complementary information for more accurate detection of early neoplasia. Kara et al. performed a cross-sectional study in 20 patients with BE using endoscopic video AFI followed by NBI [89]. AFI identified all HGIN lesions (100% sensitivity); however, the false-positive rate was high (19 in 47 lesions, or 40%). Using NBI, the false-positive rate dropped to 10% (5 in 47). Color Plate 6 shows an example of the detection of HGIN lesions using the combined modality. This result motivates the development of a multimodal system that incorporates HRE, AFI, and NBI in a single endoscope for better coregistration and easier operation.

3.4 Cross-Sectional Imaging

Compared to point-probe spectroscopy or wide-field imaging, cross-sectional imaging modalities, such as endoscopic ultrasound (EUS) and optical coherence tomography (OCT), can provide depth-resolved images revealing subsurface tissue architecture. These features are particularly important for the detection of neoplasia underneath normal-appearing squamous epithelium [90] and determination of submucosal tumor invasion. EUS has been used for the staging of advanced Barrett's esophagus with high-grade dysplasia or intramucosal carcinoma [91]. The sensitivity, specificity, and NPV for submucosal invasion were 100%, 94%, and 100%, respectively. However, EUS has limited resolution of 100 to 200 μm [92]; therefore, it is difficult to detect dysplasia [93]. In contrast, OCT provides 10 to 100 times higher resolution than EUS and has great potential for identifying early neoplasia and for guiding excisional biopsy to reduce sampling errors.

3.4.1 Endoscopic Optical Coherence Tomography

Optical coherence tomography (OCT) enables micron-scale, cross-sectional imaging of the microstructures of biological tissues in situ and in real time [94]. OCT is analogous to ultrasound B-mode imaging, except that OCT imaging is performed by measuring the intensity of backscattered light rather than sound. Cross-sectional, tomographic images are generated in a manner similar to radar. An optical beam is scanned across the tissue, and the backscattered light is measured as a function of axial range (depth) and transverse position. OCT is based on a technique known as low-coherence interferometry (LCI) [95–97]. Color Plate 7(a) shows a schematic of the OCT system. Measurements are performed using a Michelson interferometer with a low coherence-length (broad-bandwidth) light source. One arm of the interferometer is a modular probe that directs light onto the sample and collects the retroreflected signal. A second interferometer arm includes a reference mirror that generates a reference signal. The interference between the sample and reference signals can be detected by either time-domain or Fourier-domain techniques. In time-domain OCT, the reference mirror is scanned back and forth, and the interference signal is measured by a photodiode detector. Optical interference between the light from the sample and reference mirror occurs only when the optical distances traveled by the light in both the tissue sample and reference paths match to within the coherence length of the light [98]. Low-coherence interferometry permits the echo delay time (or optical path length) and magnitude of the light reflected from internal tissue microstructures to be measured with extremely high accuracy and sensitivity. The maximum imaging depth in most tissues (other than the eye) is limited by optical attenuation and scattering and is up to 2 to 3 mm, depending on the tissue's optical properties. This depth is comparable to that typically sampled by excisional biopsy and is sufficient for the evaluation of most early neoplastic changes in epithelial cancers.

With fiber-optic components, OCT can be readily integrated with a wide range of imaging devices such as catheters, which enable imaging inside the body [100]. In vivo OCT imaging of the human GI tract has been demonstrated clinically using time-domain OCT systems with axial resolutions of 10 to 20 μm and imaging speeds of approximately 0.3 to 6.7 frames per second [101–106]. Barrett's esophagus was clearly differentiated from normal esophageal mucosa, and esophageal adenocarcinoma could also be distinguished from nonneoplastic tissues. Furthermore, endoscopic Doppler OCT has been shown to reveal distinct blood flow patterns in normal esophagus, Barrett's esophagus, and esophageal adenocarcinoma [107].

OCT has been demonstrated for the detection of specialized intestinal metaplasia in Barrett's esophagus patients [108, 109] and transmural inflammation in inflammatory bowel disease (IBD) patients [110]. OCT also shows potential to distinguish hyperplastic from adenomatous polyps in the colon [111]. Recently, OCT has shown the promise for detection of high-grade dysplasia in Barrett's esophagus. Evans et al. reported a sensitivity of 83% and specificity of 75% for detecting high-grade dysplasia and intramucosal carcinoma with blinded scoring of OCT images from 55 patients using a numeric scoring system based on surface maturation and glandular architecture [112]. Isenberg et al. reported a sensitivity of 68% and a specificity of 82%, with an accuracy of 78% for the detection of dysplasia in biopsies from 33 patients with Barrett's esophagus [113]. They also suggested that further improvement in the spatial resolution would improve the diagnosis. With a computer-aided diagnosis (CAD) approach, Qi et al. found an increased sensitivity of 82%, a specificity of 74%, and an accuracy of 83% in 13 patients [114]. They used image-analysis algorithms based on texture features from OCT images acquired by the same system reported by Isenberg et al. in the aforementioned study.

3.4.2 Ultrahigh-Resolution OCT (UHROCT)

The axial image resolution of OCT is determined by the coherence length (ΔL) of the light source, which is inversely proportional to the bandwidth ($\Delta \lambda$). The axial resolution is given by the equation $\Delta L = 2\ln(2)\lambda_0^2/(\Delta \lambda)$, where ($\Delta \lambda$) is the bandwidth and ($\lambda_0$) is the median wavelength of the light source. In order to achieve high resolution, broad-bandwidth light sources are required. Most of the reported endoscopic OCT clinical studies were performed with standard axial resolution (approximately 10 to 20 μm) using superluminescent diode (SLD) light sources. With recent advances in broadband laser light sources, OCT image resolutions approaching a few microns have been achieved [115]. When compared to standard-resolution OCT images, UHR OCT images exhibited reduced speckle size and improved overall image quality [116]. By using a compact, broadband Cr:Forsterite laser at 1,300 nm, 4 μm axial resolution has been achieved in endoscopic OCT, which is a two- to threefold improvement in axial resolution when compared to standard-resolution systems [117]. Recently, UHR endoscopic OCT with approximately 3 μm axial resolution using a Ti:Sapphire laser at 800 nm has also been demonstrated in an animal model [118].

UHR endoscopic OCT imaging has been demonstrated clinically in a cross-sectional study of 50 patients [99]. Real-time endoscopic OCT imaging at four frames per second was performed by using a 1.8 mm diameter OCT catheter probe introduced into the accessory channel of a standard endoscope. Color Plate 7(b) shows a representative UHR OCT image of normal esophagus, which exhibits a characteristic layered architecture. Color Plate 7(c) shows a representative UHR OCT image of Barrett's esophagus. The layered architecture in normal esophagus is replaced by glandular structures. Low-backscattering Barrett's glands are frequently observed within the mucosa, with interlaced regions of high-backscattering connective tissue corresponding to the lamina propria. Color Plate 7(d) shows a UHR OCT image of high-grade dysplasia. OCT images of high-grade dysplasia are characterized by irregular, distorted, and cribriform, or villiform, glandular architecture, and they are more heterogeneous than in nondysplastic Barrett's epithelium. Ultrahigh-resolution OCT images showed good correlation with architectural morphology in histological findings. Enhanced image resolution and reduced speckle size enable ultrahigh-resolution OCT to visualize the tissue architectural heterogeneity correlated with the pathology more clearly than standard-resolution OCT. Future clinical studies are needed to investigate the role of ultrahigh-resolution OCT in the detection of early neoplastic lesions in the GI tract.

3.4.3 Three-Dimensional OCT

Three-dimensional-OCT imaging enables the virtual manipulation of tissue geometry, synthesis of *en face* views similar to those in wide-field endoscopic images, and quantitative measurements of tissue morphological features. Since 3D-OCT imaging in vivo requires the collection of a large amount of data (e.g., 512 × 512 × 512 pixels) in a short time period (approximately a few seconds), imaging speed becomes one of the most critical parameters for performing 3D-OCT imaging in clinical settings. The desired 3D imaging speeds would be on the order of several hundreds frames per second, whereas time-domain OCT imaging is usually performed at fewer than 10 frames per second (for a typical image with 512 axial lines); therefore, it is not sufficient for 3D imaging in vivo. Since 2003, OCT imaging speeds have been revolutionized by the development of Fourier-domain detection techniques [119–121]. Fourier-domain OCT measures the spectrum of the interference signal and produces each axial image line by Fourier transformation of the spectrum. While this requires an additional signal-processing step when compared to time-domain OCT systems, the reference path can be kept at one fixed distance, and the entire depth scan can be acquired at one time. In contrast to time-domain OCT, where each axial pixel at a different depth is acquired only when the reference mirror scans through the equidistant point in the reference arm, all axial pixels are acquired at the same time in Fourier-domain OCT. Therefore, compared to time-domain OCT, Fourier-domain OCT has a sensitivity advantage given by the ratio of the axial scan depth to the axial resolution, which is typically several hundredfold [119–121]. The enhanced sensitivity in Fourier-domain OCT enables a corresponding approximately hundredfold increase in imaging speed hundredfold. The increased speed of Fourier-domain detection enables in vivo 3D-OCT imaging [122–124] and promises new applications for OCT.

Fourier-domain OCT imaging can be performed in two ways, typically referred to as *spectral OCT* and *swept-source OCT*. Spectral OCT uses a diffraction-grating, a spectrometer, and a line-scanning CCD array in the detection arm to record the interference spectrum in parallel. Spectral OCT systems typically operate at speeds of 29,000 to 75,000 axial lines per second [125, 126]. Swept-source OCT uses a wavelength-swept laser as the light source and a photodetector in the detection arm to record the interference spectrum as the wavelength is swept [127–130]. Using swept-source OCT, imaging speeds of up to 370,000 axial lines per second have recently been demonstrated [131].

Endoscopic 3D-OCT imaging in vivo has recently been demonstrated using Fourier-domain OCT. Tumlinson et al. demonstrated ultrahigh-resolution, spectral endoscopic OCT with 2.4 μm axial resolution using a Ti:Sapphire laser with 20,000 axial lines per second in the mouse colon [132]. Using swept-source OCT (also termed *optical frequency-domain imaging*, or OFDI), Yun et al. and Vakoc et al. demonstrated 3D volumetric imaging of the porcine esophagus and artery in vivo at an imaging speed of 10,000 axial lines per second and 50,000 axial lines per second, respectively [123, 133]. Using a Fourier-domain mode-locked (FDML) laser, a novel laser technology that enables high-speed, wavelength-swept operation, Adler et al. demonstrated in vivo 3-D endoscopic OCT imaging in the rabbit colon at a record speed of 100,000 axial lines per second [124]. Figure 3.3 shows the schematic of the swept-source OCT system and representative 3D volumetric images acquired in vivo. The increased sweep speed enabled imaging of an approximately 9-mm segment of colon in less than 18 seconds. Tissue microstructure, such as colonic crypt pattern, was visualized with a resolution of 7 μm (axial) and 9 μm (transverse). With further technology refinement, higher resolution and imaging speed will be available in the near future. Suter et al. have reported the in vivo imaging of human esophagus using Fourier-domain OCT [134]. The unique capability of high-resolution imaging with a large field of view promises a more complete characterization of tissue microscopic features and open new possibilities for improving the identification of early neoplastic changes.

3.4.4 Multimodality Imaging with OCT

3.4.4.1 OCT and EUS

OCT and EUS have complementary imaging scales. OCT image penetration ranges from 1 to 2 mm with approximately 10 μm resolution, thus enabling the visualization of microscopic structures such as esophageal glands, gastric pits, intestinal villi, colonic crypts, and blood vessels. EUS penetration ranges from 10 to 20 mm with approximately 100 μm resolution, thereby enabling the visualization of major layers surrounding the GI tracts. Endoscopic OCT has been shown to provide complementary information to EUS for potential applications in the staging of GI tumors [135, 136]. Visualization of submucosal features is an important advantage for cross-sectional imaging modalities such as EUS and OCT, when compared to

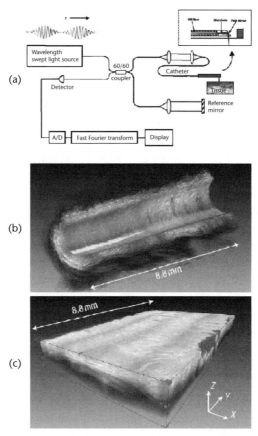

Figure 3.3 (a) Schematic diagram of Fourier-domain (swept-source) endoscopic OCT system with inset showing the schematic of OCT imaging catheter. (b, c) Volumetric endoscopic OCT imaging of rabbit colon in vivo: (b) cutaway view of the rendered volume, and (c) unfolded data set showing the cylindrical volume as a rectangular tissue slab. The entire volume was acquired in 17.7 seconds. (*From:* [124]. Reprinted with permission.)

standard white-light endoscopy. Color Plate 8 shows a case of esophageal adenocarcinoma underneath benign squamous neoepithelium in a patient 15 months after photodynamic therapy (PDT). The in vivo UHR endoscopic OCT image of adenocarcinoma shows irregularly shaped and crowded glandular architecture buried underneath the smooth squamous epithelium, as confirmed by histology. Color Plate 8(c) shows an EUS image from the same location for comparison. OCT imaging demonstrates a higher imaging resolution for epithelial morphology than EUS. However, EUS has deeper image penetration, thus enabling assessment of the depth of tumor invasion. This example suggests that the two modalities may be complementary to each other in the detection and staging of GI cancers.

3.4.4.2 OCT and Fluorescence

Since OCT can provide morphological information, the combination of fluorescence spectroscopy and OCT would also improve the diagnostic capability for early cancer in a manner similar to trimodal spectroscopy, where morphological information is revealed by scattering spectroscopy. Kuranov et al. and Sapozhnikova et al. combined OCT and LIF using ALA to improve the identification of tumor boundaries in the cervix [137, 138]. It was found that the tumor boundary detected by optical methods coincides with the morphological boundary and extends beyond the colposcopically determined boundary by about 2 mm. Tumlinson et al. developed a combined OCT and LIF imaging catheter for the in vivo imaging of mouse colon [139, 140]. Figure 3.4 shows the combined system diagram and representative OCT images and LIF spectra. This miniaturized 2-mm-diameter catheter has been applied to monitor disease progression longitudinally in the mouse colon and is able to identify colorectal adenomas in murine models [141]. In an ex vivo study of murine GI tracts, Hariri et al. showed that OCT and LIF provided complementary information for the detection of dysplasia and inflammatory bowel disease (IBD) of the intestines [142]. Another example of combining high-resolution structural information from OCT images with lower resolution metabolic information

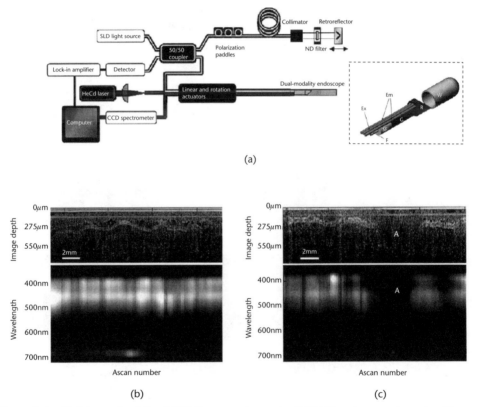

Figure 3.4 (a) Schematic of the OCT-LIF system. Inset: the OCT-LIF endoscope tip optics. The OCT channel consists of a single-mode fiber (F), a silica ferrule (SF), and a GRIN lens (G). The GRIN lens focuses the light into a rod prism (R) that bends the beam at 90° through the silica window (W) and into the tissue. The LIF channel consists of three multimode fibers with one excitation channel (Ex) and two emission channel fibers (Em). (b) OCT image (top) and corresponding LIF spectra (bottom) of healthy colon taken from a high-chlorophyll-diet mouse. The LIF emission peaks at approximately 390 and 450 nm, with an absorption dip at 420 nm that is typical of healthy tissue. The presence of a distinct peak at approximately 680 nm is visible throughout the colon as well. (c) OCT-LIF spectra of adenoma. The adenoma can be visualized in the OCT image (a). The corresponding LIF signal shows a significant reduction in the 390 and 450 nm signals and a peak in the 680 nm signal over the adenomatous region. (*From:* [140]. © 2006 Optical Society of America. Reprinted with permission.)

was demonstrated by using a hybrid positron-detection and OCT system in a rabbit atherosclerotic model [143, 144].

OCT can also be combined with wide-field fluorescence imaging in a similar way as in the case of AFI and NBI. AFI can perform large-area imaging to identify suspicious lesions, and OCT can provide detailed morphological information for further inspection. Pan et al. showed that ALA fluorescence-guided endoscopic OCT could enhance the efficiency and sensitivity of early bladder cancer diagnosis [145]. Figure 3.5 shows the schematic of the combined endoscopic imaging system and representative images. In a rat model study, they demonstrated that the specificity of fluorescence detection of transitional cell carcinoma was significantly enhanced by fluorescence-guided OCT (53% versus 93%), and the sensitivity of fluorescence detection was improved by combining it with OCT (79% versus 100%) [146]. With further technology development, 3D-OCT will be able to generate *en face* mucosal patterns in vivo, similar to those shown in magnification endoscopy

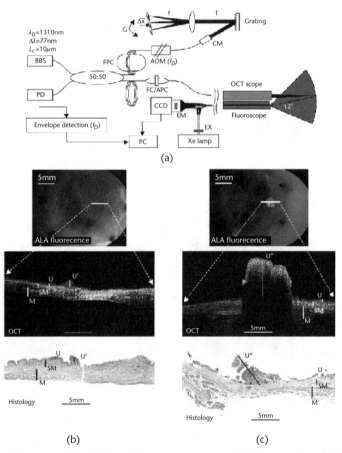

Figure 3.5 (a) Schematic of the OCT and fluorescence system (BBS = broadband light source, PD = photodiode, CM = fiber-optic collimator, FPC = fiber polarization controller, EX = blue excitation filter, EM = red emission filter, AOM = acousto-optic modulator, G = grating, FC/APC = connector). (b) ALA fluorescence, OCT, and histology of a precancer (hyperplastic) lesion in a Fischer 344 rat bladder (U = normal uroepithelium, SM = submucosa, M = muscularis layer, U′ = precancerous uroepithelium). (c) ALA fluorescence, OCT, and histology of an early cancer (neoplastic) lesion in a Fischer 344 rat bladder (U″ = cancerous uroepithelium). (*From*: [145]. © 2003 Optical Society of America. Reprinted with permission.)

(ME). However, other than ME, 3D-OCT can provide depth-resolved information beneath the mucosal surface. Therefore, the combination of AFI and 3D-OCT is a promising technology for GI cancer imaging.

These studies suggest that the high-resolution tissue morphology revealed by OCT and the biochemical and metabolic information provided by fluorescence can provide complementary diagnostic information, which, if interpreted appropriately, can enhance the sensitivity and specificity in diseases diagnosis.

3.5 Summary

The advances in endoscopic optical imaging and spectroscopy described in this chapter provide an overview of many promising technologies that may enhance the diagnostic capabilities of conventional endoscopy. The emerging optical modalities offer improved image resolution, image contrast, and tissue penetration depth, and they provide biochemical and molecular information for the diagnosis of disease. Each modality has its own unique strengths and limitations. However, by proper combination, multimodality approaches can effectively utilize the strengths of individual modalities, while compensating for each other's shortcomings. This array of optical imaging and spectroscopy technologies could be translated to a wide spectrum of clinical applications and could improve the prognosis of patients through earlier diagnosis and more accurate staging of disease.

Acknowledgments

We would like to acknowledge the contributions from Franz Kaertner, Robert Huber, Joseph Schmitt, Paul Herz, Pei-Lin Hsiung, Marcos Pedrosa, James Connolly, and Qin Huang for the OCT results presented here. This research was sponsored in part by the National Science Foundation BES-0522845 and ECS-0501478; the National Institutes of Health R01-CA75289-11 and R01-EY11289-20; the Air Force Office of Scientific Research FA9550-040-1-0011 and FA9550-040-1-0046; and the Cancer Research and Prevention Foundation.

References

[1] Zonios, G., et al., "Diffuse reflectance spectroscopy of human adenomatous colon polyps in vivo," *Appl. Opt.* 38 (1999): 6628–6637.

[2] Bigio, I. J., and J. R. Mourant, "Ultraviolet and visible spectroscopies for tissue diagnostics: Fluorescence spectroscopy and elastic-scattering spectroscopy," *Phys. Med. Biol.* 42 (1997): 803–814.

[3] Perelman, L. T., et al., "Observation of periodic fine structure in reflectance from biological tissue: A new technique for measuring nuclear size distribution," *Phys. Rev. Lett.* 80 (1998): 627–630.

[4] Backman, V., et al., "Detection of preinvasive cancer cells," *Nature* 406 (2000): 35–36.

[5] Mourant, J. R., et al., "Predictions and measurements of scattering and absorption over broad wavelength ranges in tissue phantoms," *Appl. Opt.* 36 (1997): 949–957.

[6] Reif, R., O. A'Amar, and I. J. Bigio, "Analytical model of light reflectance for extraction of the optical properties in small volumes of turbid media," *Appl. Opt.* 46 (2007): 7317–7328.

[7] Lovat, L. B., et al., "Elastic scattering spectroscopy accurately detects high-grade dysplasia and cancer in Barrett's oesophagus," *Gut* 55 (2006): 1078–1083.

[8] Dhar, A., et al., "Elastic scattering spectroscopy for the diagnosis of colonic lesions: Initial results of a novel optical biopsy technique," *Gastrointest. Endosc.* 63 (2006): 257–261.

[9] Georgakoudi, I., et al., "Fluorescence, reflectance, and light-scattering spectroscopy for evaluating dysplasia in patients with Barrett's esophagus," *Gastroenterology* 120 (2001): 1620–1629.

[10] Wallace, M. B., et al., "Endoscopic detection of dysplasia in patients with Barrett's esophagus using light-scattering spectroscopy," *Gastroenterology* 119 (2000): 677–682.

[11] Gurjar, R. S., et al., "Imaging human epithelial properties with polarized light-scattering spectroscopy," *Nat. Med.* 7 (2001): 1245–1248.

[12] Yu, C. C., et al., "Assessing epithelial cell nuclear morphology by using azimuthal light scattering spectroscopy," *Opt. Lett.* 31 (2006): 3119–3121.

[13] Kim, Y. L., et al., "Simultaneous measurement of angular and spectral properties of light scattering for characterization of tissue microarchitecture and its alteration in early precancer," *IEEE J. Sel. Top. Quant. Electron.* 9 (2003): 243–256.

[14] Roy, H. K., et al., "Four-dimensional elastic light-scattering fingerprints as preneoplastic markers in the rat model of colon carcinogenesis," *Gastroenterology* 126 (2004): 1071–1081.

[15] Wali, R. K., et al., "Increased microvascular blood content is an early event in colon carcinogenesis," *Gut* 54 (2005): 654–660.

[16] Panjehpour, M., et al., "Endoscopic fluorescence detection of high-grade dysplasia in Barrett's esophagus," *Gastroenterology* 111 (1996): 93–101.

[17] Cothren, R. M., et al., "Detection of dysplasia at colonoscopy using laser-induced fluorescence: A blinded study," *Gastrointest. Endosc.* 44 (1996): 168–176.

[18] Zonios, G. I., et al., "Morphological model of human colon tissue fluorescence," *IEEE Trans. Biomed. Eng.* 43 (1996): 113–122.

[19] Schomacker, K. T., et al., "Ultraviolet laser-induced fluorescence of colonic tissue—basic biology and diagnostic potential," *Lasers Surg. Med.* 12 (1992): 63–78.

[20] Dacosta, R. S., B. C. Wilson, and N. E. Marcon, "New optical technologies for earlier endoscopic diagnosis of premalignant gastrointestinal lesions," *J. Gastroent. Hepatol.* 17 Suppl. (2002): S85–S104.

[21] Bourg-Heckly, G., et al., "Endoscopic ultraviolet-induced autofluorescence spectroscopy of the esophagus: Tissue characterization and potential for early cancer diagnosis," *Endoscopy* 32 (2000): 756–765.

[22] Izuishi, K., et al., "The histological basis of detection of adenoma and cancer in the colon by autofluorescence endoscopic imaging," *Endoscopy* 31 (1999): 511–516.

[23] Pfau, P. R., and M. V. Sivak, "Endoscopic diagnostics," *Gastroenterology* 120 (2001): 763–781.

[24] Wu, J., M. S. Feld, and R. P. Rava, "Analytical model for extracting intrinsic fluorescence in turbid media," *Appl. Opt.* 32 (1993): 3585–3595.

[25] Zhang, Q. G., et al., "Turbidity-free fluorescence spectroscopy of biological tissue," *Opt. Lett.* 25 (2000): 1451–1453.

[26] Mayinger, B., et al., "Light-induced autofluorescence spectroscopy for the endoscopic detection of esophageal cancer," *Gastrointest. Endosc.* 54 (2001): 195–201.

[27] Mayinger, B., et al., "Evaluation of in vivo endoscopic autofluorescence spectroscopy in gastric cancer," *Gastrointest. Endosc.* 59 (2004): 191–198.

[28] Richards-Kortum, R., et al., "Spectroscopic diagnosis of colonic dysplasia," *Photochem. Photobiol.* 53 (1991): 777–786.

[29] Mayinger, B., et al., "Endoscopic light-induced autofluorescence spectroscopy for the diagnosis of colorectal cancer and adenoma," *J. Photochem. Photobiol. B—Biology* 70 (2003): 13–20.

[30] Peng, Q., et al., "5-aminolevulinic acid-based photodynamic therapy—clinical research and future challenges," *Cancer* 79 (1997): 2282–2308.

[31] Wilson, B. C., "Detection and treatment of dysplasia in Barrett's esophagus: A pivotal challenge in translating biophotonics from bench to bedside," *J. Biomed. Opt.* 12 (2007): 051401.

[32] Messmann, H., et al., "Endoscopic fluorescence detection of dysplasia in patients with Barrett's esophagus, ulcerative colitis, or adenomatous polyps after 5-aminolevulinic acid-induced protoporphyrin IX sensitization," *Gastrointest. Endosc.* 49 (1999): 97–101.

[33] Brand, S., et al., "Detection of high-grade dysplasia in Barrett's esophagus by spectroscopy measurement of 5-aminolevulinic acid-induced protoporphyrin IX fluorescence," *Gastrointest. Endosc.* 56 (2002): 479–487.

[34] Ortner, M. A., et al., "Time gated fluorescence spectroscopy in Barrett's oesophagus," *Gut* 52 (2003): 28–33.

[35] Hanlon, E. B., et al., "Prospects for in vivo Raman spectroscopy," *Phys. Med. Biol.* 45 (2000): R1–R59.

[36] Bigio, I. J., and S. G. Bown, "Spectroscopic sensing of cancer and cancer therapy: Current status of translational research," *Cancer Biol. Ther.* 3 (2004): 259–267.

[37] Shim, M. G., et al., "In vivo near-infrared Raman spectroscopy: Demonstration of feasibility during clinical gastrointestinal endoscopy," *Photochem. Photobiol.* 72 (2000): 146–150.

[38] Utzinger, U., et al., "Near-infrared Raman spectroscopy for in vivo detection of cervical precancers," *Appl. Spectroscopy* 55 (2001): 955–959.

[39] Motz, J. T., et al., "Real-time Raman system for in vivo disease diagnosis," *J. Biomed. Opt.* 10 (2005): 031113.

[40] Kendall, C., et al., "Raman spectroscopy, a potential tool for the objective identification and classification of neoplasia in Barrett's oesophagus," *J. Pathol.* 200 (2003): 602–609.

[41] Huang, Z., et al., "Near-infrared Raman spectroscopy for optical diagnosis of lung cancer," *Int. J. Canc.* 107 (2003): 1047–1052.

[42] Nelson, D. B., et al., "High resolution and high-magnification endoscopy: September 2000," *Gastrointest. Endosc.* 52 (2000): 864–866.

[43] Wang, T. D., et al., "Fluorescence endoscopic imaging of human colonic adenomas," *Gastroenterology* 111 (1996): 1182–1191.

[44] Zeng, H. S., et al., "Real-time endoscopic fluorescence imaging for early cancer detection in the gastrointestinal tract," *Bioimaging* 6 (1998): 151–165.

[45] Haringsma, J., et al., "Autofluorescence endoscopy: Feasibility of detection of GI neoplasms unapparent to white light endoscopy with an evolving technology," *Gastrointest. Endosc.* 53 (2001): 642–650.

[46] Kara, M. A., et al., "Endoscopic video autofluorescence imaging may improve the detection of early neoplasia in patients with Barrett's esophagus," *Gastrointest. Endosc.* 61 (2005): 679–685.

[47] Wang, T. D., et al., "In vivo identification of colonic dysplasia using fluorescence endoscopic imaging," *Gastrointest. Endosc.* 49 (1999): 447–455.

[48] Lam, S., et al., "Localization of bronchial intraepithelial neoplastic lesions by fluorescence bronchoscopy," *Chest* 113 (1998): 696–702.

[49] Niepsuj, K., et al., "Autofluorescence endoscopy for detection of high-grade dysplasia in short-segment Barrett's esophagus," *Gastrointest. Endosc.* 58 (2003): 715–719.

[50] Kara, M. A., et al., "A randomized crossover study comparing light-induced fluorescence endoscopy with standard videoendoscopy for the detection of early neoplasia in Barrett's esophagus," *Gastrointest. Endosc.* 61 (2005): 671–678.

[51] Endlicher, E., et al., "Endoscopic fluorescence detection of low- and high-grade dysplasia in Barrett's esophagus using systemic or local 5 aminolaevulinic acid sensitisation," *Gut* 48 (2001): 314–319.

[52] Messmann, H., et al., "Fluorescence endoscopy for the detection of low- and high-grade dysplasia in ulcerative colitis using systemic or local 5-aminolaevulinic acid sensitisation," *Gut* 52 (2003): 1003–1007.

[53] Stepinac, T., et al., "Endoscopic fluorescence detection of intraepithelial neoplasia in Barrett's esophagus after oral administration of aminolevulinic acid," *Endoscopy* 35 (2003): 663–668.

[54] Weissleder, R., and U. Mahmood, "Molecular imaging," *Radiology* 219 (2001): 316–333.

[55] Contag, C. H., and M. H. Bachmann, "Advances in vivo bioluminescence imaging of gene expression," *Ann. Rev. Biomed. Eng.* 4 (2002): 235–260.

[56] Massoud, T. F., and S. S. Gambhir, "Molecular imaging in living subjects: Seeing fundamental biological processes in a new light," *Genes Develop.* 17 (2003): 545–580.

[57] Mahmood, U., and R. Weissleder, "Near-infrared optical imaging of proteases in cancer," *Mo. Canc. Therapeut.* 2 (2003): 489–496.

[58] Blasberg, R. G. "Molecular imaging and cancer," *Mol. Canc. Therapeut.* 2 (2003): 335–343.

[59] Achilefu, S. "Lighting up tumors with receptor-specific optical molecular probes," *Technol. Canc. Res. Treat.* 3 (2004): 393–409.

[60] Weissleder, R. "Molecular imaging in cancer," *Science* 312 (2006): 1168–1171.

[61] Kelly, K., et al., "Detection of invasive colon cancer using a novel, targeted, library-derived fluorescent peptide," *Canc. Res.* 64 (2004): 6247–6251.

[62] Marten, K., et al., "Detection of dysplastic intestinal adenomas using enzyme-sensing molecular beacons in mice," *Gastroenterology* 122 (2002): 406–414.

[63] Koblinski, J. E., M. Ahram, and B. F. Sloane, "Unraveling the role of proteases in cancer," *Clin. Chim. Acta* 291 (2000): 113–135.

[64] Emmertbuck, M. R., et al., "Increased gelatinase A (Mmp-2) and cathepsin-B activity in invasive tumor regions of human colon-cancer samples," *Am. J. Pathol.* 145 (1994): 1285–1290.

[65] Hazen, L. G. M., et al., "Comparative localization of cathepsin B protein and activity in colorectal cancer," *J. Histochem. Cytochem.* 48 (2000): 1421–1430.

[66] Herszenyi, L., et al., "The role of cysteine and serine proteases in colorectal carcinoma," *Cancer* 86 (1999): 1135–1142.

[67] Funovics, M. A., R. Weissleder, and U. Mahmood, "Catheter-based in vivo imaging of enzyme activity and gene expression: Feasibility study in mice," *Radiology* 231 (2004): 659–666.

[68] Zhu, B. H., et al., "Development of a near infrared fluorescence catheter: Operating characteristics and feasibility for atherosclerotic plaque detection," *J. Phys. D—Appl. Phys.* 38 (2005): 2701–2707.

[69] Peitz, U., and P. Malfertheiner, "Chromoendoscopy: From a research tool to clinical progress," *Dig. Dis.* 20 (2002): 111–119.

[70] Bergman, J. J. G. H. M., "Gastroesophageal reflux disease and Barrett's esophagus," *Endoscopy* 37 (2005): 8–18.

[71] Canto, M. I., et al., "Methylene blue-directed biopsies improve detection of intestinal metaplasia and dysplasia in Barrett's esophagus," *Gastrointest. Endosc.* 51 (2000): 560–568.

[72] Wo, J. M., et al., "Comparison of methylene blue-directed biopsies and conventional biopsies in the detection of intestinal metaplasia and dysplasia in Barrett's esophagus: A preliminary study," *Gastrointest. Endosc.* 54 (2001): 294–301.

[73] Ragunath, K., et al., "A randomized, prospective cross-over trial comparing methylene blue-directed biopsy and conventional random biopsy for detecting intestinal metaplasia and dysplasia in Barrett's esophagus," *Endoscopy* 35 (2003): 998–1003.

[74] Lim, C. H., et al., "Randomized crossover study that used methylene blue or random 4-quadrant biopsy for the diagnosis of dysplasia in Barrett's esophagus," *Gastrointest. Endosc.* 64 (2006): 195–199.

[75] Sharma, P., et al., "Magnification chromoendoscopy for the detection of intestinal metaplasia and dysplasia in Barrett's oesophagus," *Gut* 52 (2003): 24–27.

[76] Kara, M. A., et al., "High-resolution endoscopy plus chromoendoscopy or narrow-band imaging in Barrett's esophagus: A prospective randomized crossover study," *Endoscopy* 37 (2005): 929–936.

[77] Kiesslich, R., et al., "Methylene blue-aided chromoendoscopy for the detection of intraepithelial neoplasia and colon cancer in ulcerative colitis," *Gastroenterology* 124 (2003): 880–888.

[78] Kudo, S. E., et al., "Diagnosis of colorectal tumorous lesions by magnifying endoscopy," *Gastrointest. Endosc.* 44 (1996): 8–14.

[79] Rutter, M. D., et al., "Pancolonic indigo carmine dye spraying for the detection of dysplasia in ulcerative colitis," *Gut* 53 (2004): 256–260.

[80] Hurlstone, D. P., et al., "Further validation of high-magnification chromoscopic-colonoscopy for the detection of intraepithelial neoplasia and colon cancer in ulcerative colitis," *Gastroenterology* 126 (2004): 376–378.

[81] Hurlstone, D. P., et al., "Indigo carmine-assisted high-magnification chromoscopic colonoscopy for the detection and characterisation of intraepithelial neoplasia in ulcerative colitis: A prospective evaluation," *Endoscopy* 37 (2005): 1186–1192.

[82] Kiesslich, R., P. R. Galle, and M. F. Neurath, "Endoscopic surveillance in ulcerative colitis: Smart biopsies do it better," *Gastroenterology* 133 (2007): 742–745.

[83] Yoshida, T., et al., "Narrow-band imaging system with magnifying endoscopy for superficial esophageal lesions," *Gastrointest. Endosc.* 59 (2004): 288–295.

[84] Gono, K., et al., "Appearance of enhanced tissue features in narrow-band endoscopic imaging," *J. Biomed. Opt.* 9 (2004): 568–577.

[85] Kara, M. A., and J. J. G. H. M. Bergman, "Autofluorescence imaging and narrow-band imaging for the detection of early neoplasia in patients with Barrett's esophagus," *Endoscopy* 38 (2006): 627–631.

[86] Hamamoto, Y., et al., "Usefulness of narrow-band imaging endoscopy for diagnosis of Barrett's esophagus," *J. Gastroenterol.* 39 (2004): 14–20.

[87] Sharma, P., et al., "The utility of a novel narrow band imaging endoscopy system in patients with Barrett's esophagus," *Gastrointest. Endosc.* 64 (2006): 167–175.

[88] Kara, M. A., et al., "Detection and classification of the mucosal and vascular patterns (mucosal morphology) in Barrett's esophagus by using narrow band imaging," *Gastrointest. Endosc.* 64 (2006): 155–166.

[89] Kara, M. A., et al., "Endoscopic video-autofluorescence imaging followed by narrow band imaging for detecting early neoplasia in Barrett's esophagus," *Gastrointest. Endosc.* 64 (2006): 176–185.

[90] Berenson, M. M., et al., "Restoration of squamous mucosa after ablation of Barrett esophageal epithelium," *Gastroenterology* 104 (1993): 1686–1691.

[91] Scotiniotis, I. A., et al., "Accuracy of EUS in the evaluation of Barrett's esophagus and high-grade dysplasia or intramucosal carcinoma," *Gastrointest. Endosc.* 54 (2001): 689–696.

[92] Fockens, P. "Future developments in endoscopic imaging," *Best Prac. Res. Clin. Gastroenterol.* 16 (2002): 999–1012.

[93] Adrain, A. L., et al., "High-resolution endoluminal sonography is a sensitive modality for the identification of Barrett's metaplasia," *Gastrointest. Endosc.* 46 (1997): 147–151.

[94] Huang, D., et al., "Optical coherence tomography," *Science* 254 (1991): 1178–1181.

[95] Takada, K., et al., "New measurement system for fault location in optical waveguide devices based on an interferometric technique," *Appl. Opt.* 26 (1987): 1603–1608.

[96] Gilgen, H. H., et al., "Submillimeter optical reflectometry," *IEEE J. Lightwave Technol.* 7 (1989): 1225–1233.

[97] Youngquist, R., S. Carr, and D. Davies, "Optical coherence-domain reflectometry: A new optical evaluation technique," *Opt. Lett.* 12 (1987): 158–160.

[98] Swanson, E. A., et al., "High-speed optical coherence domain reflectometry," *Opt. Lett.* 17 (1992): 151–153.

[99] Chen, Y., et al., "Ultrahigh resolution optical coherence tomography of Barrett's esophagus: Preliminary descriptive clinical study correlating images with histology," *Endoscopy* 39 (2007): 599–605.

[100] Tearney, G. J., et al., "In vivo endoscopic optical biopsy with optical coherence tomography," *Science* 276 (1997): 2037–2039.

[101] Sergeev, A. M., et al., "In vivo endoscopic OCT imaging of precancer and cancer states of human mucosa," *Opt. Exp.* 1 (1997): 432–440.

[102] Bouma, B. E., et al., "High-resolution imaging of the human esophagus and stomach in vivo using optical coherence tomography," *Gastrointest. Endosc.* 51(4) Pt. 1 (2000): 467–474.

[103] Sivak, M. V., Jr., et al., "High-resolution endoscopic imaging of the GI tract using optical coherence tomography," *Gastrointest. Endosc.* 51(4) Pt. 1 (2000): 474–479.

[104] Jäckle, S., et al., "In vivo endoscopic optical coherence tomography of the human gastrointestinal tract—toward optical biopsy," *Endoscopy* 32 (2000): 743–749.

[105] Li, X. D., et al., "Optical coherence tomography: Advanced technology for the endoscopic imaging of Barrett's esophagus," *Endoscopy* 32 (2000): 921–930.

[106] Zuccaro, G., et al., "Optical coherence tomography of the esophagus and proximal stomach in health and disease," *Am. J. Gastroent.* 96 (2001): 2633–2639.

[107] Yang, V. X., et al., "Endoscopic Doppler optical coherence tomography in the human GI tract: Initial experience," *Gastrointest. Endosc.* 61 (2005): 879–890.

[108] Poneros, J. M., et al., "Diagnosis of specialized intestinal metaplasia by optical coherence tomography," *Gastroenterology* 120 (2001): 7–12.

[109] Evans, J. A., et al., "Identifying intestinal metaplasia at the squamocolumnar junction by using optical coherence tomography," *Gastrointest. Endosc.* 65 (2007): 50–56.

[110] Shen, B., et al., "In vivo colonoscopic optical coherence tomography for transmural inflammation in inflammatory bowel disease," *Clin. Gastroenterol. Hepatol.* 2 (2004): 1080–1087.

[111] Pfau, P. R., et al., "Criteria for the diagnosis of dysplasia by endoscopic optical coherence tomography," *Gastrointest. Endosc.* 58 (2003): 196–202.

[112] Evans, J. A., et al., "Optical coherence tomography to identify intramucosal carcinoma and high-grade dysplasia in Barrett's esophagus," *Clin. Gastroent. Hepatol.* 4 (2006): 38–43.

[113] Isenberg, G., et al., "Accuracy of endoscopic optical coherence tomography in the detection of dysplasia in Barrett's esophagus: A prospective, double-blinded study," *Gastrointest. Endosc.* 62 (2005): 825–831.

[114] Qi, X., et al., "Computer-aided diagnosis of dysplasia in Barrett's esophagus using endoscopic optical coherence tomography," *J. Biomed. Opt.* 11 (2006): 10.

[115] Drexler, W., et al., "Ultrahigh-resolution ophthalmic optical coherence tomography," *Nat. Med.* 7 (2001): 502–507.

[116] Hsiung, P. L., et al., "Ultrahigh-resolution and 3-dimensional optical coherence tomography ex vivo imaging of the large and small intestines," *Gastrointest. Endosc.* 62 (2005): 561–574.

[117] Herz, P. R., et al., "Ultrahigh resolution optical biopsy with endoscopic optical coherence tomography," *Opt. Exp.* 12 (2004): 3532–3542.

[118] Tumlinson, A. R., et al., "In vivo ultrahigh-resolution optical coherence tomography of mouse colon with an achromatized endoscope," *J. Biomed. Opt.* 11 (2006): 06092RR.

[119] Choma, M. A., et al., "Sensitivity advantage of swept source and Fourier domain optical coherence tomography," *Opt. Exp.* 11 (2003): 2183–2189.

[120] de Boer, J. F., et al., "Improved signal-to-noise ratio in spectral-domain compared with time-domain optical coherence tomography," *Opt. Lett.* 28 (2003): 2067–2069.

[121] Leitgeb, R., C. K. Hitzenberger, and A. F. Fercher, "Performance of Fourier domain vs. time domain optical coherence tomography," *Opt. Exp.* 11 (2003): 889–894.

[122] Wojtkowski, M., et al., "Three-dimensional retinal imaging with high-speed ultrahigh-resolution optical coherence tomography," *Ophthalmology* 112 (2005): 1734–1746.

[123] Yun, S. H., et al., "Comprehensive volumetric optical microscopy in vivo," *Nat. Med.* 12 (2006): 1429–1433.

[124] Adler, D. C., et al., "Three-dimensional endomicroscopy using optical coherence tomography," *Nat. Photon.* 1 (2007): 709–716.

[125] Nassif, N., et al., "In vivo human retinal imaging by ultrahigh-speed spectral domain optical coherence tomography," *Opt. Lett.* 29 (2004): 480–482.

[126] Zhang, Y., et al., "High-speed volumetric imaging of cone photoreceptors with adaptive optics spectral-domain optical coherence tomography," *Opt. Exp.* 14 (2006): 4380–4394.

[127] Fercher, A. F., et al., "Measurement of intraocular distances by backscattering spectral interferometry," *Opt. Commun.* 117 (1995): 43–48.

[128] Chinn, S. R., E. A. Swanson, and J. G. Fujimoto, "Optical coherence tomography using a frequency-tunable optical source," *Opt. Lett.* 22 (1997): 340–342.

[129] Golubovic, B., et al., "Optical frequency-domain reflectometry using rapid wavelength tuning of a Cr4+:forsterite laser," *Opt. Lett.* 22 (1997): 1704–1706.

[130] Yun, S. H., et al., "High-speed wavelength-swept semiconductor laser with a polygon-scanner-based wavelength filter," *Opt. Lett.* 28 (2003): 1981–1983.

[131] Huber, R., D. C. Adler, and J. G. Fujimoto, "Buffered Fourier domain mode locking: Unidirectional swept laser sources for optical coherence tomography imaging at 370,000 lines/s," *Opt. Lett.* 31 (2006): 2975–2977.

[132] Tumlinson, A. R., et al., "Endoscope-tip interferometer for ultrahigh resolution frequency domain optical coherence tomography in mouse colon," *Opt. Exp.* 14 (2006): 1878–1887.

[133] Vakoc, B. J., et al., "Comprehensive esophageal microscopy by using optical frequency-domain imaging (with video)," *Gastrointest. Endosc.* 65 (2007): 898–905.

[134] Suter, M. J., et al., "In vivo 3D comprehensive microscopy of the human distal esophagus," *Gastrointest. Endosc.* 65 (2007): AB154–AB154.

[135] Das, A., et al., "High-resolution endoscopic imaging of the GI tract: A comparative study of optical coherence tomography versus high-frequency catheter probe EUS," *Gastrointest. Endosc.* 54 (2001): 219–224.

[136] Cilesiz, I., et al., "Comparative optical coherence tomography imaging of human esophagus: How accurate is localization of the muscularis mucosae?" *Gastrointest. Endosc.* 56 (2002): 852–857.

[137] Kuranov, R. V., et al., "Combined application of optical methods to increase the information content of optical coherent tomography in diagnostics of neoplastic processes," *Quant. Electron.* 32 (2002): 993–998.

[138] Sapozhnikova, V. V., et al., "Capabilities of fluorescence spectroscopy using 5-ALA and optical coherence tomography for diagnosis of neoplastic processes in the uterine cervix and vulva," *Laser Phys.* 15 (2005): 1664–1673.

[139] Tumlinson, A. R., et al., "Miniature endoscope for simultaneous optical coherence tomography and laser-induced fluorescence measurement," *Appl. Opt.* 43 (2004): 113–121.

[140] McNally, J. B., et al., "Task-based imaging of colon cancer in the Apc(Min/+) mouse model," *Appl. Opt.* 45 (2006): 3049–3062.

[141] Hariri, L. P., et al., "Endoscopic optical coherence tomography and laser-induced fluorescence spectroscopy in a murine colon cancer model," *Lasers Surg. Med.* 38 (2006): 305–313.

[142] Hariri, L. P., et al., "Ex vivo optical coherence tomography and laser-induced fluorescence spectroscopy imaging of murine gastrointestinal tract," *Comp. Med.* 57 (2007): 175–185.

[143] Zhu, Q., et al., "Simultaneous optical coherence tomography imaging and beta particle detection," *Opt. Lett.* 28 (2003): 1704–1706.

[144] Piao, D. Q., et al., "Hybrid positron detection and optical coherence tomography system: Design, calibration, and experimental validation with rabbit atherosclerotic models," *J. Biomed. Opt.* 10 (2005): 044010.

[145] Pan, Y. T., et al., "Enhancing early bladder cancer detection with fluorescence-guided endoscopic optical coherence tomography," *Opt. Lett.* 28 (2003): 2485–2487.

[146] Wang, Z. G., et al., "Fluorescence guided optical coherence tomography for the diagnosis of early bladder cancer in a rat model," *J. Urol.* 174 (2005): 2376–2381.

CHAPTER 4
Diffuse Optical Techniques: Instrumentation

Daqing Piao

4.1 Introduction: Deterministic "Diffuse" Detection of Probabilistic Photon Propagation

The term *diffuse optical technique* refers to the use of photons undergoing many scattering events to obtain the measurement of optical properties in deep tissue volumes for the ultimate purpose of investigating tissue physiology [1–5]. When depth-resolved cross-sectional image is the endpoint of visualization, it is specified as diffuse optical tomography (DOT) [6–10]. DOT is becoming increasingly interesting and important for functional imaging in biological tissues [11]. DOT relies on noninvasive or minimally invasive administration of light in the near-infrared (NIR) spectral window. The diagnostic premises of NIR light have been established from at least three physical pieces of evidence. First, the relatively weak NIR absorption in water allows photon propagation into deep tissue volumes. Second, the stronger NIR absorption of hemoglobin as compared to other tissue constituents such as water provides intrinsic contrast between blood and parenchymal tissues [12–24]. Third, the distinct crossover feature of NIR absorption by hemoglobin between oxygenated and deoxygenated states enables direct quantification of tissue oxygenation [25–27]. The integrative outcome of utilizing NIR light is thus directed to obtaining optically expressed physiological contrasts, such as differences in microvessel density and tissue oxygenation, in deep tissue volumes by nonionizing optical interrogation. Such physiological contrasts offer specific and often sensitive indications of tissue metabolic changes and malignancies at both macroscopic and microscopic scales.

Although biological tissue is a weak absorber of NIR light due to the large water content, it is a strong NIR scatterer owing predominantly to the micrometer-scale intracellular organelles. NIR light becomes essentially diffuse a few millimeters away from the point of a directional launching in typical soft biological tissue wherein a single scattering event may occur at a scale of 100 μm or less [28]. The NIR diffuse propagation makes it feasible to interrogate tissue volume that is much wider than the direct geometric sensing region between light illumination and collection positions and much deeper than the depth achieved by optical imaging methods in which the coherent photons are utilized, as such optical coherence tomography [29] and low-coherence enhanced backscattering [30].

Although DOT is not a choice of whole-body imaging for human due to NIR's limited penetration of several centimeters in soft tissue and strong attenuation by bone, in many cases it can perform relatively large-scale imaging of tissues or organs comparable to the size of breast. When compared with imaging modalities that employ ballistic illumination-detection path for organ-level imaging, such as X-ray CT, DOT requires fewer illumination and measurement channels in order to measure the same volume of tissue. However, due to the loss of intrinsic information in DOT related to where the photon was launched when it is detected, the sensing of a photon that transpasses or originates from a specific spatial location becomes a probabilistic matter. The direct information that DOT measurement seeks to acquire is the tissue optical property, such as the absorption coefficient and reduced scattering coefficient upon which the relevant contrast of physiological parameters may be retrieved. Since these optical properties are coupled with probabilistic propagation of NIR light in the imaging volume, the deterministic detection of the trajectory of diffuse photons becomes one of the preeminent issues in DOT techniques.

The aims of DOT instrumentation in performing deterministic "diffuse" detection of probabilistic photon propagation may be specified into the flowing three categories: (1) to identify the position of where the photon is launched from, (2) to determine the path along which the photon is diffused, and (3) to locate the target by which the photon is perturbed. These three objectives are resolved in principle by individual or combined solutions of following tasks: (1) encoding source-detector pairs for signal discrimination among many channels, (2) separating absorption and scattering contributions to the photon attenuation, and (3) obtaining tomographic image reconstruction of the heterogeneity in optical properties without or with prior information. The advancement in these three tasks may foster new DOT applications; at the same time, the drive to apply NIR methods to new imaging regimes may prompt novel approaches in DOT techniques, in particular, the instrumentation. The first part of this chapter is intended to provide a brief overview of some fundamental technological issues of DOT that have evolved over the time. Detailed discussion covering these technological advances in more breadth and depth can be found in many outstanding review papers [7–11, 28]. The second part of this chapter introduces in detail some of the latest unconventional approaches in DOT instrumentation for the aim of extending DOT to previously unattempted or difficult applications. These unconventional approaches may also infer potential future directions of DOT instrumentation.

4.2 Methods of Differentiating the Origin of Diffuse Photons

NIR imaging uses diffused photons as measured through transmission of significant volumes of tissue and after they have undergone many scattering events. The intrinsic information related to where the photon was launched from is thus lost when it is detected. NIR DOT as a tomographic imaging modality requires measurements from multiple source and detector channels; therefore, a mechanism of differentiating the signals corresponding to specific source and detector pairs must be implemented.

4.2.1 The Source-Encoding Requirement in DOT

The measurements by multiple detectors when multiple sources are launched may be expressed by the following equation (it is derived by assuming a linear model for simplicity; however, the derivation can also be applied to a nonlinear model):

$$D_{M\times 1} = \Psi_{M\times N} S_{N\times 1} \tag{4.1}$$

where D denotes the assembly of detector outputs, M is the number of detector channels, S represents the assembly of source inputs, N is the number of source channels, and Ψ is the weight matrix governed by the imaging geometry and the medium optical property. The output of the individual detector is then represented by

$$d_m = \sum_{n=1}^{N} \psi_{mn} s_n, \quad m = 1, 2, \ldots, M, n = 1, 2, \ldots, N \tag{4.2}$$

which indicates that the output of each single detector contains a mixture of signals originating from all source channels. The separation of individual source-detector signals of diffuse photon propagation as a requirement of DOT image formation can only be implemented through encoding of the source-detector channels at the source side and proper decoding of the channels at the measurement. This may not be as explicit as it seems without the analysis of two simplified configurations. When considering the geometry of an imaging array with only one source and multiple detectors, the detector outputs are

$$D_{M\times 1} = \Psi_{M\times 1} S_{1\times 1} \tag{4.3}$$

or

$$d_m = \psi_m s \tag{4.4}$$

where it is clear that there is a unique correspondence of the signal from the single source to each detector by $1 \rightarrow m$. For the other geometry with multiple sources and only one detector, the detector output becomes

$$D_{1\times 1} = \Psi_{1\times N} S_{N\times 1} \tag{4.5}$$

or

$$d = \sum_{n=1}^{N} \psi_{1n} s_n \tag{4.6}$$

where the multiple-source information is coupled in the output of the single detector. Equation (4.6) implies that the source origination of diffuse photons cannot be tracked unless the photons are differentiated prior to launching into the medium, or, in other words, unless the source channels are properly encoded.

When the sources in DOT are properly encoded, the discriminated signals corresponding to all source-detector pairs can be described intuitively by

$$D_{M \times N} = \Psi_{M \times N} E_{N \times 1} S_{1 \times N} \qquad (4.7)$$

where $E = <encod>$ represents the encoding operation applied to the source channels:

$$<encod_i> s_j = \begin{cases} <s_j> & i = j \\ 0 & i \neq j \end{cases} \qquad (4.8)$$

Substituting (4.8) into (4.7) for E gives

$$\begin{bmatrix} d_{11} & d_{12} & \cdots & d_{1N} \\ d_{21} & d_{22} & \cdots & d_{2N} \\ \vdots & \vdots & \cdots & \vdots \\ d_{M1} & d_{M2} & \cdots & d_{MN} \end{bmatrix} = \begin{bmatrix} <\psi_{11} s_1> & <\psi_{12} s_2> & \cdots & <\psi_{1N} s_N> \\ <\psi_{11} s_1> & <\psi_{22} s_2> & \cdots & <\psi_{2N} s_N> \\ \vdots & \vdots & \cdots & \vdots \\ <\psi_{11} s_1> & <\psi_{M2} s_2> & \cdots & <\psi_{MN} s_N> \end{bmatrix} \qquad (4.9)$$

Equation (4.9) indicates that under a proper detector decoding that matches with the source-encoding method, the signals corresponding to all source-detector pairs can be discriminated thoroughly.

4.2.2 Methods of Source Encoding and Detector Decoding for Diffuse Optical Tomography

Many source-encoding and detector-decoding methods have been demonstrated [31]. These methods fall into one or a combination of the following three categories.

4.2.2.1 Time-Based Multiplexing

Perhaps the most straightforward method of source encoding is sequentially turning on the sources, or time-series multiplexing [32, 33]. This time-based multiplexing is valid if the multiplexing interval is much greater than the time of photon flight, which is obviously obeyed for all biological tissues of finite size. This encoding technique can be described based on (4.7) as

$$D^\tau_{M \times N} = \Psi_{M \times N} T_{N \times 1} S_{1 \times N} \qquad (4.10)$$

The $T_{N \times 1}$ in (4.10) is an operator representing the time-based multiplexing of

$$T_{N \times 1} = \begin{bmatrix} <\delta(\tau - 1)> \\ <\delta(\tau - 2)> \\ \vdots \\ <\delta(\tau - N)> \end{bmatrix} \qquad (4.11)$$

where the discrete time impulse function δ is used to denote the turning-on sequencing of the source from 1 to N. The output of each detector at each multiplexing sequence is then

$$d_{mn} = \sum_{\tau=1}^{N} \psi_{m\tau} s_\tau \delta(\tau - n) = \psi_{mn} s_n \qquad (4.12)$$

Equation (4.12) gives the decoded signal for a specific source-detector pair $n \to m$, which also means that the time-based multiplexing operation performs both source encoding and detector decoding instantaneously. The advantage of this time-based multiplexing technique for source encoding and detector decoding is that at any instance of source sequencing, each detector receives only the signal illuminated from one source; therefore, the maximum dynamic range of each photodetector (denoted by I_{max}) is devoted exclusively to the detection of signals from a single source-detector pair. The disadvantage of this encoding/decoding technique is the potentially lengthy data acquisition for entire source-detector pairs at a total period of $(N-1) \cdot \Delta t_0$, where Δt_0 is the multiplexing timing for each step, under the condition that the signal-to-noise ratio integrated over the time of Δt_0 is sufficient. The vast majority of all optical tomography methods use this approach either to deliver light of single-band to multiple-source channels or to distribute light of multiple bands to a single-source channel.

4.2.2.2 Frequency-Based Multiplexing

Modulation frequency-based multiplexing is another commonly used source-encoding method [34–37]. In frequency-based multiplexing, the source intensities are modulated at different frequencies of $\omega_n = \omega_0 + \delta\omega_n$ upon the same base band of ω_0, under the valid assumption that the intensity modulation frequency does not vary when propagating through diffuse medium.

Similar to (4.10), the frequency-encoded signal at the detector output can be expressed by

$$D^{\omega}_{M \times N} = \Psi_{M \times N} F_{N \times 1} S_{1 \times N} \qquad (4.13)$$

where $F_{N \times 1}$ is an operator representing the frequency multiplexing of

$$F_{N \times 1} = \begin{bmatrix} <\cos[(\omega_0 + \delta\omega_1)t]> \\ <\cos[(\omega_0 + \delta\omega_2)t]> \\ \vdots \\ <\cos[(\omega_0 + \delta\omega_N)t]> \end{bmatrix} \qquad (4.14)$$

and the output of each detector is approximately

$$d_m = \sum_{n=1}^{N} \psi_{mn} s_n \cos[(\omega_0 + \delta\omega_n)t] + k_{nm} \qquad (4.15)$$

Note that the exact signal is not precisely a pure cosine wave for the response of the laser, and the detector to modulation is not entirely linear with the applied current. Here $\psi_{mn}s_n$ is the modulation depth and k_{nm} is the dc bias offset due to the fact that the laser must operate with a positive output. For frequency-based source encoding, the detector decoding of source-detector pair $n \to m$ is obtained by demodulation of d_m at ω_0 and bandpass filtering at $\delta\omega_n$, that is,

$$d_{mn} = \psi_{mn} s_n \cos[\delta\omega_n t] \qquad (4.16)$$

The advantage of source encoding and detector decoding by frequency multiplexing/demultiplexing is the gain in sampling speed by simultaneous measurement of signals from all source-detector pairs as a result of parallel light delivery. However, the frequency-encoded source signals must be directed to the same photodetector for photoelectronic conversion prior to applying any demodulation operation for signal decoding. When one detector collects signals from N source channels in parallel, the average dynamic range corresponding to one source-detector pair reduces to

$$I_{n \to m} = \frac{\sum_{n=1}^{N}(\psi_{mn} s_n)^2}{N} = \frac{I_{\max}}{N} \qquad (4.17)$$

Therefore the average dynamic range available for each source-detector signal is linearly reduced with adding on of more source channels, and the lowest-level signals are potentially buried under the noise present in the higher-intensity signals. This is particularly problematic if the tissue volume being imaged is large, the absorption of the tissue is strong, and the distances between optodes have big variations. To fully understand the limiting factors in this type of system, an analysis of signal to noise would be required where the limiting contribution to noise in the ideal case is shot noise.

4.2.2.3 Wavelength-Based Multiplexing or Spectral Encoding

A wavelength-based multiplexing method for source encoding was introduced recently [38, 39]. This method of source encoding refers to operating the sources at different wavelengths. The encoded signal after transmitting through the medium thus becomes

$$D^{\lambda}_{M \times N} = \Psi_{M \times N} \Gamma_{N \times 1} S_{1 \times N} \qquad (4.18)$$

where $\Gamma_{N \times N}$ is the wavelength-multiplexing or spectral-encoding operator having the structure of

$$\Gamma_{N \times 1} = \begin{bmatrix} <\lambda_1> \\ <\lambda_2> \\ \vdots \\ <\lambda_N> \end{bmatrix} \qquad (4.19)$$

with $<\lambda_n>$, $n = 1, 2, ..., N$ representing the operating wavelength of the source. When a spectrometer is used at the detection side, the spectrally encoded signals can be spatially spread or decoded to provide measurement of

$$d_{mn} = \psi_{mn} s_n(\lambda_n) \tag{4.20}$$

for a source-detector pair $n \to m$. If the orientation of the detector array is set orthogonal to the spectral-spread direction, all source-detector pairs can be decoded completely in a two-dimensional pattern and acquired simultaneously by parallel photodetectors such as CCD. This approach performs decoding of all source-detector pairs prior to the photoelectronic conversion as compared with either time-based multiplexing or frequency-based multiplexing where the photoelectronic detection is performed along with or prior to the decoding. This feature of parallel light delivery renders the advantage that adding on more sources will not cause reduction in the signal dynamic range of an individual source-detector channel. This is valid so long as the source spectra can be differentiated by the spectrometer and the number of photoelectronic conversion channels in the detector is greater than that of source channels. This configuration ensures that different photoelectronic detector elements sense different signals, and each detector's full dynamic range is maintained.

The major advantage of this wavelength-based source-encoding and detector-decoding method is the data-acquisition speed it could potentially reach without compromising the dynamic range of each detection channel. However, attention should be paid to the overall wavelength range used for source encoding. Contrary to time-based and frequency-based multiplexing methods, in which all source channels are detected at a single wavelength, the source channels in wavelength-based multiplexing experiences wavelength-dependent light propagation. This is due to the fact that in the NIR band of 650 to 900 nm, the absorption of hemoglobin is stronger and more wavelength variant in comparison to the water, even though the scattering may not be as wavelength-dependent for both hemoglobin and water. Therefore, in the spectral-encoding approach, the overall source wavelength band should be within a small range, ideally less than 5 nm, in order to maintain relatively uniform tissue absorption among different source channels. This poses a limitation on source channels that can be encoded within the spectrometer resolution.

4.3 Techniques of Decoupling the Absorption and Scattering Contributions to the Photon Remission

Source encoding and detector decoding assure the discrimination of photons transported from a specific source to a detector. Microscopically, the photons could take any path from the source to the detector due to the strong scattering of NIR photons in biological tissue. Yet, statistical analyses demonstrate that macroscopically the highest probability of photon propagation takes a banana-shaped path connecting the source and the detector [40]. The banana shape gives a rough estimation of the path length of the majority of the photons arriving at the detector. The optical properties that DOT expects to retrieve contain both absorption and reduced- or transport-scattering coefficients. This requires knowledge not only of the actual photon path length but also the method of differentiating absorption and scattering contributions to the photon loss, both being evaluated by surface measurement of remitted photons. Theoretical breakthroughs and instrumentation advancements have demonstrated that time-resolved or time-domain detection and frequency-domain detection methods are capable of determining the photon path length and differentiating or decoupling absorption and reduced-scattering properties of the medium.

4.3.1 Time-Domain Detection

When a short light pulse (typically 2 to 5 ps for NIR DOT) is delivered to a purely absorptive tissue, the pulse detected after propagation will change in only the amplitude due to the attenuation, as depicted in Figure 4.1(a). When the same pulse is

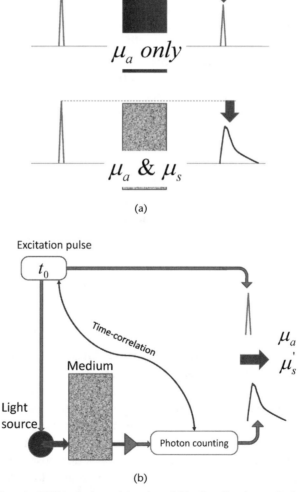

Figure 4.1 Time-domain DOT technique: (a) pulse width alteration by scattering medium compared with pulse attenuation by purely absorptive medium, and (b) schematic illustration of time-domain detection of light pulse propagating through a turbid medium.

4.3 Techniques of Decoupling the Absorption and Scattering Contributions

delivered to an absorptive and highly scattering tissue, the family of photon paths produced by scattering leads to broadening of the pulse in addition to the amplitude attenuation of the pulse. The time $<t>$ of the temporal point spread function (TPSF) at which the maximum detected intensity occurs relative to the input pulse is the mean arrival time of photons, and this may be used, together with velocity of light c in tissue to calculate a mean optical path length of $<ct>$ [28]. Use of the measurement of time gives the method its alternative name, *time-resolved* or *time-of-flight detection*.

When the diffusion approximation is incorporated into the radiative transport equation, the time-domain photon-diffusion equation may be written as [41]

$$\frac{1}{c}\frac{\partial}{\partial t}\phi(\vec{r},t) = \vec{\nabla}\cdot\left(D\vec{\nabla}\phi(\vec{r},t)\right) - \mu_a\phi(\vec{r},t) + S(\vec{r},t) \quad (4.21)$$

where $\phi(\vec{r},t)$ is the diffuse photon fluence rate, c is the speed of light in the tissue, D is the diffusion coefficient,

$$D = \frac{1}{3[\mu_a + (1-g)\mu_s]} \quad (4.22)$$

where μ_a is the absorption coefficient, μ_s is the scattering coefficient, g is the mean cosine of the scattering angle, and $S(\vec{r},t)$ is the photon source. The term $(1-g)\mu_s$ is often denoted by a reduced scattering coefficient of μ_s' to represent the assembled equivalent isotropic scattering property of tissue if each scattering event is anisotropic.

For a short pulse from a point source, $S(\vec{r},t) = \delta(0,0)$, it may be shown that the mean photon path length for a tissue slab of thickness d is [28]

$$<ct> = \left(4\pi_a D\right)^{-1/2}\frac{(d-z_0)\exp\left(2z_0\sqrt{\mu_a/D}\right) - (d+z_0)}{\exp\left(2z_0\sqrt{\mu_a/D}-1\right)} \quad (4.23)$$

where $z_0 = [(1-g)\mu_s]^{-1}$ is the depth between the actual source location of initial directional launching and the position of an imaginary point from which the photons can be considered to be becoming isotropic. Equation (4.23) indicates the feasibility of determining the absorption μ_a and diffusion coefficient D (predominantly the reduced scattering) by multiple measurements of mean photon path length or by fitting to the single measurement data using "time-of-flight" estimation.

Figure 4.1(b) gives the simplified instrumentation scheme for a time-domain DOT measurement. Two fundamental requirements of the instrumentation are generation of short-pulse light and time-correlated measurement of the pulse width and amplitude after tissue propagation. Fast-streaking camera or other slower single-photon counting devices may be used for the detection. It is acknowledged that time-domain measurement leads to the richest or the most accurate information about the tissue optical properties; however, the instrumentation is typically expensive and difficult [42, 43].

4.3.2 Frequency-Domain Detection

When a light of amplitude modulation (typically 100 MHz to 1 GHz for NIR DOT) is delivered to purely absorptive tissue, both the dc and ac levels of the light after detection will be attenuated with no alteration of its phase, as depicted in Figure 4.2(a). When the same light is delivered to an absorptive and highly scattering tissue, the multiple photon scattering leads to a delay of the modulation phase in addition to the attenuation of dc and ac levels. The phase delay and ac/dc attenuation rate can also be used to calculate the mean optical path length of photons for calculation of the absorption and scattering contribution to the diffuse photon propagation [44].

The Fourier transform of the time-domain diffusion equation (4.21) will lead to the frequency-domain diffusion equation of [43, 44]

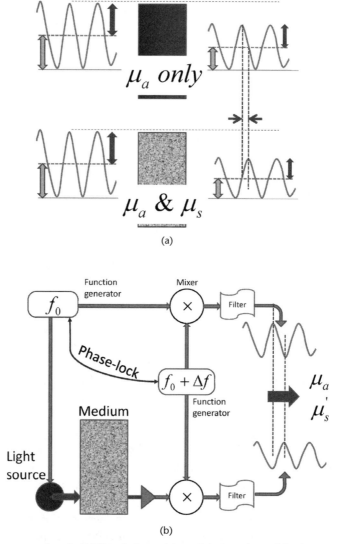

Figure 4.2 Frequency-domain DOT technique: (a) modulation phase delay by scattering medium compared with modulation amplitude attenuation by purely absorptive medium, and (b) schematic illustration of frequency-domain detection of light propagating through a turbid medium.

4.3 Techniques of Decoupling the Absorption and Scattering Contributions

$$\frac{1}{c}\frac{\partial}{\partial t}\phi(\vec{r},\omega) = \vec{\nabla}\cdot\left(D\vec{\nabla}\phi(\vec{r},\omega)\right) - \left(\mu_a + i\frac{\omega}{c}\right)\phi(\vec{r},\omega) + S(\vec{r},\omega) \qquad (4.24)$$

where ω is the angular frequency of the light modulation. For infinite medium and an amplitude modulation of the light at

$$I = I_{dc} + I_{ac}\sin(\omega t - \Phi) = I_{dc} + I_{ac}\sin(2\pi\nu t - \Phi) \qquad (4.25)$$

it is found that the detector measurement of steady-state photon density, the amplitude of photon-density modulation, and the phase shift of the photon-density modulation can be expressed by [28]

$$U_{dc} = \frac{S}{4\pi D}\frac{\exp\left[-r\left(\frac{\mu_a}{D}\right)^{1/2}\right]}{r} \qquad (4.26)$$

$$U_{ac} = \frac{S\frac{I_{ac}}{I_{dc}}}{4\pi\nu D}\frac{\exp[r\,\text{Re}(k)]}{r} \qquad (4.27)$$

$$\Phi = r\,\text{Im}(k) + \Phi_s \qquad (4.28)$$

where

$$k = -\left(\frac{\mu_a - i2\pi\nu}{D}\right)^{1/2} \qquad (4.29)$$

and r is the source-detector separation. More complicated expression of similar measurements for a semiinfinite medium can be found in [44–46]. By single measurement of the changes in both the phase and modulation, the absorption and reduced-scattering properties of the bulk tissue can be retrieved.

Frequency-domain instrumentation involves amplitude modulation of the light at frequencies on the order of hundreds of megahertz, by which the phase change of photon density caused by tissue scattering over several centimeters of tissue volume may be resolved. In practice, the frequency-domain measurement is usually done by downshifting the frequency to the kilohertz or tens-of-kilohertz range to take advantage of much-reduced sampling requirements. This requires demodulation of the light propagating through the medium by a phase-locked local oscillator signal. The downshifted signal passing through the scattering medium is compared with a reference signal that is demodulated directly from the source modulation frequency to retrieve the phase shift and ac/dc attenuation. The light source used for frequency-domain detection is usually laser diode, which can be conveniently modulated, and the photodetector is most frequently chosen between photomultiplier tube (PMT) and avalanche photodiode (APD). PMT is known to have excellent sensitivity and gain, while APD generally has better performance in terms of dynamic range.

4.3.3 Continuous-Wave Detection

The continuous-wave DOT detection method can be considered the extreme case of time-domain measurement in (4.21) when $t \to \infty$; therefore, the photon density becomes time invariant. The continuous-wave DOT method can also be considered the special case of frequency-domain measurement in (4.24) when $\omega \to 0$; thus, the photon density contains only the dc component. Instrumentation for continuous-wave DOT measurement is the simplest since it needs only source and detector running at steady state or at low-frequency kilohertz range modulation [36, 47–49].

At one time, it was generally argued that CW measurement provides limited information regarding tissue optical properties and cannot reliably recover the absolute values of absorption and reduced-scattering properties of the tissue even with very careful calibration due to lack of phase information which is critical to the determination of photon path length. However, recent studies have demonstrated that when a complicated image-reconstruction method is used, the absorption and reduced-scattering properties may be reconstructed separately from continuous-wave measurement [50, 51].

4.4 Principles of Determining the Heterogeneity of Optical Properties

When the launching position and path of the photons can be determined, the global optical properties along the photon trajectory may be quantified. However, without a tomographic visualization of the optical properties of the tissue volume, the physiological information that diffuse photon detection can provide is limited since the potential existence of optical heterogeneity within a bulky tissue volume is not localized; therefore, correlating the abnormal optical properties with physiological malfunctions tends to be inexplicit.

4.4.1 Tomographic Image Reconstruction and Prior Utilization

Tomographic imaging or cross-sectional mapping of optical heterogeneity in DOT can be achieved by integration of projection measurements at multiple angles as illustrated in Figure 4.3. The image reconstruction may be conducted by assuming linear projection of the measurement data as in X-ray tomography [52] or by use of a model-based iterative approach [6, 8, 9]. Model-based DOT image reconstruction involves solving the photon-diffusion equation with numerical methods such as the finite-element method and iteratively minimizing the error between the measurement and the model prediction to recover the piecewise optical properties within a given imaging volume [53–55]. The flow chart of a typical model-based image-reconstruction routine is sketched in Figure 4.4(a).

The forward estimation task based on the light-propagation model is known to be sensitive to small perturbations in the light measurements (which is the basis of superior contrast in DOT imaging), not all of which may be caused by the heterogeneity changes in tissue optical properties. The ill-posed and underdetermined features of the DOT inverse problem, coupled with this ill-conditioning, imply that the accuracy of retrieving optical heterogeneity (including location, size, and contrast) inside the tissue volume is dependent upon many issues such as the stability of

4.4 Principles of Determining the Heterogeneity of Optical Properties

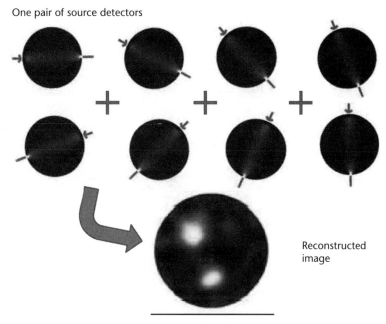

Figure 4.3 Illustration of image reconstruction in DOT where integration of the multiple-angle projection measurements leads to the localization of optical heterogeneity in the imaging volume, similar to back-projection in CT. (Courtsey of Brian W. Pogue.)

surface measurement and the number of iterations. Investigations demonstrated that significant improvement in the stability and accuracy of the reconstruction process can be obtained by including prior information in the iterative minimization process [56–61]. Studies have shown that anatomical information from other modalities, such as ultrasound, MRI, or CT, when used in the reconstruction procedure, can improve the stability of the reconstruction and result in faster convergence, better localization, more accurate optical properties, and higher spatial resolution [62–65].

The spatial (also known as structural or anatomic) prior information can be utilized within the NIR DOT image-reconstruction scheme in two forms. The hard prior illustrated in Figure 4.4(b), also known as region-based (or parameter-reduction) reconstruction, utilizes the prior anatomic regions information to reduce the large number of unknown parameters into a few unknown parameters by assuming that the optical distribution within each region is constant [61]. Since the number of the unknowns is dramatically reduced, the computation becomes efficient. In the soft prior, the spatial information is instead incorporated within the image-reconstruction algorithm in a form of regularization [see Figure 4.4(b)]. This type of a priori information in effect relates the recovery of each unknown parameter within the reconstruction to other unknowns within the same defined region [61].

Another type of prior for DOT reconstruction when multispectral measurement is performed incorporates the known spectral behavior of tissue chromophores and Mie scattering theory as constraints. This type of prior-guided NIR image reconstruction uses multiwavelength measurements simultaneously to compute images of constituent parameters without intermediate recovery of optical properties.

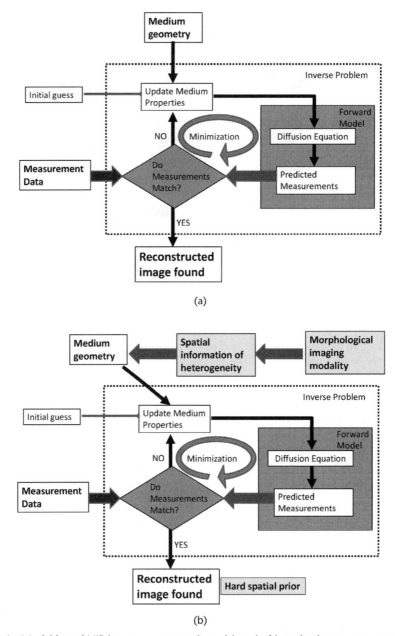

Figure 4.4 Model-based NIR image reconstructions: (a) typical iterative image reconstruction based on photon propagation model, (b) NIR image reconstruction by use of hard spatial prior, (c) NIR image reconstruction by use of soft spatial prior, and (d) NIR image reconstruction by use of spectral prior.

Simulation studies have shown that the combination of spatial and spectral priors improves the accuracy and quality of NIR images [49, 66]. The spectral prior obtained by including the intrinsic behavior of tissue chromophores and scattering plays a more important role in preserving quantitative functional parameter estimates by DOT. It has been demonstrated that a synergy between these two priors

4.4 Principles of Determining the Heterogeneity of Optical Properties

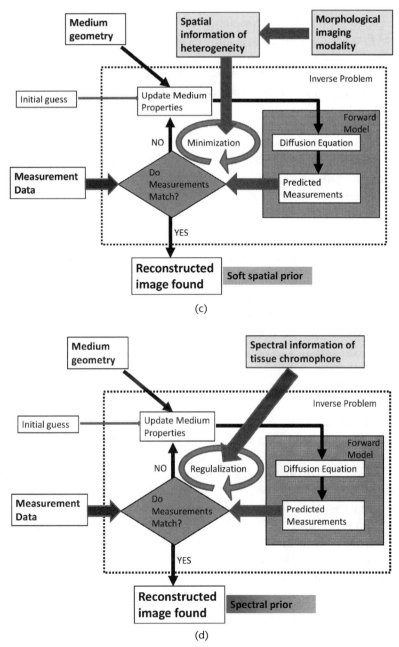

Figure 4.4 (continued)

yields the most accurate characterization of absolute tissue optical properties currently available [49, 67, 68].

4.4.2 Diffuse Optical Tomography Imaging in the Context of Multimodality Imaging

The functional or spectroscopic information of near-infrared DOT is often compromised by the limitations inherent to the ill-posed iterative image reconstruction required for diffuse photon detection. Combining DOT with other imaging modalities that are anatomically accurate can not only correlate the DOT functional contrast with the spatial anatomy of the lesion but also use the structural delineation of the lesion to guide and constrain the DOT image reconstruction. In terms of the morphological imaging modalities that can be cohesively integrated with DOT for complimentary imaging as well as the prior-guided DOT reconstruction, there have been a few choices out of some standard techniques mainly used for anatomic imaging, but arguably the most-successful modalities may be US [69–73] and MRI [59, 63–65, 74–76]. The following section briefly reviews the instrumentations leading to the integration of DOT with US and MRI for breast cancer imaging, which are the representative examples of the DOT instrumentation advancement and the growing impact of DOT technology in multimodality clinical imaging.

4.4.2.1 Diffuse Optical Tomography Integrated with Ultrasound

Ultrasound imaging is frequently used as an adjunct tool to mammography in differentiating cysts from solid lesions. Ultrasound also plays an important role in guiding interventional procedures such as needle aspiration, core needle biopsy, and prebiopsy needle localization [69].

Several studies have been reported on the instrumentation technology of combining DOT with US [69–72]. The system developed at the University of Connecticut is implemented by simultaneously deploying optical sensors and a commercial US transducer mounted on a handheld probe and utilizing coregistered lesion structure information provided by US to improve the inverse optical imaging reconstruction. The handheld hybrid probe consists of a commercial US transducer located in the center and the NIR source-detector fibers distributed at the periphery [see Figure 4.5(a)]. The NIR imager consists of 12 pairs of dual-wavelength (780 and 830 nm) laser diodes and eight photomultiplier tubes (PMTs) for detection. The laser diodes' outputs were amplitude modulated at 140 MHz, and the detector outputs were demodulated to 20 kHz. The demodulated signals were further amplified and bandpass filtered at 20 kHz. A reference signal of 20 kHz was also generated by directly mixing the detected radiofrequency (RF) signals with the RF signal generated from the oscillator.

The NIR reconstruction takes advantages of US localization of lesions and segments the imaging volume into a finer grid in lesion region L and a coarser grid in nonlesion background region B [see Figure 4.5(b)]. A modified Born approximation is used to relate the scattered field measured at each source and detector pair to total absorption variations at wavelength in each volume element of two regions within the sample. The absorption distribution at each wavelength is obtained by dividing total absorption distribution changes of lesion and background regions, respectively, by different voxel sizes in lesion and background tissue regions. This dual-mesh scheme results in well-conditioned inversion and convergence of the image reconstruction in a few iterations [69, 71, 73].

An example of a DOT/US image is given in Figure 4.5(c, d) for an early-stage invasive ductal carcinoma [69]. US showed a nodular mass with internal echoes, and the lesion was considered suspicious. The estimated lesion diameter measured from the US image was 8 mm. US-guided core needle biopsy revealed intraductal and

4.4 Principles of Determining the Heterogeneity of Optical Properties

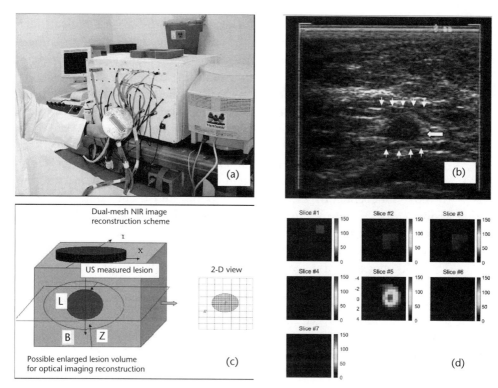

Figure 4.5 (a) Prototype of the handheld combined NIR/US imager developed at the University of Connecticut is shown. (b) The entire imaging volume is segmented into lesion (L) and background (B) regions. The fine imaging grid is used for the lesion region, and the coarse grid is used for the background. (c) NIR/US images of a nonpalpable lesion in a 55-year-old woman are shown. US showed a nodular mass with internal echoes, and the lesion was considered suspicious. (d) The maps of total hemoglobin concentration distribution correspond to slices from 0.7 cm underneath the skin surface to the chest wall, with 0.5 cm spacing. The lesion is well resolved in slice 5. (*From:* [69]. © 1998 Elsevier. Reprinted with permission.)

infiltrating ductal carcinoma. The total hemoglobin concentration distribution computed from optical absorption maps at 780 and 830 nm wavelengths are shown, with the first slice 0.7 cm deep into the breast tissue from the skin surface and the last slice closer to the chest wall at slice spacing of 0.5 cm. The horizontal and vertical axes of each slice are spatial x and y optical probe dimensions of 9 cm. The lesion is well resolved in slice 5, and the measured maximum total hemoglobin concentration for the lesion is 122 mmol/L, the average measured within full width and half maximum (FWHM) is 91 mmol/L, and the measured average background hemoglobin concentration is 14 mmol/L.

4.4.2.2 Diffuse Optical Tomography Integrated with Magnetic Resonance Imaging

The NIR/MRI imaging system [Color Plate 9(a)] developed at Dartmouth College [74] consisted of six laser diodes (660 to 850 nm), which were amplitude modulated at 100 MHz. The bank of laser tubes was mounted on a linear translation stage that sequentially coupled the activated source into 16 bifurcated optical-fiber bundles. The central seven fibers delivered the source light, while the remaining fibers collected transmitted light and were coupled to photomultiplier tube (PMT) detectors. For each source, measurements of the amplitude and phase shift of the 100 MHz signal were acquired from 15 locations around the breast. The fibers extended 13m [Color Plate 9(b)] into a 1.5-T whole-body MRI (GE Medical Systems), and the two data streams (i.e., NIR and MRI) were acquired simultaneously. The open architecture breast array coil (Invivo, Orlando, Florida) houses the MR-compatible fiber-positioning system [Color Plate 9(c)]. Two fiber-breast interface prototypes were constructed. The first, pictured in Color Plate 9(d), allows each of the 16 fibers to move independently in a radial direction, and tissue contact is enforced with bronze compression springs. The second, shown in Color Plate 9(e), maintains a circular breast circumference and allows more user control.

One set of MRI-guided NIR reconstruction images is shown in Color Plate 9(f). The MRI images are axial and coronal T1-weighted slices of a breast. Reconstructed images of chromophores and scatter parameters from simultaneously acquired NIR measurements (left to right) are as follows: total hemoglobin concentration ([HbT], μM), hemoglobin oxygen saturation (S_tO_2, %), water fraction (H_2O, %), scattering amplitude (A), and scattering power. Interestingly, the spatial distributions in the NIR images do not exactly match the segmented MRI regions in all cases, and some heterogeneity occurs, although the predominant effect is the significant change in optical properties that results between the adipose and fibroglandular boundaries. The technique provides high-resolution images of both tissue structure through MRI and tissue function through NIR contrast.

The combined NIR/US and NIR/MRI modalities demonstrated the increasing probability that DOT will provide high sensitivity and specificity values to diagnostics when combined with other imaging systems.

4.5 Novel Approaches in Instrumentation of Diffuse Optical Tomography: Source Spectral Encoding

4.5.1 Discrete Spectral Encoding by Use of Multiple Laser Diodes

The principle of parallel source delivery based on wavelength multiplexing or spectral encoding is initially demonstrated by use of multiple laser diodes (LDs) [38, 39]. In this approach, each LD operates at a unique wavelength as shown in Color Plate 10 and Figure 4.6(a). The unique wavelength corresponds to $<\lambda_n>$ ($n = 1, 2, ..., N$) in (4.19). It is imperative to maintain small wavelength separation among the source channels as discussed previously. Actually, the LDs can be spectrally encoded at close wavelength separation, simply and effectively, by use of a number of single-mode diodes manufactured for the same spectral band whose emission wavelengths can be varied slightly by adjusting the laser operating temperature. The wavelength of the LD is a function of both operating temperature and driving current. The wavelength stability of the LD against temperature and current may be expressed by

4.5 Novel Approaches in Instrumentation of Diffuse Optical Tomography

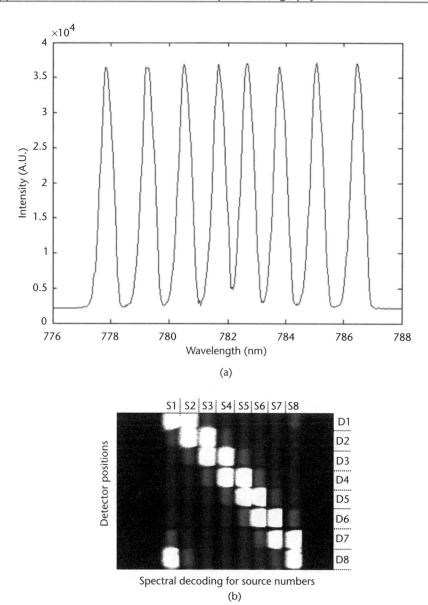

Figure 4.6 The spectral-encoding NIR tomography system developed by Dartmouth NIR imaging group: (a) the source spectral-encoding profile, where the emission wavelengths of eight laser diodes are operated at approximately 1.25 nm separation, and (b) the completely decoded signals acquired by CCD after spectrometer corresponding to eight sources and eight detectors in Color Plate 10.

$$\frac{d\lambda}{dT} = a_1 - \frac{a_2}{T_0} \qquad (4.30)$$

where a_1 corresponds to a red shift in wavelength with temperature at constant current, and a_2 corresponds to a blue shift in wavelength with current at constant temperature. By operating the LD in constant current mode and adjusting the LD temperature, the emission wavelength can be adjusted with a typical tuning sensitivity of 0.1 to 0.3 nm/°C [77]. In this LD-based spectral-encoding system, a source spectral separation of 1.25 nm is achieved among eight source channels. The source spectral separation can be reduced if the precision of LD temperature control is improved and mode hopping of LD can be suppressed.

The parallel source illumination and complete decoding of all source-detector pairs allow rapid acquisition of the DOT data by imaging devices like CCD. Figure 4.6(b) shows the data pattern of parallel source-detector decoding that is available for CCD detection. This LD-based spectral-encoding system has achieved a 35-Hz frame rate of data acquisition in a medium of 27 mm in diameter, which is believed as the first DOT system of performing video-rate sampling.

4.5.2 Imaging Examples of Spectral-Encoding Rapid NIR Tomography

Video-rate NIR imaging allows real-time sampling of transient changes in tissue optical properties that may be linked to fast physiological responses such as tissue permeability variation. One example is given in Figure 4.7, where the images were taken when diluted ink as an optical absorber was continuously injected to Intralipid solution contained within a hole of solid tissue phantom. The instantaneous absorption coefficients of the solution over 10 seconds are plotted with the inset showing the images of the phantom at six discrete timings. Slow ink injection started after 2 seconds and stopped at 9 seconds. A total of 350 frames were taken over 10 seconds. The gradual increasing of the absorption coefficient after the ink injection and the reaching of a plateau before stopping the ink injection are very

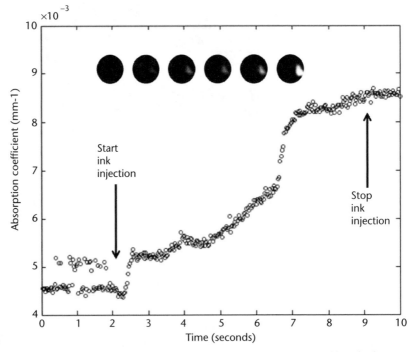

Figure 4.7 Examples of video-rate NIR tomography imaging. Images of diluted-ink injection into the Intralipid solution held in a hole of a solid phantom. Continuous changes of the light absorption during ink injection have been successfully captured. The inset shows the images at 2, 3, 4, 5, 6, and 7 seconds.

clearly captured. Such "snapshot" capturing of spatial absorption variations and time-resolved measurements of localized transient absorption changes is critical for dynamic imaging of rapid perfusion changes in biological tissues by DOT.

Figure 4.8 shows in vivo imaging of tumor and hemodynamic responses by this video-rate NIR system. A tumor-bearing rat leg was imaged in Figure 4.8(a), where the bigger and brighter spot at the bottom was the implanted solid prostate tumor, and the smaller spot at the top was the tail. The implanted tumor has clear elevated contrast compared with the normal tissue. In Figure 4.8(b), a mouse leg was utilized to image the blood pulsation in the muscle. Both legs were imaged successively, with one leg having compromised blood flow due to blockage of the iliac artery, while the other leg had normal blood flow. The tomographic images of these legs are shown in Figure 4.8(b), with each pair of images being one of a sequence of images at 1/35th of a second. The blood flow pulsation in the left leg can be seen between images 3 and 4 as a successive decrease in overall intensity, whereas the intensity of pulsation is significantly less in the right leg [78].

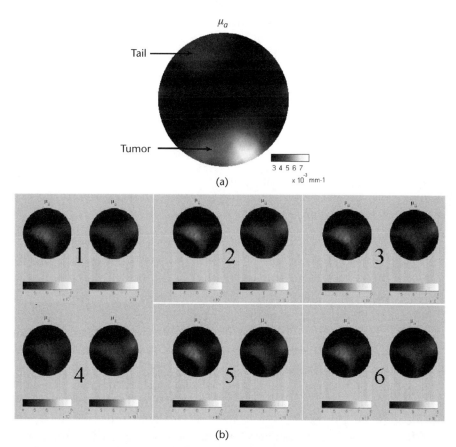

Figure 4.8 In vivo images taken with this spectral-encoding video-rate NIR system. (a) Image of rat tumor. The tumor was at the lower half of the FOV, and the tail was at the top.
(b) Tomographic images of the two legs of a mouse at successive time points, with one frame every 1/35th of a second. The leg at left in each pair of frames was normal, and the leg at right in each pair of images had the iliac artery blocked. The lower overall absorption coefficient is apparent in the leg at right, and the pulsation in the leg at left is more apparent between frames 3, 4, and 5. This pulsation is due to blood flow.

4.5.3 Spread Spectral Encoding by Use of Single Wideband Light Source

Alternately, spectral encoding can be implemented by use of a low-coherence (implying a finite or wide-bandwidth) light source. The spectrum of a wideband light source can be dispersed by optical components, such as a grating, and collimated thereafter to form a one-dimensional spatial spectral distribution (see Color Plate 11). The linear spatial distribution of dispersed spectral components can be coupled to a fiber bundle within which the light delivered to each fiber has a small wavelength offset from the neighboring ones. This configuration gives a spread spectral encoding of the source channels in comparison to the discrete spectral encoding from multiple LDs. In spread spectral encoding, the dimension of the collimated beam strip at the fiber bundle facet plane is determined by

$$L_{FWHM} = 2f \tan(\Delta\beta) \approx \frac{f \cdot \Delta\lambda_{FWHM}}{p\sqrt{1-(\lambda_0/p - \sin\alpha)^2}} \quad (4.31)$$

where f is the focal length of the collimating lens following the grating dispersion, $\Delta\beta$ is the half of the angular dispersion of the low-coherence source by the grating, $\Delta\lambda_{FWHM}$ is the FWHM spectral bandwidth of the source, λ_0 is the center wavelength of the source, p is the grating period, and α is the beam incident angle with respect to the grating normal. For a linear fiber bundle consisting of N fibers aligned side by side, the total spectral band coupled to the fiber bundle is

$$\Delta\lambda_{bundle} = N \cdot \Delta\lambda_{fiber} = N \cdot \frac{d_{fiber}}{L_{FWHM}} \cdot \Delta\lambda_{FWHM} = N \frac{d_{fiber}}{f} p\sqrt{1-(\lambda_0/p - \sin\alpha)^2} \quad (4.32)$$

where $\Delta\lambda_{fiber}$ is the bandwidth coupled to one fiber, and d_{fiber} is the diameter of one fiber. The spread-spectral-encoding operator can be expressed by (4.19) with argument $<\lambda_n>$ being represented by

$$<\lambda_n> = <\lambda_0 + \left[n - \frac{N+1}{2}\right] \cdot \Delta\lambda_{fiber}> \quad (4.33)$$

where the total number of the bundled fibers N is assumed to be even, and the overall spectral band coupled to the fiber bundle is assumed to be centered at λ_0.

The use of a low-coherence source gives a "spread" spectral encoding among the fibers for parallel illumination unto the tissue. A single light source is used to couple to all these channels; therefore, a potential trade-off exists between the number of channels and the power coupled to each channel. On the other hand, the use of a single light source for spread spectral encoding provides several unique characteristics in comparison to the LD-based spectral-encoding approach. First, the wavelength difference between the neighboring channels is generated by the grating dispersion of a single light source; therefore, the spectral encoding coupled to the fibers is always constant, and none of the coupled bands will cross over to the neighboring ones, which may happen in LD based spectral encoding due to spontaneous mode hopping of each individual LD. The spread spectral encoding is thus a shift-free configuration that ensures the decoding of the source-detector signal at all times. Second, the interchannel intensity profile always follows the source power spectrum; therefore, the spontaneous channel-to-channel intensity fluctuation can be minimized compared with LD-based configuration, wherein the intensity of each LD is spontaneously fluctuating. This may lead to substantially confined or reduced uncertainty in reconstruction. Third, the linear fiber bundle used for source coupling can be fabricated with bare or thinly coated fibers, which makes it feasible to arrange the fibers into a circular array inside a small probe for endoscopic interrogation that extends NIR tomography to imaging of internal organs [79]. The implementation of NIR optical tomography to endoscopic mode would have been difficult with conventional methods, including the LD-based spectral-encoding technique, because the separate coupling of each LD to a connector-terminated fiber or light guide is rather bulky, and integrating many channels of such jacketed fibers inside an endoscopic probe is difficult.

4.5.4 Light Sources for Spread Spectral Encoding

There are at least three parameters to consider for the use of a low-coherence or wideband source in spread spectral encoding: (1) the center wavelength, (2) the spectral bandwidth, and (3) the power. A center wavelength around 800 nm is required as NIR tomography operates in the neighborhood of this band. A narrow bandwidth of less than 10 nm is preferred for coupling to the fiber bundle to minimize the wavelength-dependent absorption variation that would occur among the source channels. A high power of tens of milliwatts is needed to provide sufficient illumination to each channel following the segmentation of the light power among fibers by spectral encoding. A number of low-coherence sources are available on the market. Among these sources, the light-emitting diode (LED) can provide hundreds of milliwatts in a narrow bandwidth of several nanometers, but the collimation and coupling of LED emission into a fiber for grating illumination is rather difficult. A white-light source like a tungsten or halogen lamp provides tens of watts across hundreds of nanometers; however, coupling such a source into small fibers is always highly problematic. A fiber-based stimulated-emission-amplifier source may provide high power for low-coherent light illumination; nevertheless, this type of source is mostly centered around 1,300 or 1,550 nm. A pulsed-light source like the femtosecond Ti:sapphire laser is perhaps the most powerful within a narrow bandwidth, but this type of source is still currently quite expensive or bulky, although future generations may be more attractive.

Superluminescent diode (SLD) [or superluminescent LED (SLED)] is a light-emitting diode in which there is stimulated emission with amplification but insufficient feedback for oscillations to build up to achieve lasing action [80]. SLDs have similar geometry to LDs but no built-in optical feedback mechanism as required by an LD to achieve lasing action for amplification of narrow modes. SLDs have structural features similar to the edge-emitting LED (ELED) that suppresses lasing action by reducing the reflectivity of the facets. An SLD is essentially a combination of LD and ELED [81, 82].

An idealized LED emits incoherent spontaneous emission over a wide spectral range into a large solid angle. The unamplified light emerges in one pass from a depth limited by the material absorption. The LED output is unpolarized and increases linearly with input current. An idealized LD emits coherent stimulated emission (and negligible spontaneous emission) over a narrow spectral range and solid angle. The light emerges after many passes over an extended length with intermediate partial mirror reflections. The LD output is usually polarized and increases abruptly at a threshold current that provides just enough stimulated gain to overcome losses along the round-trip path and at the mirrors. In an idealized SLD, however, the spontaneous emission experiences stimulated gain over an extended path and, possibly, one mirror reflection, but no feedback is provided. The output is low coherent compared with an LD due to the spontaneous emission; on the other hand, it is at high power with respect to an LED because of the stimulated gain. The SLD output, which may be polarized, increases superlinearly versus current with a knee occurring when a significant net positive gain is achieved [83].

In the last decade, SLDs at several wavelength options have been implemented extensively in low-coherence interferometry [84–89] and optical coherence tomography techniques [29, 90–93] owing to its relatively high power available on the order of 10 mW and a bandwidth of tens of nanometers that corresponds to a low temporal coherence on the order of 10 μm. The spread-spectral-encoding method presented in this work demonstrates that SLD sources are also applicable to NIR diffuse optical tomography.

4.5.5 Characteristics of Spread Spectral Encoding

4.5.5.1 The Spectral Band and Power Coupled into the Linear Fiber Bundle

Because single source is used, the spectral bandwidth and power coupled to the fibers are associated. Consider an SLD source with a Gaussian spectrum profile of

$$S_0(\lambda) = \frac{2\sqrt{\ln 2/\pi}}{\Delta\lambda_{FWHM}} \exp\left[-4\ln 2\left(\frac{\lambda - \lambda_0}{\Delta\lambda_{FWHM}}\right)^2\right] \quad (4.34)$$

and assume that only the middle portion of the dispersed beam is coupled to the fiber bundle and that the coupled spectrum profile is essentially a Gaussian spectrum truncated on both sides. The percentage of the spectrum power remaining in this truncated Gaussian spectrum with respect to the SLD source power is determined by

$$\frac{P_{bundle}}{P_{source}} = erf\left(\sqrt{\ln 2} \cdot \frac{\Delta\lambda_{bundle}}{\Delta\lambda_{FWHM}}\right) \quad (4.35)$$

where erf is the error function defined as

$$erf(\lambda) = \frac{2}{\sqrt{\pi}} \int_0^\lambda \exp(-x^2)dx \quad (4.36)$$

Equation (4.35) indicates that reducing the bandwidth coupling to the fiber bundle to further minimize the wavelength-dependent absorption among the source channels would cause a major reduction in the total power delivered to the tissue. This, however, can be improved if a source with higher power concentrated at a narrower bandwidth can be employed.

4.5.5.2 The Shift-Free Encoding and Minimized Reconstruction Uncertainty

In the LD-based discrete-spectral-encoding system, the instantaneous wavelength-intensity fluctuation of each channel was independent of the others. In the SLD-based spread-spectral-encoding system, the spectral encoding was from the single source; therefore, the instantaneous intensity change of each coupled channel was always correlated with those of other channels. Moreover, the use of dispersion to create spectral encoding also prevented the coupling profile from wavelength shifting. These two features imply a more stable NIR tomography measurement.

The use of multiple LDs for spectral encoding introduced an average of 1.0% and 1.2% signal intensity fluctuations over 1-minute and 30-minute periods, respectively [39]. The average wavelength shift observed for the LD-based system in a well-controlled situation was 0.027 and 0.21 nm over 1- and 30-minute periods, respectively. The long-term wavelength shift over the course of 30 minutes is greater than the spectrometer resolution of 0.1 nm, and a 1.2% standard deviation in the intensity fluctuation over this period introduced a 4.8% standard deviation in the reconstructed absorption coefficient value over the time. Quantitative measurements similar to those for an LD-based discrete-spectral-encoding system have been conducted for an SLD-based spread-spectral-encoding system. It is found that the short-term and long-term wavelength shifts of the SLD-based system were on the order of 0.02 nm, or about one-fifth of the spectrometer resolution. This subresolution shift more likely resulted from the digitization of the signal rather than the occurrence of actual wavelength shift. Compared with the LD-based system where the long-term wavelength shift was substantially higher than the short-term shift, there is no meaningful difference between the long-term and short-term wavelength shifts in this SLD-based measurement. This validates that the use of a single wideband source via dispersion provides virtually shift-free spectral encoding among the channels. The interchannel intensity fluctuation of this system was less than, yet close to, that of the LD-based system. The variation of the reconstructed μ_a value in the 300 frames acquired in 30 minutes is calculated. Compared with the similar experiments in the LD-based system, however, the measurement is less clustered, and the uncertainty of the μ_a value was 1.49% standard deviation, a value less than one-third of that observed in the LD-based system. Considering that the intensity fluctuation was a perturbation to the image reconstruction, the uncertainty of reconstructed μ_a values appears to be an amplification of the data uncertainty. In the LD-based system, the 1.2% perturbation caused a fourfold amplification of 4.8% in the reconstructed absorption coefficient value, whereas in this SLD-based system, the 0.86% perturbation ended up with only 1.49% of uncertainty in reconstruction, an amplification factor less than 2. The significantly reduced amplification of the intensity fluctuation in the SLD-based system implies that the intensity fluctuation in this configuration might be due to the measurement noise rather than any systematic factor and validates the notion that a more accurate and stable measurement could be made. The relatively small 1.49% reconstruction standard deviation of this rapid NIR tomography system constructed based on a single wideband source indicated that there was good likelihood of discerning subtle and rapid absorption variations in biological tissues.

4.5.6 Hemodynamic Imaging by Spread-Spectral-Encoding NIR Tomography

A 5 Hz frame-rate NIR DOT system based on the spread spectral encoding of a single SLD source was constructed at Oklahoma State University. The typical resting heart rate (HR) of an adult is between about 60 and 100 beats per minute (bpm); therefore, the 5 Hz NIR tomography should be sufficient for measuring the absorption changes when induced by normal heart rate pulsation in the capillaries, as measured by pulse oximetry. An example is given in Figure 4.9 to evaluate the feasibility of imaging hemodynamic responses with this system. A male volunteer with resting HR of 72 bpm was imaged. The volunteer positioned his little finger against the lower-left surface of the imaging array and practiced voluntary breath holding, starting from when the image acquisition begun, to provide a hemoglobin variation signal that was not contaminated by breathing variation and motion artifact. A total of 50 frames were acquired in 10 seconds. One frame of the reconstructed image is

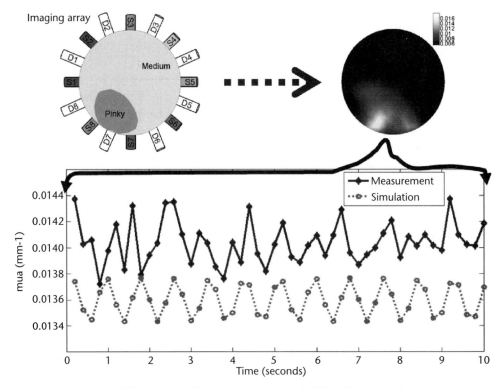

Figure 4.9 Imaging of finger during 10 seconds of breath holding. The curve shows near-periodic variation of the global absorption value of the finger, and it is correlated to the heart rate of the subject. The global absorption variation is 5.0% at the beginning of the acquisition and reduces to 2.9% at the end of the 10 second imaging period.

displayed. The cross section of the imaged finger was approximately 13 mm, which corresponds well with the higher absorption area in the image. In order to assess the time-resolved absorption changes of the finger, the absorption coefficients within 15% difference from the peak value were averaged for each frame. The global absorption changes in 50 frames of acquisition were compared with a simple simulated response by assuming 12 pulsations in 10 seconds. The simulation curve was placed under the curve of measurement to assess if there was a periodic variation of the responses; therefore, the absolute value of the simulated curve is chosen arbitrarily. It is interesting to notice that the variance of the global absorption values follows the simulated periodic pattern quite well except for the jittering between about 1 and 2 seconds. The mean value of the global absorption coefficient was 0.014 mm^{-1}, which is close to the expected value for human tissue [94]. The variance of the global absorption coefficient at the beginning of the breath holding was 5.0% and reduced gradually to 2.9% during the 10 seconds of breath holding. Both are above the measured system reconstruction uncertainly of 1.5%.

4.6 Novel Approaches in Instrumentation of Diffuse Optical Tomography: Transrectal Applicator

Near-infrared DOT has been shown to be particularly useful over the past decades for functional imaging of biological tissues where scattering of the photons dominates and where NIR contrast based on intrinsic chromophore content or exogenous probe can be linked to tissue physiology such as angiogenesis, oxygen deprivation, or overexpression of specific biomarkers. Despite the considerably promising outcome of NIR optical tomography in the diagnosis of breast cancer, the understanding of cortex response [11], and the characterization of rheumatologic dysfunction [95–97], where all the tissues under imaging are interrogated externally by noninvasive methods, there is limited information regarding the practice of NIR tomography in internal imaging regimes. Since similar physiological conditions may be found valuable for diagnostics in internal organs, an extension of DOT to imaging internally applicable tissue/organs becomes imperative. Interstitial measurement by use of diffuse or near-diffuse photons has been employed for monitoring photodynamic responses in organs such as the prostate [98]. From the diagnostic perspective, the most appealing feature of NIR tomography may arguably be its unique functional contrast that is obtained noninvasively. It is thereby not surprising to see that significant interest has developed recently in understanding the challenges and benefits of noninvasive NIR optical tomography of internal organs, particularly imaging the prostate [99, 100].

There is evidence that prostate cancer development is associated with angiogenesis [101], and NIR imaging may provide noninvasive assessment of prostate cancer. Noninvasive prostate imaging by optical means will enable the study of prostate optical properties and augment current diagnostics if the optical properties of prostate cancer are found to have substantial contrast with respect to those of normal prostate tissues. In this section, the instrumentation involved in developing an internal or endoscopic applicator array for DOT of the prostate or potentially other internal organs is presented.

4.6.1 Transrectal Applicator for Transverse DOT Imaging

Although the principle of near-infrared tomography of internal organs, specifically the prostate, is similar to that of breast, noninvasive internal DOT imaging faces unique challenges. In NIR optical tomography of breast, either planar-shaped or ring-type applicators of minimum restriction in size can be applied at either reflection or transmission geometry. In prostate imaging, there is only limited space inside the rectum for transrectal probing of deep tissue volumes. Special consideration must be incorporated into the design of the internal applicator. Figure 4.10 shows the schematic diagram of the first approach to the internal transverse (axial) imaging NIR probe. It utilizes the above-mentioned spread spectral encoding, where the spectrum of a broadband source is dispersed and coupled to a linear fiber bundle. The linear fiber bundle coupling the source light is rearranged to circular geometry at the distal end of the endoscope probe, and a conic lens is used to deflect the light circumferentially. The detector fibers are cocentric to and interspersed with the source fibers, and the proximal end of the detector fiber is linearly aligned to adapt to the spectrometer entrance slit. This outward-imaging geometry gave the first DOT image that is in endoscopic view [79].

Figure 4.11 shows a transverse-imaging NIR probe having a 20-mm diameter. This probe consists of 16 fibers of 1.0 mm in core diameter evenly spaced with interspersing source and detector channels. Each fiber is parallel to the longitudinal axis of the probe and is aligned to a 45° rod lens 2 mm in diameter. The beam is deflected transversely for side firing. A 2 mm drum lens is then used to provide a sealed optical

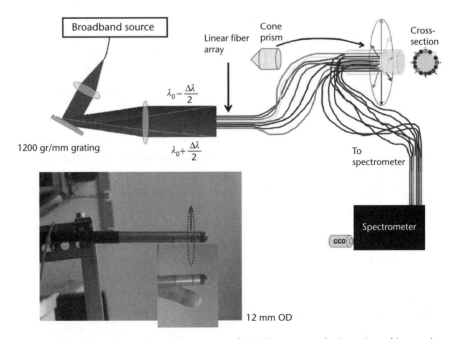

Figure 4.10 The first endoscopic applicator array for NIR tomography imaging of internal organs. A direct comparison with Figure 4.8 shows that the fiber bundle consisting of bare fibers can be integrated into a circular array inside the endoscopic probe. Circumferential illumination and detection is done by using a conic lens. The inset is the photograph of a 12 mm diameter endosocpic NIR tomography probe having eight source channels and eight detector channels.

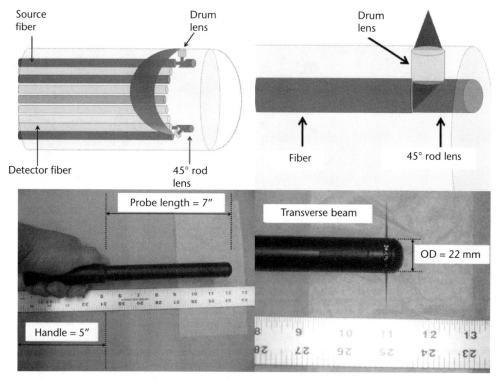

Figure 4.11 The transverse-imaging transrectal NIR tomography probe of 20 mm diameter. Each source/detector channel consists of a 1 mm fiber; a 2 mm, 45° rod lens; and a 2 mm drum lens. The light beam is delivered and focused transversely. Photograph of the probe shows the dimensions of 20 mm in diameter, 7" in probing length, 5" handle, and the two fiber bundles 3m long for source and detector coupling.

aperture for illumination as well as beam focusing. All eight source and eight detector channels have used the same light-delivering configuration. The eight source fibers and eight detector fibers are aligned to form a linear source fiber bundle and detector fiber bundle. The illumination light is coupled to the source fiber bundle by the spread-spectral-encoding technique, and the detector fiber bundle is adapted to the spectrometer for acquisition of NIR surface-measurement data.

The internal-application NIR tomography images taken by this 20 mm transverse-imaging NIR probe are given in Figure 4.12. The imaging geometry is now opposite to what is done for most NIR imaging of breast, as the optodes are distributed noninvasively and internally to the tissue volume. We incorporated the outward imaging finite-element mesh as shown to reconstruct the NIR tomography images. The annular image is taken from a highly absorptive phantom over an intralipid background medium by use of the 20 mm transverse-imaging probe. The semiannular image was taken from a sample of avian rectum tissue with injected NIR absorption contrast by use of the 12 mm transverse-imaging NIR probe shown in Figure 4.10. Both sets of images demonstrate that NIR contrast of heterogeneous targets can be acquired successfully by these probes at internal-imaging geometry.

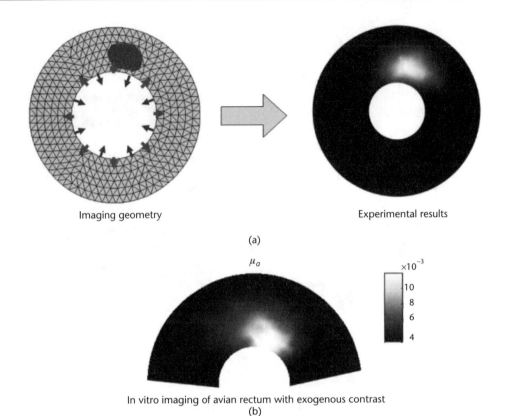

Figure 4.12 The transverse-imaging examples by transrectal NIR probe. (a) The top row demonstrates the relative positions of optodes in the imaging volume as well as the reconstructed images of a contrast occlusion embedded in background Intralipid medium. (b) The bottom image was taken by transrectal imaging of an avian rectum sample with connecting tissues, where the contrast was from a small amount of diluted ink to introduce exogenous contrast to the homogenous rectal tissue.

4.6.2 Transrectal Applicator for Sagittal DOT Imaging

We have lately developed a sagittal-imaging NIR probe to attach to a commercial biplane TRUS transducer for multimodality imaging [102]. The NIR applicator can perform stand-alone DOT imaging or utilize the spatial prior information from ultrasound. The design, dimension, and completed probe are detailed in Figure 4.13. This probe is capable of acquiring sagittal NIR images concurrently with TRUS. The source/detector channels are placed at 1 cm separation, and the source array is placed 2 cm from the detector array. The array dimension of 60×20 mm is designed to couple to the 60×10 mm TRUS transducer performing sagittal imaging at the middle plane of the NIR array.

4.6.2.1 Simulation for the Sagittal Transrectal DOT Applicator

Simulations for the sagittal NIR probe are given in Figure 4.14 for a 10 mm diameter inclusion located at middle plane and 5 mm longitudinal shift from the center of the probe. The transrectal NIR probe is placed at the bottom of the imaging volume,

4.6 Novel Approaches in Instrumentation of Diffuse Optical Tomography: Transrectal Applicator

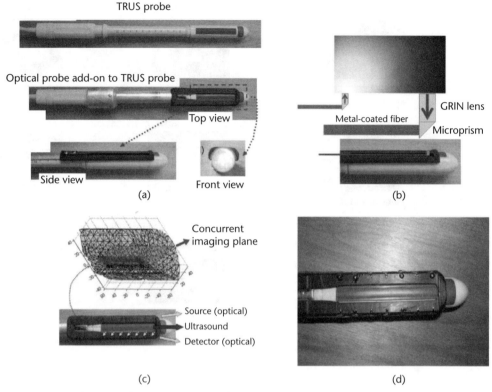

Figure 4.13 The sagittal-imaging transrectal NIR tomography probe for coupling with TRUS. (a) The overall assembly of transrectal NIR attached to TRUS is shown. (b) The probe has one source array and one detector array, each having seven channels. Each channel consists of a 600 μm metal-coated fiber coupled to a 1 mm coated microprism for 90° deflection and a 1 mm gradient-index (GRIN) lens for coupling to and from the tissue surface. (c) The NIR imaging reconstruction is taken at the middle sagittal plane of source and detector arrays, which falls identically with the sagittal TRUS. (d) Photograph of completed transrectal NIR probe attached to TRUS is shown.

and the depth is counted upward. Homogenous background is set at $\mu_a = 0.002$ mm^{-1}, $\mu'_s = 0.8$ mm^{-1}, and the target has $\mu_a = 0.025$ mm^{-1}, $\mu'_s = 1.0$ mm^{-1}. A noise level of 1% has been added to the forward calculation.

The NIR-only reconstruction (uniform mesh density throughout the imaging volume) is conducted for the target at depths of 1, 2, and 3 cm. The second row of Figure 4.14 shows that the target is reconstructed accurately for 1 cm depth and closer to the probe surface for 2 cm depth. This is expected due to the sensitivity that degrades along with the depth. The third row of Figure 4.14 gives the images reconstructed with spatial prior information, which is available from TRUS, using a denser mesh in the target location and at a size double that of the target [103]. The images reconstructed with this guided-reconstruction approach locate the lesion correctly. The accuracy of recovering lesions in the longitudinal dimension is given in Figure 4.15 for a lesion of 2 cm depth that is placed at 2, 4, and 6 cm in axial dimension. Their positions are correctly reconstructed.

90   Diffuse Optical Techniques: Instrumentation

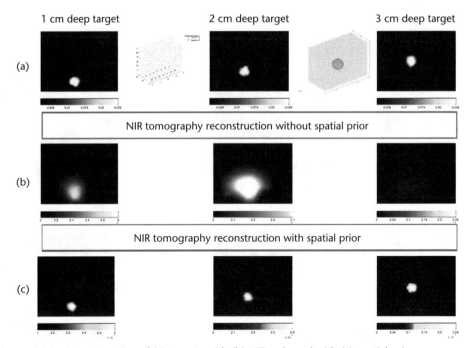

Figure 4.14 Reconstruction of (a) targets with (b) NIR only and with (c) spatial prior.

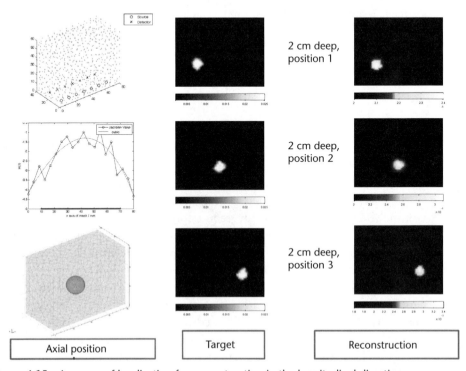

Figure 4.15 Accuracy of localization for reconstruction in the longitudinal direction.

4.6.2.2 Experimental Results of the Sagittal Transrectal DOT Applicator

Figure 4.16 gives the images reconstructed from experimental data for a highly absorbing cylindrical occlusion positioned at the left side, middle, and right side. The bottom of the cylinder is roughly 7 mm away from the probe surface, giving a 15-mm depth of the occlusion. The left column is reconstructed with NIR information only, and the right column is reconstructed by knowing the location and approximate size of the occlusion as the hard spatial prior. The images reconstructed with a priori information show the occlusion closer to true positions. The image for the occlusion at the right end of the probe is quite interesting, where the two-blob artifact shown for NIR-only image reconstruction is corrected when the reconstruction is guided by prior information.

Color Plate 12 presents the images reconstructed from experimental data using avian breast tissue as the background medium and an inclusion. The inclusion is a cylinder 15 mm in diameter and 15 mm in height made of black plastic material to simulate an absorption target. The TRUS image obtained in Color Plate 12(a) has a field of view of 50×50 cm. Using the information of target location and approximate size, dual-mesh NIR tomography reconstruction is performed with a sagittal field of view of 80×60 cm, where the size of denser mesh for the target doubles the approximate size of the target shown on TRUS. The reconstructed sagittal NIR image is displayed at a field of view of 60×30 cm, and the active US transducer of 5 cm long is indicated underneath for comparison. The NIR image with TRUS guidance clearly reconstructs the target identified by TRUS. In Color Plate 12(b), no inclusion is embedded in the avian breast medium; yet, the dual-mesh identical to

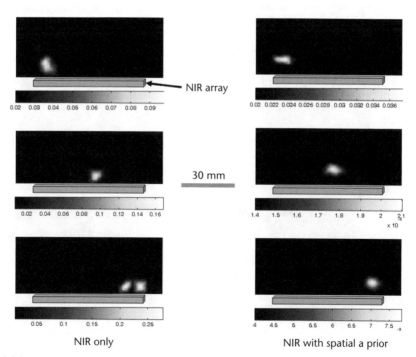

Figure 4.16 Image reconstructed from experimental data without and with a priori location information.

that in Color Plate 12(a) is used. The reconstructed NIR image does not show a target in the denser mesh region, which demonstrates that NIR measurement of the target amid the background medium is reliable. In Color Plate 12(c), the target is shifted longitudinally, and in Color Plate 12(d), the target is moved approximately 5 mm deeper. In both cases, the NIR image reconstruction resolves the target.

Figure 4.17 presents a very interesting result. In the left column, the background medium is avian breast only; therefore, a homogenous mesh is used for NIR image reconstruction since there is no spatial prior information for any target available from TRUS. The reconstructed NIR image does not show a target. In the right column, a cube of avian breast tissue was immerged in absorbing solution (diluted ink) for 20 minutes and then embedded in the middle of the tissue at a depth of approximately 1.5 cm. The TRUS image does not identify a target in the manipulated region. NIR reconstruction is again performed by use of homogenous mesh, assuming that no spatial prior from TRUS is available. The target shows up in NIR image at the correct longitudinal position but shallower depth. The shallower depth is caused by the reduced sensitivity along the depth as indicated previously when only NIR information is used for reconstruction. This example demonstrates that transrectal NIR is capable of detecting target that is nonsensitive to TRUS. The clinical outcome of integrating transrectal NIR and TRUS is mainly directed at providing optical contrast for the lesions that are suspicious to US; nevertheless, this example proved that transrectal NIR tomography could localize lesions to which US is blind. This is potentially very important for biopsy guidance and diagnostics since

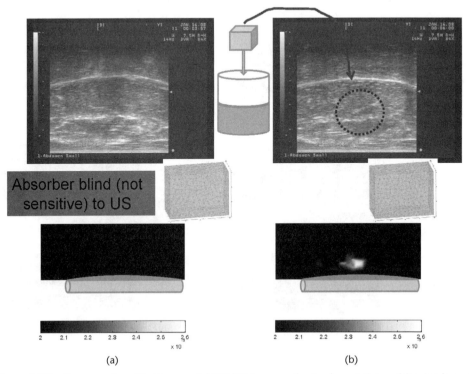

Figure 4.17 Concurrent sagittal transrectal NIR/US images of avian breast tissue: (a) avian breast tissue only, and (b) a cube of avian breast immerged in diluted ink for approximately 20 minutes, then embedded in the medium. The absorptive surface of the tissue cube is insensitive to US. NIR image reconstruction without prior information located the target.

a malignant lesion that may be missed by TRUS could be identified by transrectal NIR.

4.7 Potential Directions of Instrumentation for Diffuse Optical Measurements

The advancement of biomedical-oriented optical imaging technology, including diffuse optical techniques, is dependent largely upon the progresses in photonics instruments, including a variety of coherent, low-coherent, or incoherent light sources and high-speed, high-sensitivity, high-dynamic range detectors. Meanwhile, the special need of optical imaging application, such as optical coherence tomography, has been a driving force behind some important advancement in photonic devices. It is certain that novel applications and advancements in optical imaging and optical instrumentation will foster each other over a long period of time.

The applicator array for external imaging in DOT has evolved from rigid single modality to flexible modality [11], from rigid multimodality [62] to adaptive multimodality [74]. Recently, the applicator array for internal imaging has evolved from rigid single modality [100] to rigid multimodality for prostate imaging [102]. If there comes the demand of applying DOT techniques to internal organs other than the prostate, flexible internal applicator array may be necessary for single-modality or multimodality imaging.

So far, the varieties of sources used for diffuse optical imaging include noncoherent source like tungsten light [51], coherent source like laser diode [62], and low-coherent sources like superluminiscenet diode and the mode-locked Ti:sapphire laser [79]. The mode-locked pulsed-laser source is particularly interesting for DOT. First, it may be used for time-domain measurement by taking advantage of its short pulse operation. Second, it has been used in spread-spectral-encoding-based DOT systems for its low coherence or wideband feature. Third, it may also be used in frequency-domain measurement if the repetition timing can serve as the modulation base frequency. Other light sources like swept laser have found exciting applications in OCT [104], and it is anticipated that swept source may find novel application in DOT if the wavelength band is appropriate.

Applying DOT to noninvasive imaging of internal organs presents unprecedented benefits and challenges. For external imaging of DOT, no matter whether for breast, brain, or joints, there isn't much limitation for placing the bulky source and detector fibers, except for some multimodality imaging requirements. Internal imaging in small spaces is, however, different. A small-diameter fiber, such as a single-mode fiber, is sufficient for delivering tens of milliwatts of light power to the tissue for a point-source illumination. For detection, however, even though the orientation of the fiber is not important, the dimension of the fiber detection aperture is critical for collecting sufficient photons. If the small-diameter fiber needs to be implemented, it is likely that the fiber tip will need microoptics to improve the total detection power. Another option may be to fabricate microphotosensors directly to the applicator if the interference of electrical signals can be resolved. Direct multimodality sensing on the applicator may also be performed if a monolithic multimodality sensor/detector can be engineered.

4.8 Conclusions

The diffuse optical technique is continuously evolving as a viable biomedical imaging modality owing to its unique spectroscopic functional contrast. Near-infrared light probes tissue absorption as well as scattering properties by means of diffuse photon measurement. Although the spatial resolution of diffuse optical detection is limited due to indefinite photon path when compared with other imaging modalities such as MRI and CT, DOT provides access to a variety of physiological parameters that are otherwise not accessible [9]. Other appealing features of DOT include noninvasive or minimally invasive imaging; nonionizing radiation, eliminating the concern of repeated dose; and compactness, relatively low cost, and appropriateness for continuous use in office or at the bedside [9]. The exciting applications of DOT in diagnostics over the past decades have been led by several key advancements in instrumentation techniques that are briefly reviewed in this chapter. The emerging interest in DOT for coupling with other diagnostic modalities as well as application to different organ levels presents new challenges for DOT instrumentation principles as well as device techniques.

Acknowledgments

This work has been supported in part by the Prostate Cancer Research Program of the U.S. Army Medical Research Acquisition Activity (USAMRAA), 820 Chandler Street, Fort Detrick, MD, 21702-5014, through grant W81XWH-07-1-0247, and the Health Research Program of the Oklahoma Center for the Advancement of Science and Technology (OCAST) through grant HR06-171. The content of the information does not necessarily reflect the position or policy of the USAMRAA or OCAST, and no official endorsement should be inferred.

The graduate students who contributed to this work include Zhen Jiang, Guan Xu, Cameron H. Musgrove, and Hao Xie. I acknowledge collaborations with Drs. Charles F. Bunting, Jerzy S. Kransiski, and Weili Zhang in my department. Drs. Kenneth E. Bartels, Jerry Ritchey, and G. Reed Holyoak from Oklahoma State University Vet-Med College, Dr. Gennady Slobodov of the University of Oklahoma Health Sciences Center, and Dr. Sreenivas Vemulapalli of Tri-Valley Urology are acknowledged for their suggestions. Finally, this work would not have been possible without the encouragement of many experts in the DOT field, including Drs. Brian W. Pogue, Quing Zhu, and Bruce J. Tromberg.

References

[1] Yodh, A. G., and B. Chance, "Spectroscopy and imaging with diffusing light," *Phys. Today* 48(3) (1995): 34–40.

[2] Benaron, D. A., G. Müller, and B. Chance, "Medical perspective at the threshold of clinical optical tomography," in G. Müller, et al., (eds.), *Medial Optical Tomography: Functional Imaging and Monitoring*, 3–9, Bellingham, WA: SPIE—International Society for Optical Engineering, 1993.

[3] Tromberg, B., A. Yodh, E. Sevick, and D. Pine, "Diffusing photons in turbid media: introduction to the feature," *Appl. Opt.* 36(1) (1997): 9–9.

[4] Boas, D. A., et al., "Imaging the body with diffuse optical tomography," *IEEE Sign. Process. Mag.* 18(6) (2001): 57–85.

[5] Miller, E., "Focus issue: diffuse optical tomography—introduction," *Opt. Exp.* 7(13) (2000): 461–461.

[6] Pogue, B. W., et al., "Image analysis methods for diffuse optical tomography," *J. Biomed. Opt.* 11(3) (2006): 033001.

[7] Gibson, A. P., J. C. Hebden, and S. R. Arridge, "Recent advances in diffuse optical imaging," *Phys. Med. Biol.* 50(4) (2005): R1–R43.

[8] Hielscher, A. H., "Optical tomographic imaging of small animals," *Curr. Opin. Biotechnol.* 16(1) (2005): 79–88.

[9] Hielscher, A. H., et al., "Near-infrared diffuse optical tomography," *Dis. Mark.* 18, Nos. 5–6 (2002): 313–337.

[10] Ntziachristos, V., and B. Chance, "Probing physiology and molecular function using optical imaging: applications to breast cancer," *Breast Canc. Res.* 3(1) (2001): 41–46.

[11] Hillman, E. M., "Optical brain imaging in vivo: techniques and applications from animal to man," *J. Biomed. Opt.* 12(5) (2007): 051402.

[12] Hebden, J. C., and T. Austin, "Optical tomography of the neonatal brain," *Eur. Radiol.* 17(11) (2007): 2926–2933.

[13] Zhang, X., V. Toronov, and A. Webb, "Spatial and temporal hemodynamic study of human primary visual cortex using simultaneous functional MRI and diffuse optical tomography," *Proc. 27th Ann. Conf. IEEE Eng. Med. Biol. Soc.*, Shanghai, China, September 1–4, 2005, 727–730.

[14] Wang, X., et al., "Imaging of joints with laser-based photoacoustic tomography: an animal study," *Med. Phys.* 33(8) (2006): 2691–2697.

[15] Srinivasan, S., et al., "In vivo hemoglobin and water concentrations, oxygen saturation, and scattering estimates from near-infrared breast tomography using spectral reconstruction," *Acad. Radiol.* 13(2) (2006): 195–202.

[16] Diamond, S. G., et al., "Dynamic physiological modeling for functional diffuse optical tomography," *NeuroImage* 30(1) (2006): 88–101.

[17] Rinneberg, H., et al., "Scanning time-domain optical mammography: detection and characterization of breast tumors in vivo," *Technol. Canc. Res. Treat.* 4(5) (2005): 483–496.

[18] Zhao, H., et al., "Time-resolved diffuse optical tomographic imaging for the provision of both anatomical and functional information about biological tissue," *Appl. Opt.* 44(10) (2005): 1905–1916.

[19] Taga, G., et al., "Brain imaging in awake infants by near-infrared optical topography," *Proc. Natl. Acad. Sci. USA* 100(19) (2003): 10722–10727.

[20] Durduran, T., et al., "Bulk optical properties of healthy female breast tissue," *Phys. Med. Biol.* 47(16) (2002): 2847–2861.

[21] Barbour, R. L., et al., "Optical tomographic imaging of dynamic features of dense-scattering media," *J. Opt. Soc. Am. A* 18(12) (2001): 3018–3036.

[22] Hintz, S. R., et al., "Bedside functional imaging of the premature infant brain during passive motor activation," *J. Perinat. Med.* 29(4) (2001): 335–343.

[23] Boas, D. A., et al., "The accuracy of near infrared spectroscopy and imaging during focal changes in cerebral hemodynamics," *NeuroImage* 13(1) (2001): 76–90.

[24] Van Houten, J. P., D. A. Benaron, S. Spilman, and D. K. Stevenson, "Imaging brain injury using time-resolved near infrared light scanning," *Pediat. Res.* 39(3) (1996): 470–476.

[25] Srinivasan, S., et al., "Interpreting hemoglobin and water concentration, oxygen saturation, and scattering measured in vivo by near-infrared breast tomography," *Proc. Natl. Acad. Sci. USA* 100(21) (2003): 12349–12354.

[26] Heffer, E., et al., "Near-infrared imaging of the human breast: complementing hemoglobin concentration maps with oxygenation images," *J. Biomed. Opt.* 9(6) (2004): 1152–1160.

[27] Zhu, Q., S. Tannenbaum, and S. H. Kurtzman, "Optical tomography with ultrasound localization for breast cancer diagnosis and treatment monitoring," *Surg. Oncol. Clin. N. Am.* 16(2) (2007): 307–321.

[28] Rolfe, P., "In vivo near-infrared spectroscopy," *Ann. Rev. Biomed. Eng.* 2 (2000): 715–754.

[29] Huang, D., et al., "Optical coherence tomography," *Science* 254(5035) (1991): 1178–1181.

[30] Kim, Y. L., et al., "Low-coherence enhanced backscattering: review of principles and applications for colon cancer screening," *J. Biomed. Opt.* 11(4) (2006): 0411250.

[31] Yodh, A. G., and D. A. Boas, "Functional imaging with diffusing light," in T. Vo-Dinh (ed.), *Biomedical Photonics Handbook*, Ch. 21, Boca Raton, FL: CRC Press, 2003.

[32] Schmitz, C. H., et al., "Instrumentation for fast functional optical tomography," *Rev. Sci. Instr.* 73(2) (2002): 429–439.

[33] Nissilä, I., et al., "Instrumentation and calibration methods for the multichannel measurement of phase and amplitude in optical tomography," *Rev. Sci. Instr.* 76(4) (2005): 044302–044302-10.

[34] Fantini, S., et al., "Frequency-domain optical mammography: edge effects correction," *Med. Phys.* 23(1) (1996): 149–157.

[35] Franceschini, M. A., et al., "Frequency-domain techniques enhance optical mammography: initial clinical results," *Proc. Natl. Acad. Sci. USA* 94(12) (1997): 6468–6473.

[36] Siegel, A. M., J. J. A. Marota, and D. A. Boas, "Design and evaluation of a continuous-wave diffuse optical tomography system," *Opt. Exp.* 4(8) (1999): 287–298.

[37] Cerussi, A. E., and B. J. Tromberg, "Photon migration spectroscopy frequency-domain techniques," in T. Vo-Dinh (ed.), *Biomedical Photonics Handbook*, Ch. 22, Boca Raton, FL: CRC Press, 2003.

[38] Piao, D., et al., "Video-Rate Near-Infrared Optical Tomography Using Spectrally Encoded Parallel Light Delivery," *Opt. Lett.* 30(19) (2005): 2593–2595.

[39] Piao, D., et al., "Instrumentation for video-rate near-infrared diffuse optical tomography," *Rev. Sci. Instr.* 76(12) (2005): 124301–124301-13.

[40] Hillman, E. M. C., *Experimental and Theoretical Investigations of Near-Infrared Tomographic Imaging Methods and Clinical Applications*, Ph.D. Dissertation, University College London, UK, 2002, 15–26.

[41] Patterson, M. S., B. Chance, and B. C. Wilson, "Time resolved reflectance and transmittance for the noninvasive measurement of tissue optical properties," *Appl. Opt.* 28(12) (1989): 2331–2336.

[42] Grosenick, D., et al., "Development of a time-domain optical mammograph and first in vivo applications," *Appl. Opt.* 38(13) (1999): 2927–2943.

[43] Hawrysz, D. J., and E. M. Sevick-Muraca, "Developments toward diagnostic breast cancer imaging using near-infrared optical measurements and fluorescent contrast agents," *Neoplasia* 2(5) (2000): 388–417.

[44] Fantini, S., and M. A. Franceschini, "Frequency-domain techniques for tissue spectroscopy and imaging," in V. T. Tuchin (ed.), *Handbook of Optical Biomedical Diagnostics*, 405–453, Bellingham, WA: SPIE Press, 2002.

[45] Pogue, B. W., et al., "Instrumentation and design of a frequency-domain diffuse optical tomography imager for breast cancer detection," *Opt. Exp.* 1(13) (1997): 391–403.

[46] Fantini, S., M. A. Franceschini, and E. Gratton, "Semi-infinite geometry boundary problem for light migration in highly scattering media: a frequency-domain study in the diffusion approximation," *J. Opt. Soc. Am. B* 11(10) (1994): 2128–2138.

[47] Intes, X., et al., "In Vivo Continuous-Wave Optical Breast Imaging Enhanced with Indocyanine Green," *Med. Phys.* 30(6) (2003): 1039–1047.

[48] Su, J., H. Shan, H. Liu, and M. V. Klibanov, "Reconstruction method with data from a multiple-site continuous-wave source for three-dimensional optical tomography," *J. Opt. Soc. Am. A* 23(10) (2006): 2388–2395.

[49] Corlu, A., et al., "Uniqueness and wavelength optimization in continuous-wave multispectral diffuse optical tomography," *Opt. Lett.* 28(23) (2003): 2339–2341.

[50] Jiang, H., Y. Xu, and N. Iftimia, "Experimental three-dimensional optical image reconstruction of heterogeneous turbid media from continuous-wave data," *Opt. Exp.* 7(5) (2000): 204–209.

[51] Xu, H., *MRI-Coupled Broadband Near-Infrared Tomography for Small Animal Brain Studies*, Ph.D. Dissertation, Dartmouth College, Hanover, NH, 2005, 36–36.

[52] Walker, S. A., S. Fantini, and E. Gratton, "Image reconstruction using back-projection from frequency-domain optical measurements in highly scattering media," *Appl. Opt.* 36(1) (1997): 170–179.

[53] Arridge, S. R., and M. A. Schweiger, "A Gradient-Based Optimisation Scheme for Optical Tomography," *Opt. Exp.* 2(6) (1998): 213–226.

[54] Saquib, S. S., K. M. Hanson, and G. S. Cunningham, "Model-Based Image Reconstruction from Time-Resolved Diffusion Data," *Proc. SPIE* 3034 (1997): 369–380.

[55] Hielscher, A. H., A. D. Klose, and K. M. Hanson, "Gradient-based iterative image reconstruction scheme for time resolved optical tomography," *IEEE Trans. Med. Imag.* 18(3) (1999): 262–271.

[56] Brooksby, B., et al., "Combining near infrared tomography and magnetic resonance imaging to study in vivo breast tissue: implementation of a Laplacian-type regularization to incorporate magnetic resonance structure," *J. Biomed. Opt.* 10(5) (2005): 051504.

[57] Arridge, S. R., and M. Schweiger, "Sensitivity to prior knowledge in optical tomographic reconstruction," *Proc. SPIE* 2389 (1995): 378–388.

[58] Brooksby, B., et al., "Magnetic resonance-guided near-infrared tomography of the breast," *Rev. Sci. Instr.* 75(12) (2004): 5262–5270.

[59] Ntziachristos, V., X. H. Ma, and B. Chance, "Time-correlated single photon counting imager for simultaneous magnetic resonance and near-infrared mammography," *Rev. Sci. Instr.* 69(12) (1998): 4221–4233.

[60] Dehghani, H., et al., "Three-dimensional optical tomography: resolution in small object imaging," *Appl. Opt.* 42(16) (2003): 3117–3128.

[61] Dehghani, H., et al., "Structural a Priori Information in Near-Infrared Optical Tomography," *Proc. SPIE* 6431 (2007): 64310B.

[62] Zhu, Q., "Optical tomography with ultrasound localization: initial clinical results and technical challenges," *Technol. Canc. Res. Treat.* 4(3) (2005): 235–244.

[63] Ntziachristos, V., A. G. Yodh, M. Schnall, and B. Chance, "Concurrent MRI and diffuse optical tomography of breast after indocyanine green enhancement," *Proc. Natl. Acad. Sci. USA* 97(6) (2000): 2767–2772.

[64] Gulsen, G., et al., "Congruent MRI and near-infrared spectroscopy for functional and structural imaging of tumors," *Technol. Canc. Res. Treat.* 1(6) (2002): 497–505.

[65] Strangman, G., J. P. Culver, J. H. Thompson, and D. A. Boas, "A quantitative comparison of simultaneous BOLD fMRI and NIRS recordings during functional brain activation," *NeuroImage* 17(2) (2002): 719–731.

[66] Li, A., et al., "Reconstructing chromosphere concentration images directly by continuous-wave diffuse optical tomography," *Opt. Lett.* 29(3) (2004): 256–258.

[67] Brooksby, B., et al., "Spectral priors improve near-infrared diffuse tomography more than spatial priors," *Opt. Lett.* 30(15) (2005): 1968–1970.

[68] Corlu, A., et al., "Diffuse optical tomography with spectral constraints and wavelength optimization," *Appl. Opt.* 44(11) (2005): 2082–2093.

[69] Zhu, Q., S. Tannenbaum, and S. H. Kurtzman, "Optical Tomography with ultrasound localization for breast cancer diagnosis and treatment monitoring," *Surg. Oncol. Clin. N. Am.* 16(2) (2007): 307–321.

[70] Zhu, Q., et al., "Benign versus malignant breast masses: optical differentiation with US-guided optical imaging reconstruction," *Radiology* 237(1) (2005): 57–66.

[71] Zhu. Q., et al., "Utilizing optical tomography with ultrasound localization to image heterogeneous hemoglobin distribution in large breast cancers," *Neoplasia* 7(3) (2005): 263–270.

[72] Holboke, M. J., et al., "Three-dimensional diffuse optical mammography with ultrasound localization in a human subject," *J. Biomed. Opt.* 5(2) (2000): 237–247.

[73] Zhu, Q., et al., "Ultrasound-guided optical tomographic imaging of malignant and benign breast lesions," *Neoplasia* 5(5) (2003): 379–388.

[74] Brooksby, B., et al., "Imaging breast adipose and fibroglandular tissue molecular signatures by using hybrid MRI-guided near-infrared spectral tomography," *Proc. Natl. Acad. Sci. USA* 103(23) (2006): 8828–8833.

[75] Shah, N., et al., "Combined diffuse optical spectroscopy and contrast-enhanced magnetic resonance imaging for monitoring breast cancer neoadjuvant chemotherapy: a case study," *J. Biomed. Opt.* 10(5) (2005): 051503.

[76] Huppert, T. J., et al., "Quantitative spatial comparison of diffuse optical imaging with blood oxygen level–dependent and arterial spin labeling–based functional magnetic resonance imaging," *J. Biomed. Opt.* 11(6) (2006): 064018.

[77] Kondow, M., T. Kitatani, K. Nakahara, and T. Tanaka, "Temperature dependence of lasing wavelength in a GaInNAs laser diode," *IEEE Photon. Technol. Lett.* 12(7) (2000): 777–779.

[78] Pogue, B. W., D. Piao, H. Dehghani, and K. D. Paulsen, "Demonstration of video-rate diffuse optical tomography in phantoms and tissues," *Proc. 2006 IEEE Int. Symp. Biomed. Imag.*, Arlington, VA, April 6–9, 2006, 1196–1199.

[79] Piao, D., et al., "Endoscopic, rapid near-infrared optical tomography," *Opt. Lett.* 31(19) (2006): 2876–2878.

[80] Shidlovski, V., "Superluminescent diodes: short overview of device operation principles and performance parameters," 2004, http://www.superlumdiodes.com/pdf/sld_overview.pdf (accessed February 2008).

[81] Holtmann, C., P. A. Besse, and H. Melchior, "High-power superluminescent diodes for 1.3 μm," *Electron. Lett.* 32(18) (1996): 1705–1706.

[82] Li, L. H., et al., "Wide emission spectrum from superluminescent diodes with chirped quantum dot multilayers," *Electron. Lett.* 41(1) (2005): 41–42.

[83] Kaminow, I. P., G. Eisenstein, L. W. Stulz, and A. G. Dentai, "Lateral confinement InGaAsP superluminescent diode at 1.3 μm," *IEEE J. Quant. Electron.* QE-19(1) (1983): 78–82.

[84] Youngquist, R. C., S. Carr, and D. E. N. Davies, "Optical coherence domain reflectometry: a new optical evaluation technique," *Opt. Lett.* 12(3) (1987): 158–160.

[85] Swanson, E. A., et al., "High-resolution optical coherence domain reflectometry," *Opt. Lett.* 17(2) (1992): 151–153.

[86] Chiang, H. P., W. S. Chang, and J. Wang, "Imaging through random scattering media by using CW broadband interferometry," *Opt. Lett.* 18(7) (1993): 546–548.

[87] Wang, X. J., et al., "Characterization of human scalp hairs by optical low-coherence reflectometry," *Opt. Lett.* 20(6) (1995): 524–526.

[88] Podoleanu, A. G., G. M. Dobre, D. J. Webb, and D. A. Jackson, "Simultaneous en-face imaging of two layers in the human retina by low-coherence reflectometry," *Opt. Lett.* 22(13) (1997): 1039–1041.

[89] Choi, H. S., H. F. Taylor, and C. E. Lee, "High-performance fiber-optic temperature sensor using low-coherence interferometry," *Opt. Lett.* 22(23) (1997): 1814–1816.

[90] Tearney, G. J., et al., "Determination of the refractive index of highly scattering human tissue by optical coherence tomography," *Opt. Lett.* 20(21) (1995): 2258–2260.

[91] de Boer, J. F., T. E. Milner, M. J. C. can Gemert, and J. S. Nelson, "Two-dimensional birefringence imaging in biological tissue by polarization-sensitive optical coherence tomography," *Opt. Lett.* 22(12) (1997): 934–936.

[92] Everett, M. J., K. Schoenenberger, B. W. Colston Jr., and L. B. Da Silva, "Birefringence characterization of biological tissue by use of optical coherence tomography," *Opt. Lett.* 23(3) (1998): 228–230.

[93] Jiao, S., and L. V. Wang, "Two-dimensional depth-resolved Mueller matrix of biological tissue measured with double-beam polarization sensitive optical coherence tomography," *Opt. Lett.* 27(2) (2002): 101–103.

[94] Cheong, W. F., S. A. Prahl, and A. J. Welch, "A review of the optical properties of biological tissues," *IEEE J. Quant. Electron.* 26(12) (1990): 2166–2185.

[95] Scheel, A. K., et al., "First clinical evaluation of Sagittal laser optical tomography for detection of synovitis in arthritic finger joints," *Ann. Rheum. Dis.* 64(2) (2005): 239–245.

[96] Yuan, Z., Q. Zhang, E. Sobel, and H. Jiang, "Three-dimensional diffuse optical tomography of osteoarthritis: initial results in the finger joints," *J. Biomed. Opt.* 12(3) (2007): 034001.

[97] Xu, Y., et al., "Three-dimensional diffuse optical tomography of bones and joints," *J. Biomed. Opt.* 7(1) (2002): 88–92.

[98] Yu, G., et al., "Real-time in situ monitoring of human prostate photodynamic therapy with diffuse light," *Photochem. Photobiol.* 82(5) (2006): 1279–1284.

[99] Li, C., R. Liengsawangwong, H. Choi, and R. Cheung, "Using a priori structural information from magnetic resonance imaging to investigate the feasibility of prostate diffuse optical tomography and spectroscopy: a simulation study," *Med. Phys.* 34(1) (2007): 266–274.

[100] Piao, D., et al., "Near-infrared optical tomography: endoscopic imaging approach," *Proc. SPIE* 6431 (2007): 643103.

[101] Padhani, A. R., C. J. Harvey, and D. O. Cosgrove, "Angiogenesis imaging in the management of prostate cancer," *Nat. Clin. Prac., Urol.* 2(12) (2005): 596–607.

[102] Piao, D., et al., "Approach on trans-rectal optical tomography probing for the imaging of prostate with trans-rectal ultrasound correlation," *Proc. SPIE* 6850 (2008): 68500E.

[103] Huang, M, and Q. Zhu, "Dual-mesh optical tomography reconstruction method with a depth correction that uses a priori ultrasound information," *Appl. Opt.* 43(8) (2004): 1654–1662.

[104] Choma, M., M. Sarunic, C. Yang, and J. Izatt, "Sensitivity advantage of swept source and Fourier domain optical coherence tomography," *Opt. Exp.* 11(18) (2003): 2183–2189.

CHAPTER 5
Multimodal Diffuse Optical Tomography: Theory

Simon Arridge, Christos Panagiotou, Martin Schweiger, and Ville Kolehmainen

5.1 Introduction

By optical tomography we mean the measurement of transmitted and/or reflected light in the visible or near-infrared part of the spectrum, after traversal of biological tissue. When the length of path is many orders of magnitude greater than the mean free path between photon scattering events, a random-walk or diffusionlike process becomes quite an accurate description of the light propagation process, which has led to the term diffuse optical tomography (DOT) for this type of imaging. A variety of measurement techniques are available which are broadly classified into time domain and frequency domain, with the so-called DC measurement being the zero modulation frequency component of the latter. DC systems provide the simplest mode of measurement, but the DC data suffer from an inherent loss of ability to distinguish between absorption and scattering processes, unless additional information such as multispectral measurements is employed. The image reconstruction in DOT is a highly ill-posed inverse problem, whose solution requires the use of regularization to transform the problem into a well-posed form. Typically, regularization is carried out by augmenting the inverse problem with a side constraint that is chosen based on a priori information or assumptions about the properties of the unknown solution.

During recent years, there has been significant progress in development of multimodality DOT imaging, which combines optical tomography with other imaging modalities to produce anatomical and physiological information in a complimentary manner. Examples include coregistered DOT with magnetic resonance imaging (MRI-DOT), with computed tomography (CT-DOT), and with ultrasound imaging (US-DOT). It is well established that in such cases the quality of the DOT reconstructions can be significantly improved if image information from the higher-resolution modality is suitably utilized as prior information in the regularization of the DOT problem.

In this chapter, we concentrate on the theory behind image reconstruction for multimodality DOT. We give a review of previous work on multimodality DOT and then describe two techniques for the incorporation of the multimodality information in terms of prior information into the regularization of the DOT problem.

The first approach is based on structural priors, and the second, on information-theoretic metrics based on mutual information. We present the theory in the framework of the frequency-domain DOT approach. Since the inverse problem is inherently nonlinear we concentrate on computation methods drawn from large-scale optimization.

The rest of the chapter is organized as follows. In Section 5.2 we describe both the forward model and the inverse problem and their discrete implementations. In Section 5.3 we review the approaches that involve multimodality systems. In Section 5.4 we discuss the incorporation of multimodality information in terms of prior information and the development of regularization schemes, together with some examples. In Section 5.5 we draw some conclusions and suggest topics for future research.

5.2 Diffuse Optical Tomography

Like all indirect imaging methods (i.e., methods in which the image has to be inferred from the data rather than being imaged directly), diffuse optical tomography (DOT) is posed as an inverse problem. It is known to be ill-posed in the sense of Hadamard [1], implying that the solution to the problem is unstable with respect to the measurement errors or that the problem may not even have a unique solution.

As a general context to image reconstruction, we discuss an optimization-based approach in which we seek the image x that minimizes an objective functional:

$$E(y^{meas}, F(x)) = \ell(y^{meas}, F(x)) + \Psi(x) \to \min \tag{5.1}$$

where y^{meas} denotes data, x denotes the solution, and F denotes the forward mapping. The functional $\ell(y^{meas}, F(x))$ is a data residual term that penalizes the residual between the measured data and the forward mapping, and functional $\Psi(x)$ is the regularization term that is used to transform the ill-posed minimization of the term $\ell(y^{meas}, F(x))$ into a well-posed problem.

We note that within the Bayesian framework, (5.1) can be interpreted as a maximum a posteriori (MAP) estimation problem. The first term in (5.1), the likelihood term, is equivalent to the negative log of the probability of obtaining data y^{meas} given image x. The second term in (5.1), the regularization functional Ψ, is equivalent to the negative log of the prior probability distribution for x:

$$\Psi(x) = -\log \pi_\psi(x) \tag{5.2}$$

The most widely used form of the problem (5.1) in DOT is the regularized output least squares formulation:

$$\|y^{meas} - F(x)\|_W^2 + \Psi(x) \to \min \tag{5.3}$$

where $\|v\|_W^2 := \langle v, Wv \rangle$ is the weighted L^2-norm, W being a symmetric positive definite weighting matrix.

Within the Bayesian interpretation, the choice of the square norm for the data misfit $\ell(y^{meas}, F(x))$ is tantamount to assuming a Gaussian noise model for the distribution of measurements around the noise free model:

$$e = y^{meas} - F(x) \sim N(0, \mathbf{W}^{-1}) \tag{5.4}$$

where x and e are statistically independent and $\mathbf{W}^{-1}$ models the covariance of the measurement noise process.

Although we will discuss in the first instance the problem from the deterministic, optimization-based viewpoint, it should be noted that in the Bayesian paradigm, all variables, x included, are redefined as random variables with associated probability distribution models. This will become more relevant when we discuss information-theoretic approaches for the utilization of prior information in Section 5.4.2.

5.2.1 The Forward Problem and Linearization

The most commonly used forward model for optical diffusion tomography is the diffusion approximation (DA) to the radiative transfer equation (RTE), and it is the one employed herein. The issue of how well the diffusion model approximates the radiative transfer equation or the actual DOT measurements is not considered in this chapter, but see, for example, [2–10]. For further details on derivation and properties of the forward models and boundary conditions, see [11–14].

Let $\Omega \subset R^n$ be a simply connected domain containing two real positive scalar functions $\mu_a(r)$, $\kappa(r)$. Let $f(m; \omega)e^{i\omega t}$ be a time-harmonic incoming-radiation boundary condition. We define the operators

$$D(a, b; \omega) := \left\{ -\nabla \cdot b\nabla + a + \frac{i\omega}{c} \right\} \tag{5.5}$$

$$B(s) := I + s\frac{\partial}{\partial \nu} \tag{5.6}$$

where c is the speed of light (assumed constant), and ν is the outward normal of the boundary $\partial\Omega$ at m; then the photon density $\Phi(r; \omega)$ inside the domain satisfies

$$D(\mu_a, \kappa; \omega)\Phi(r; \omega) = 0 \quad r \in \Omega/\partial\Omega \tag{5.7}$$

$$B(2\zeta\kappa)\Phi(m; \omega) = f(m; \omega) \quad m \in \partial\Omega \tag{5.8}$$

where ζ is a boundary term which incorporates the refractive index mismatch at the tissue-air boundary [13, 15]. In the literature, the optical coefficients are often expressed in terms of absorption and scattering. The reduced scattering coefficient, μ'_s, is related to μ_a and κ by

$$\kappa = \frac{1}{3(\mu_a + \mu'_s)} \tag{5.9}$$

The measureable *exitance* is the (diffuse) outgoing radiation and corresponds to the Neumann data

$$z(m;\omega) = -\kappa(m)\frac{\partial \Phi(m;\omega)}{\partial \nu}, \quad m \in \partial\Omega \tag{5.10}$$

We use X to denote the function space of the parameters, Q the function space of the sources, and Y the function space of the data. Some discussion of the form of these spaces can be found in [2, 11].

5.2.1.1 The Forward Operator

$$F_j : X \to Y \tag{5.11}$$

is a nonlinear mapping from pairs of functions in the solution space to data on the boundary, for given incoming radiation f_j.

5.2.1.2 The Direct Fréchet Derivative

$$F'_j(\mu_a, \kappa; \omega) : X \to Y \tag{5.12}$$

is a linear mapping from pairs of functions in the solution space to data on the boundary, for given incoming radiation f_j. F'_j is the linearization of F_j around the solution point $\{\mu_a, \kappa\}$ that maps changes $\{\mu_a^\delta, \kappa^\delta\} \equiv \{\alpha, \beta\}$ in solution-space functions to changes z_j^δ in data. The value of the mapping

$$z_j^\delta(m;\omega) = F'_j(\mu_a, \kappa; \omega)\begin{pmatrix}\alpha\\\beta\end{pmatrix} \tag{5.13}$$

is given by

$$D(\mu_a, \kappa; \omega)\Phi_j^\delta(r;\omega) = -D(\alpha, \beta; \omega)\Phi_j(r;\omega), \; r \in \Omega/\partial\Omega \tag{5.14}$$

$$B(2\zeta\kappa)\Phi_j^\delta(m;\omega) = 0, \quad m \in \partial\Omega \tag{5.15}$$

$$z_j^\delta(m;\omega) = -\kappa(m)\frac{\partial \Phi_j^\delta(m;\omega)}{\partial \nu}, m \in \partial\Omega \tag{5.16}$$

5.2.1.3 The Adjoint Fréchet Derivative

$$F'^*_j(\mu_a, \kappa; \omega) : Y \to X \tag{5.17}$$

is a linear mapping from functions on the boundary to pairs of functions in the solution space for a given incoming radiation f_j. The value of the mapping

5.2 Diffuse Optical Tomography

$$\begin{pmatrix} \alpha \\ \beta \end{pmatrix} = F_j'^{*}(\mu_a, \kappa; \omega) z_j^{\delta}(m; \omega) \tag{5.18}$$

is given by

$$\overline{D}(\mu_a, \kappa; \omega)\Psi_j(r; \omega) = 0, \quad r \in \Omega/\Omega \tag{5.19}$$

$$B(2\zeta\kappa)\Psi_j(m; \omega) = z_j^{\delta}(m; \omega), \quad m \in \partial\Omega \tag{5.20}$$

$$\begin{pmatrix} \alpha \\ \beta \end{pmatrix} = \mathrm{Re}\begin{pmatrix} -\overline{\Psi}_j \Phi_j \\ -\nabla\overline{\Psi}_j \cdot \nabla\Phi_j \end{pmatrix}, \quad r \in \Omega/\partial\Omega \tag{5.21}$$

We assume a finite number of incoming radiation sources:

$$\mathbb{S} = \{f_j(m);\ j = 1\ldots S\}$$

where $f_j(m)$ is a function of local support on $\partial\Omega$ representing the finite width and profile of the jth source. The forward operator is now considered as a stacked set of operators:

$$z(m; \omega) = \begin{bmatrix} z_1(m; \omega) \\ z_2(m; \omega) \\ \vdots \\ z_S(m; \omega) \end{bmatrix} = \mathbf{F}(\mu_a, \kappa; \omega) = \begin{bmatrix} F_1(\mu_a, \kappa; \omega) \\ F_2(\mu_a, \kappa; \omega) \\ \vdots \\ F_S(\mu_a, \kappa; \omega) \end{bmatrix} \tag{5.22}$$

The data in (5.22) represent complex functions whose inversion would lead to a complex parameter update. For this reason, the data is usually split into real and imaginary parts with a commensurate splitting of the linearized derivative operators. In addition, when considering log of the data the splitting associates the real part with logarithmic amplitude, and the imaginary part with phase. The measurement used in practice is therefore

$$y = \begin{pmatrix} \mathrm{Re}(\log(z)) \\ \mathrm{Im}(\log(z)) \end{pmatrix} \in Y \tag{5.23}$$

Finally we consider a measurement model corresponding to the finite sampling of the outgoing distributions $z_j(m; \omega)$:

$$z_{j,i}(\omega) = M_i[z_j(m; \omega)] = \int_{\partial\Omega} w_i(m) z_j(m; \omega) dS \tag{5.24}$$

where $w_i(m)$ represents the finite aperture of a detector. In the following, we will use $\mathbb{W} = \{w_i(m);\ i = 1\ldots M\}$ to assume a finite number M of detectors, with $\mathbb{W}_j \subset \mathbb{W}$ representing the subset of size $M_j \leq M$ of detectors that see source j. Let $n_m = \Sigma_j M_j$ be the total number of measured data.

With this sampling, the data become vectors, and we have a *semidiscrete* forward mapping $F_j : X \to \mathbb{R}^{2M_j}$ whose stacked form becomes

$$y(\omega) = F(\mu_a, \kappa; \omega), \quad F: X \to \mathbb{R}^{2n_m} \tag{5.25}$$

5.2.2 Inverse Problem

To implement a computational approach to the inverse problem, the functions need to be cast into a discrete representation. We assume a finite element method (FEM) approximation, in which the domain Ω is divided into P elements Ω_ℓ, which are joined by D node points. The photon density is approximated in a finite dimensional basis

$$\Phi^h(r) = \sum_{\ell=1}^{D} \phi_\ell \varphi_\ell(r) \tag{5.26}$$

where the term φ_ℓ represents the nodal basis functions of the finite element mesh. By inserting approximation (5.26) into the variational formulation of (5.7) and (5.8) and using the basis functions φ_ℓ as the test functions, we arrive at the matrix equation

$$\left(\mathbf{K}(\kappa) + \mathbf{C}(\mu_a) + \mathbf{R} + i\omega B\right)\Phi^h = G \tag{5.27}$$

where the elements of the system matrices are given by

$$\mathbf{K}_{\ell,\ell'} = \int_\Omega \kappa \nabla \varphi_\ell \cdot \nabla \varphi_{\ell'} \, dr \tag{5.28}$$

$$\mathbf{C}_{\ell,\ell'} = \int_\Omega \mu_a \varphi_\ell \varphi_{\ell'} \, dr \tag{5.29}$$

$$\mathbf{B}_{\ell,\ell'} = \frac{1}{c}\int_\Omega \varphi_\ell \varphi_{\ell'} \, dr \tag{5.30}$$

$$\mathbf{R}_{\ell,\ell'} = \int_{\partial\Omega} 2\zeta \varphi_\ell \varphi_{\ell'} \, dS \tag{5.31}$$

and the source vector is of the form

$$G_\ell^{(j)} = \int_{\partial\Omega} f^{(j)} \varphi_\ell \, dS \tag{5.32}$$

The complex measurement vector $z^{(j)}$ containing the measured flux for the jth source is obtained by solving (5.27) and applying the discrete representation of (5.24):

$$z^{(j)} = \mathbf{M}\Phi_j^h \tag{5.33}$$

where the elements of the measurement matrix $\mathbf{M}$ are defined by

$$\mathbf{M}_{i,\ell} = \int_{\partial\Omega} \frac{w_i(m)\varphi_\ell(m)}{2\zeta} \, dS, \quad i = 1, \ldots, M \quad \ell = 1, \ldots, D \tag{5.34}$$

To complete the specification of the discretized forward model, let

5.2 Diffuse Optical Tomography

$$z = \left(z^{(1)}, \ldots, z^{(S)}\right)^T \in \mathbb{C}^{n_m}$$

denote the concatenated vector of complex data for all the S sources. The splitted data corresponding to (5.23) is then

$$y = \begin{pmatrix} \text{Re}(\log(z)) \\ \text{Im}(\log(z)) \end{pmatrix} \in \mathbb{R}^{2n_m} \tag{5.35}$$

To specify the discretization of the unknowns (μ_a, μ'_s) for the inverse problem, we define an expansion in basis coefficients:

$$\mu_a(r) = \sum_{k=1}^{n_p} \mu_{a_k} b_k(r) \tag{5.36}$$

$$\mu'_s(r) = \sum_{k=1}^{n_p} \mu'_{s_k} b_k(r) \tag{5.37}$$

where $\{b_k; k = 1 \ldots n_p\}$ represents a set of image basis functions spanning the finite dimensional parameter space X_n. For details of choices of basis function and their implementation, see [16]. The parameter vector for the inverse problem becomes

$$x = \begin{pmatrix} \mu_a \\ \mu'_s \end{pmatrix} = \left(\mu_{a_1}, \ldots, \mu_{a_{n_p}}, \mu'_{s_1}, \ldots, \mu'_{s_{n_p}}\right)^T \in \mathbb{R}^n, \quad n = 2n_p \tag{5.38}$$

The computation of the MAP estimate by the minimization of (5.3) can be carried out, for example, by a Newton algorithm:

$$x^{(n+1)} = x^{(n)} + \tau Q\left(F'^*\left(x^{(n)}\right) W\left(y^{meas} - F\left(x^{(n)}\right) - \Psi'\left(x^{(n)}\right)\right)\right) \tag{5.39}$$

where Q is a symmetric positive definite approximation to the inverse Hessian of the optimization functional and τ is a step length. In the Gauss-Newton method, we take

$$Q\left(x^{(n)}\right) = \left(F'^*\left(x^{(n)}\right) W F'\left(x^{(n)}\right) + \Psi''\left(x^{(n)}\right)\right)^{-1} \tag{5.40}$$

The discrete representation of the Fréchet derivative $F'(x^{(n)})$ is a $2n_m \times 2n_p$ matrix $\mathbf{J}_n$ whose components can be calculated by computing S forward and M adjoint solutions.

Note that when the number $2n_p$ of unknowns is large, the Gauss-Newton updates can be efficiently computed with the implicit Gauss-Newton method; see, for example, [17]. In the lagged-diffusivity Gauss-Newton method the Hessian of the prior functional is replaced by a linear operator [18],

$$\Psi''(x)v \cong \mathcal{L}(x)v \tag{5.41}$$

so that (5.39) becomes, in the discrete setting,

$$x^{(n+1)} = x^{(n)} + \tau\left(J_n^T W J_n + L\right)^{-1}\left(J_n^T W\left(y^{meas} - F\left(x^{(n)}\right)\right) - L_n x^{(n)}\right) \qquad (5.42)$$

where L_n is the discrete matrix representation of the operator $\mathcal{L}(x^{(n)})$.

5.3 Multimodality Reconstruction: Review of Previous Work

Multimodality imaging refers to the combination of the varying capacities of two or more medical imaging technologies in extracting physiological and anatomical information about organisms in a complimentary fashion in order to enable the consistent retrieval of accurate and content-rich biological information. A sample of established areas of multimodality imaging include Positron Emission Tomography (PET) imaging with Computed Tomography (CT) in PET-CT studies and, to a lesser extent, with magnetic resonance imaging (MRI); see, for example, [19–26]. Research on multimodality is also carried on magneto- and electroencephalography (MEG/EEG) where information from the high spatially resolved, but less temporarily resolved, functional MRI (fMRI) is incorporated into the EEG/MEG inverse problem [27, 28]. Attempts to combine EEG and MEG signals have also taken place [29]. The benefits of multimodality imaging have also been recognized by the optical tomography community and significant research output has been produced over the past years.

Optical tomography suffers from low spatial resolution mainly due to the diffuse nature of light propagation inside tissues. Light is detected on the boundary having followed a complex path, which renders the spatial localization of the interactions (absorbtion and scattering) that occurred along the way extremely difficult. Improved optical resolution can be achieved by introducing a priori information regarding the expected solution into the problem. One such source of a priori information is images from higher-resolution modalities where the information under discussion consists of spatially localized distinct anatomical areas and/or physiological events, which correlate with optical events. For example, it is known [30] that distinct anatomical areas of the brain, such as gray and white matter, scalp, skull, and cerebrospinal fluid (voids), are characterized by different optical absorption and scattering coefficients—at least on a baseline level, as different amounts of blood presence can locally change the literature values. In the absence of prior information, optical tomography can fail to distinguish the existing optical differences among these areas. Using prior information from higher-resolution imaging modalities such as MRI, CT, or ultrasound (US) can designate the location of such areas to the optical tomography inverse solver and enable consistently improved reconstructions, spatially and quantitatively.

Chang et al. in 1996 [31] used volumetric breast MRI data in order to simulate a realistic anatomical medium to be probed. The MRI was segmented by a simple thresholding scheme, and the obtained regions of fat and parenchyma were assigned with typical optical values. Additional features were explicitly inserted in the simulated anatomy to act as pathological regions. The reconstruction involved a difference imaging study where both target and reference images were derived from the

MRI data, although the pathological regions were not present in the reference image. The obtained reconstructions accurately retrieved the pathologies, allowing us to positively comment about the use of multimodal priors from CT or MRI in optical imaging.

Pogue and Paulsen in 1998 [32] used the information from a segmented coronal MRI slice acquired from a rat in order to create a realistic finite element mesh (FEM)–based numerical phantom to be probed. The three distinct regions of bone, muscle, and brain tissue in the phantom were assigned optical values from the literature known to correspond to each of the identifiable tissue types. The numerical phantom was then used for the simulation of the data-acquisition process. The solution of the inverse problem was regularized by restricting the reconstruction of the optical parameters in regions that would correspond to brain or bone structures. The initial guess of the optical parameters would again match the literature; however, after initialization, the algorithm would be free to reevaluate the parameter distribution. The knowledge of the regions to restrict the reconstruction comprised the a priori anatomical information.

The method also proved able to cope with local perturbations in the optical coefficients. Schweiger and Arridge [33] proposed a method that used an MRI slice of an adult, presegmented into four distinct regions corresponding to skin, bone, and gray and white matter identifiable structures. Rather than using literature values as an initialization for the inverse method, they approached the reconstruction in two separate steps. In the first step, the solver was asked to assume uniform scattering and absorption in the regions of interest and to recover the best value for each region. Thus, the solver had to recover only eight parameters in this initial step. In the second step, the reconstruction was performed on a higher-resolution basis, where the initial values of the optical parameters were supplied by the converged initial step. Thus, the prior MRI image provided information related only to the existence of separate regions, more specifically, using boundary information.

Zhu et al. [34–36] have proposed the simultaneous probing of tissue with ultrasound and optical tomography. Their apparatus consisted of a handheld probe combining on the same application surface 12 optical source fibers, 4 optical detector fibers, and 20 piezoelectric crystals comprising the ultrasound array. The combined apparatus guaranteed sufficient coregistration between the optical and ultrasound signal. While the ultrasound signal provided very accurate localization of a tumor, the optical data provided information regarding the hemoglobin concentration of the tumor, allowing classification between malignant cancers and benign lesions.

Ntizachristos et al. [37] studied the performance of MRI-guided diffuse optical spectroscopy of breast lesions. The apparatus of the system allowed scanning with both modalities without change in the positioning of the patient, thus enforcing coregistration of the involved medical signals. This allowed the voxels in the solution domain of the optical image to be labeled according to the tissue type of the breast on which they were superimposed. The determination of the tissue type was accomplished by the coregistered MRI signal. As in [33], by restricting all pixels in the optical domain belonging to the same tissue type to be completely correlated, the underdetermined problem of DOT becomes overdetermined as the number of unknowns drops dramatically.

In realistic scenarios, structural or physiological correlation between the true optical solution and a prior image from a different medical imaging modality cannot be guaranteed even in the intrasubject case. This is due to the different imaging functions governing each modality, which target different physical attributes of the probed medium. It is then expected that prior images might contain features with their corresponding analogs in the optical image being absent. The presence of such local feature space asymmetries between the true optical solution and prior image can lead to incorrect reconstructions of the former due to the incorrect bias of the latter. Guven et al. [38] proposed a method toward the incorporation of multimodal priors in optical tomography, enabling the alleviation of the incorrect bias from the regions of the prior image with no optical analog, but preserving the prior information leading toward the true solution. Based on this method, Intes et al. [39] reported results of optical absorption parameter reconstruction of a slab, mimicking typical values encountered in a human breast, assisted by MRI-derived priors.

Brooksby et al. [40] investigated the reconstruction of heterogeneities as tumors using MRI-inferred prior information. This approach involved the insertion of the prior distribution as a generalized zeroth-order Tikhonov regularization with spatially adaptive regularization weight. Prior information was inserted after an initialization guess was retrieved using a method similar to the one proposed by Schweiger and Arridge [33]. In another approach [41], Brooksby et al. investigated the incorporation of structural a priori information from MRI-based priors in phantom studies and in a healthy woman in vivo. As in most studies, regions of similar tissue type are identified prior to the reconstruction process in order to bias similar tissue type to exhibit similar optical properties. The incorporation of the prior information is accomplished by a modified Tikhonov-based approach. Effectively, the region-based prior information globally enforces smoothing inside regions of the same tissue type but not across boundaries.

Boverman et al. [42] examined the effects of imperfect structural a priori information in the quantitative spectroscopic diffuse optical tomography framework. In this study, the reconstruction is split into two steps. The first step retrieves a piecewise constant chromophore concentration distribution retrieved over distinct regions predetermined by a structural prior image. The study involved four different structural prior distributions involving the true distribution, eroded and dilated versions of the true distribution, and a homogeneous version. The second step aimed to recover an artificial heterogeneity or perturbation simulating a pathology. It was evident from the simulations that the eroded and dilated versions of the true spatial prior information produced better results than the homogeneous one. In addition, Boverman et al. comment regarding a possible asymmetric effect of the prior on the image reconstruction by comparing rates of change in bias at different regions, such as background and pathology.

Spectral priors are introduced in [43–45], where the idea is to derive direct chromophore reconstruction in contrast to the indirect inference of the chromophores via the optical absorption and scattering. Li et al. [45] proposed the use of multiple spectral and spatial priors in optical tomography. Making use of MRI Dixon images, spatial prior information for the chromophores of water and lipid could be incorporated into the optical inverse problem. The remaining chromophores targeted by OT, oxy- and deoxyhemoglobin, were retrieved by the acquired optical data. The reconstruction of the same chromophores from different optical wavelength data acquisitions comprised a form of spectral prior.

In [46, 47] the description of an apparatus for coregistered tomographic X-ray and optical imaging is presented where the high spatial resolution of X-rays and the functional information that DOT can provide are combined. Similar to other multimodality frameworks, both X-ray and optical signals are guaranteed to be registered due to the nature of the imaging system. The highly spatially resolved X-ray tomography images provide information that can be used to label tissue types in the DOT solution domain. A spatially varying regularization scheme is then adopted that enforces high regularization in regions expected to be characterized by less optical contrast, whereas the effect of regularization is reduced in regions where the optical contrast is expected to be high, such as regions identified as lesions.

Douiri et al. [48] proposed the incorporation of edge prior information in the problem of DOT. Edge prior information can be extracted via a segmentation process from anatomical priors, as is done in most studies discussed in this section. The proposed method allows locally adaptive regularization whose nature and magnitude is governed by the local distribution of the reference image gray levels. More specifically, regions of the image with homogeneously distributed gray levels are regularized with a first-order Tikhonov regularization presenting isotropic smoothing characteristics, while regions in the reconstructed image characterized by strong edge formation tendencies are mostly smoothed in a direction parallel to the edge but less across it. Edge formation in the optical image can be a combination of data-driven edge formation and explicit intervention from an edge prior image.

5.4 Multimodality Priors and Regularization

In this section, we discuss the utilization of multimodality prior information in the regularization of the DOT problem. We consider the problem in the regularized output least squares framework (5.3) and present two approaches to incorporate prior information into the regularization functional $\Psi(x)$. In both approaches, we assume that we have a reference image, such as MRI or CT reconstruction, available from the coregistered auxliary imaging modality. We denote the reference image by x_{ref}.

5.4.1 Structural Priors

Typical choices for the regularization term $\Psi(x)$ in (5.3) include, for example, first-order Tikhonov (Phillips-Twomey), total variation (TV), and generalized Gaussian Markov random field (GGMRF) functionals [49]. A common feature of these regularization functionals is that they pose assumptions about the regularity (e.g., smoothness) of the solution, the regularity being measured in terms of some norm of the solution and its differentials. Image-processing methods for computer vision offer a large set of techniques for denoising and segmentation based on anisotropic diffusion processes [50–52]. These techniques directly formulate a PDE for image flow, rather than a variational form like the Euler equation, and can be considered more general.

Consider now the multimodality DOT where we have the MRI or CT image as the reference image x_{ref}. In such a case, it is reasonable to assume that the local regularity of the optical images correlates spatially quite well with the local regularity in the reference image x_{ref}. In the structural priors, the idea is to modify the standard regularizer $\Psi(x)$, which penalizes the regularity of the solution uniformly and isotropically over the entire image domain to accommodate and reflect this prior information. In the implementation of the structural priors, we consider a particular form of the functional Ψ:

$$\Psi(x) = \alpha \int_\Omega \psi(|\nabla x|_D) dr, \; \alpha > 0 \tag{5.43}$$

where ψ is an image-to-image mapping, and

$$|\nabla x|_D := \sqrt{(\nabla x)^T D(r) \nabla x} \tag{5.44}$$

where D is a symmetric tensor function and α is a regularization parameter.

Using standard variational techniques, we obtain

$$\mathcal{L}(x) = -\nabla^T k D(r) \nabla \tag{5.45}$$

where we have defined the *diffusivity*

$$k := \frac{\psi'(|\nabla x|_D)}{|\nabla x|_D} \tag{5.46}$$

and we can interpret $\mathcal{L}(x)$ as the Fréchet derivative of ψ evaluated at x.

Choice of D allows us to control the behavior of the image update according to prior information about the image structure [48, 53]. For example, by choosing $\psi(t) = t^2$ and

$$D(r) = I - \left(1 + \|\nabla x_{ref}(r)\|^2\right)^{-1} \nabla x_{ref}(r) \nabla x_{ref}(r)^T \tag{5.47}$$

we arrive to the nonhomogeneous anisotropic smoothness regularization that was presented in [29]. On the other hand, with the choices $D(r) = I$ and $\psi(t) = t^2$ we would arrive at the standard first-order Tikhonov regularization.

In the following examples, we take the simple form

$$D = \gamma(x_{ref}) I \tag{5.48}$$

where x_{ref} is a reference image and γ is an edge-indicator function which we here take to be

$$\gamma(x_{ref}) = \exp\left\{-\left[\frac{|\nabla x_{ref}|}{T_{ref}}\right]\right\} \tag{5.49}$$

5.4 Multimodality Priors and Regularization

where T_{ref} is a threshold controlling the influence of the edges in x_{ref}.

5.4.1.1 Examples

In this section, we show some results of applying different priors to the DOT reconstruction problem. The test domain consists of a cylindrical object with $\Omega = \{r = (x, y, z) | \sqrt{x^2 + y^2} \leq 25 \wedge -25 \leq z \leq 25\}$, with all units in millimeters. This domain is represented by a finite element mesh consisting of 83,142 nodes and 444,278 four-noded tetrahedral elements, defining a piecewise linear basis φ for the fields. The optical background parameters were set to $\mu_a = 0.01$ mm^{-1} and $\mu'_s = 1$ mm^{-1}. Embedded in the homogeneous background were various ellipsoidal and spherical objects of increased absorption or scattering coefficients. The arrangement of target objects is shown in Color Plate 13. Measurement data were computed for all combinations of 80 sources and 80 detectors, arranged in 5 rings of 16 sources and 16 detectors each around the mantle of the cylinder, at elevations $z = -20, -10, 0, 10, 20$. The measurements consisted of logarithmic amplitude and phase at a source modulation frequency of $f = 100$ MHz, contaminated with 0.5% of multiplicative Gaussian-distributed random noise.

For the reconstructions, a basis of $n_p = 80 \times 80 \times 80$ bilinear voxels was used to represent the unknown distributions of optical coefficients. Image recovery was obtained by 50 iterations of the lagged-diffusivity Gauss-Newton method (5.3), combined with a one-dimensional line search for step size parameter τ. Positivity of the absorption and scatter images was ensured by carrying out the optimization using logarithmic parametrization for the unknowns. The weighting of the data residual and regularization terms was fixed for all cases. The weighting matrix $\mathbf{W}$ was chosen such that the initial value of the least squares residual functional in (5.3) was 1, $\alpha = 0.01$, and $T_{ref} = 0.1$. For the functional ψ, we used an approximation of the total variation (TV) functional:

$$\psi(x) = T\sqrt{\left[|\nabla x|^2_D + T^2\right]} - T^2, \quad \mathscr{L}(x) = \nabla \cdot \frac{T}{\sqrt{|\nabla x|^2_D + T^2}} \mathbf{D} \nabla$$

In the computations, we used value $T = 0.05$ for the smoothing parameter in the TV approximation.

Color Plate 13 and Figures 5.1 through 5.3 show cases where the γ function is chosen to reflect: (1) flat weighting $x_{ref}(r) \equiv 1$ (i.e., conventional TV-regularization), (2) the true edges of all structures in each of μ_a and μ'_s, (3) the sum of the γ function for μ_a and μ'_s, and (4) only partial information about these structures. The results show the improvement in the reconstruction quality obtained from these priors.

5.4.2 Regularization Using Mutual Information

An alternative to structural prior regularization is to take an information-theoretic measure of image similarity as the penalty term. For general references on probability theory, see Papoulis et al. [54], whereas details regarding information entropy

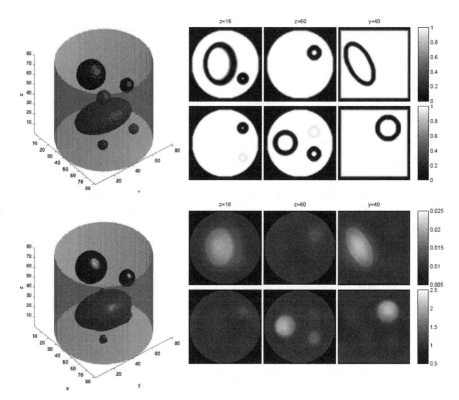

Figure 5.1 TV prior with exact edges weighting. Top: Prior image and cross sections through the resulting edge priors for absorption and scattering. Bottom: reconstructions, displayed as iso-surfaces and cross sections.

can be found in Shannon's celebrated paper of communication theory [55] and numerous recent texts, such as Cover et al. [56].

We make use of the Bayesian interpretation explained in Section 5.2 that all parameters are considered to be random variables (r.v.). The mutual information between two such r.v.s (i.e., in this context, the solution and the reference image) is given by a linear combination of entropic terms $H(\cdot)$:

$$MI(x, x_{ref}) = H(x) + H(x_{ref}) - H(x, x_{ref}) \quad (5.50)$$

More specifically, the terms $H(x)$ and $H(x_{ref})$ denote the marginal entropies for the corresponding distributions, and the term $H(x, x_{ref})$ denotes the joint entropy of x and x_{ref}. Mutual information and various normalized variants of (5.50) have found extensive use in medical imaging as the driving force for multimodal medical image registration problems [57–59], due to its inherent capacity to assess the similarity between two images, even when the gray values between intermodality corresponding objects are incommensurately related. In the context of image reconstruction, Somayajula [60, 61] proposed the application of a mutual-information-based regularization functional,

$$\Psi(x) = -MI(x, x_{ref}) \quad (5.51)$$

5.4 Multimodality Priors and Regularization

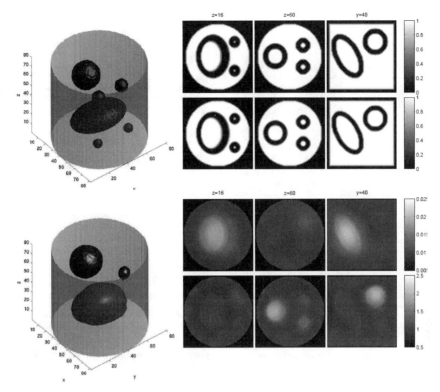

Figure 5.2 TV prior with sum edges weighting. Top: Prior image and cross sections through the resulting edge priors for absorption and scattering. Bottom: reconstructions, displayed as iso-surfaces and cross sections.

which has the attribute of being invariant to absolute intensity values.

The information entropy, defined by Shannon in 1948 [55], is defined over the space of the probabilities of random variables and not on the actual values of the variables themselves. More specifically, the information entropy H of a random variable x is defined as

$$H(x) = -\int_{-\infty}^{\infty} p_x(x) \log(p_x(x)) dx \qquad (5.52)$$

where $p_x(x)$ is the probability density function of random variable x, denoting the probability $P(x \in [x, x+\delta]) \cong p_x(x)\delta$ for small δ. The above definition renders evident the fact that two images, x and x_{ref}, can have the same entropies when the probabilities of their gray values, but not necessarily the gray values themselves, are equivalent. Entropy does not return information regarding the structure of an image that can be interpreted as the distribution of gray values in space. It rather returns information regarding the *shape* of the probability density of the gray values, which can be interpreted as the frequency at which gray values appear on the image—irrespective of their values or spatial distribution.

In practice, the true probability density function $p_x(x)$ is not known, but has to be estimated from the image x itself. Density estimation from a sample is a nontrivial task as the retrieval of accurate estimates, especially when the density is

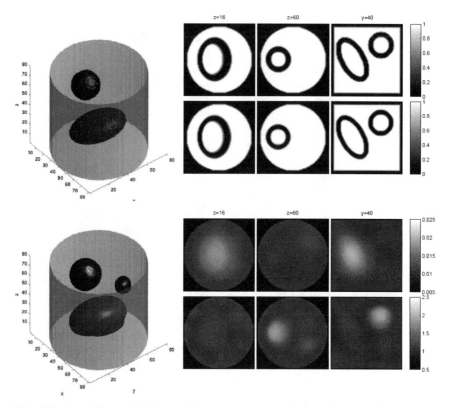

Figure 5.3 TV prior with partial edges weighting. Top: Prior image and cross sections through the resulting edge priors for absorption and scattering. Bottom: reconstructions, displayed as iso-surfaces and cross sections.

expected to have more than one mode, involves methods with computational complexity increasing, often exponentially, with the size of the available sample.

Entropy may be interpreted as a measure of randomness; highly predictable random variables have less entropy than those that involve a higher degree of randomness. An r.v. is more predictable if some outcomes are realized significantly more frequently than others. In the limit that $p_x(x)$ tends to a Dirac delta function, (5.52) tends to a limit of $-\infty$. In the case that all realizations of x are equally likely, the entropy $H(x)$ should be a monotonically increasing function of the sample length [55]. In the image analog, this translates to maximum entropy when all pixels are assigned with different gray values x_i, and $p_x(x)$ is uniform.

Joint entropy $H(x, x_{ref})$ is a measure of randomness characterizing the joint system of the two random variables x and x_{ref}. It is defined as

$$H(x, x_{ref}) = -\int_{-\infty}^{\infty} p_{x,x_{ref}}(x, x_{ref}) \log(p_{x,x_{ref}}(x, x_{ref})) dx \qquad (5.53)$$

where $p_{x,x_{ref}}(x, x_{ref})$ is the joint probability density function of the system defined by x and x_{ref}, such that the probability of a joint event $P(x \in [(x, x+\delta)])$, and $x_{ref} \in [(x_{ref}, x_{ref}+\delta)]) \cong p_{x,x_{ref}}(x, x_{ref})\delta^2$ for small δ. We obtain an estimate (discrete or continuous) of the joint probability density function of two images using the available tuples (x_i,

5.4 Multimodality Priors and Regularization

$x_{ref,i}$), where subscript i denotes the ith pixel location in both images. It is implicitly assumed that images x and x_{ref} are defined over the same spatial domain.

The interpretation of the joint entropy in the image analog is similar to that of its marginal counterpart. The joint system with the least joint entropy would be the most predictable, for example, a system in which one or few tuples are significantly more probable than others. As with the marginal case, it would involve two images with a corresponding joint probability density function resembling a 2D Dirac delta function.

On the contrary, maximum randomness would involve a system of two images where all the available gray-value tuples would be equally likely, leading to a joint 2D histogram that is nearly flat.

In an image reconstruction framework, we would like the reference image to act as a penalty function for the reconstructed image. Suppose that Image 1 in Figure 5.4 is the true solution we attempt to reconstruct, and the other three images are potential reference images. The joint entropy is the same in each case, even though Image 4, for example, is clearly less informative as a reference. In the absence of any data (no feedback from the likelihood term), the regularization should be able to produce a solution similar to the reference density. In the case of joint entropy, however, there is some ambiguity as to how effectively the prior can provide accurate support to the reconstruction. This is a motivation for using mutual information rather than simply joint entropy. A large mutual information value involves a low joint entropy value $H(\hat{x}, x_{ref})$ and, simultaneously, high individual marginal entropies $H(\hat{x})$ and $H(x_{ref})$. As the prior image is usually constant throughout the

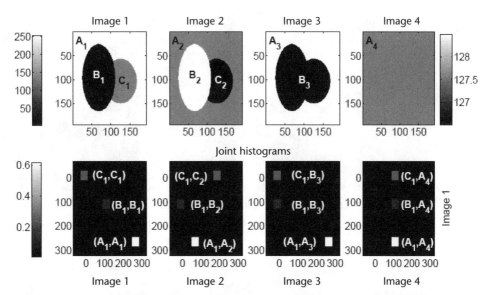

Figure 5.4 Joint entropy between images. Image 2 is a product of recoloring of image 1. Image 3 has structural similarities with Image 1 but fewer quantization levels. Image 4 is homogeneous. Bottom row shows the joint histograms between Image 1 and all other images, including itself in the first example. It is apparent that all joint histograms have the same three modes, but centered in different locations in the intensity space. Due to the equiprobability of the possible events (just three tuples in this case), the joint entropies of the defined pairs are equal with values $H(1, 1) = H(1, 2) = H(1, 3) = H(1, 4) = 0.9035$.

reconstruction process $H(x_{ref})$ is constant. We thus seek an estimate $\hat{x}$ that has low joint entropy with the prior image but also maximum marginal entropy.

5.4.2.1 Examples

Preliminary results that provide some evidence regarding the applicability of the mutual information functional as a form of regularization in optical tomography, have been obtained. The simulation corresponding to Figure 5.5 involves a FEM

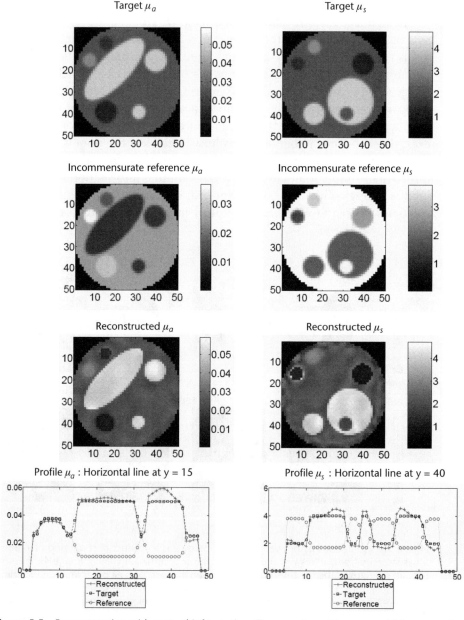

Figure 5.5 Reconstruction with mutual information. Top row: target images, middle row: reference images; bottom row: reconstructions.

mesh of $D = 3,730$ nodes, $S = 32$ sources, and $M = 32$ detectors. The reconstruction basis consists of $n_p = 50 \times 50$ bilinear pixels. As in Section 5.4.1.1, the modulation frequency is $\omega = 100$ MHz; however, the percentage of noise has been increased to 5% (Gaussian multiplicative).

The marginal and joint probability density functions in (5.52) and (5.53) are computed via a univariate binned kernel density estimator that utilizes the fast Fourier transform [62, 63] and its multivariate extensions [64, 65], thus allowing the evaluation of the mutual information within reasonable time frames. The optimization of the objective function (5.3) is accomplished via an iterative gradient descent optimization

$$x^{(n+1)} = x^{(n)} + \tau\left(F'^{*}\left(x^{(n)}\right)\mathbf{W}\left(y^{meas} - F'\left(x^{(n)}\right) - \Psi'\left(x^n\right)\right)\right) \tag{5.54}$$

where τ is a step-length parameter, which is obtained via an inexact line search based on quadratic interpolation in order to bracket the minimum at each iteration n [17]. The first-order derivative approximation of the MI prior, $\Psi'(x)$, is obtained via an analytic exression. Two reference images have been employed in the process, corresponding to μ_a and μ'_s, respectively. Both reference images (Figure 5.5, middle row) present structural characteristics identical with these of the target reconstruction. However, in order to simulate a multimodal framework, we ensure that gray values populating the prior images are incommensurately related to the ones of the corresponding target reconstructions. For implementation purposes, we scale the range of gray values to be similar to the expected reconstructed range.

5.5 Conclusions

In this chapter we gave a summary of an iterative-model-based minimization approach to multimodality DOT reconstruction. We discussed the construction of different forms of prior information for the regularization of this problem with numerical examples. There are several areas for future research including the further development of the structural and information-theoretic priors. In addition to the assumption of a fixed reference image prior, we could consider the simultaneous reconstruction of the optical and the reference image with cross-regularization. A further fruitful approach will be the combination of reconstruction with image analysis/segmentation techniques which could lead to a more robust algorithm if the expected model extraction is only of low order.

Acknowledgments

The work described in this chapter was supported by EPSRC grants EP/D502330/1 and EP/E034950/1 and by the Academy of Finland (projects 119270 and 213476). We wish to thank Professor Richard Leahy and Sangeetha Somayajula of the Signal and Image Processing Institute, University of Southern California, for help with the mutual information regularization methods.

References

[1] Hadamard, J., "Sur les problemes aux derivees partielles et leur signification physique," *Bulletin Princeton University* 13 (1902), 49–52.

[2] Dorn, O., "A transport-backtransport method for optical tomography," *Inverse Problems* 14, no. 5, (1998), 1107–1130.

[3] Hielscher, A. H., R. E. Alcouffe, and R. L. Barbour, "Comparison of finite-difference transport and diffusion calculations for photon migration in homogeneous and hetergeneous tissue," *Phys. Med. Biol.* 43 (1998), 1285–1302.

[4] Klose, A. D., and A. H. Hielscher, "Iterative reconstruction scheme for optical tomography based on the equation of radiative transfer," *Med. Phys.* 26 (1999), 1698–1707.

[5] Bal, G., and Y. Maday, "Coupling of transport and diffusion models in linear transport theory," *Math. Model. Numer. Anal.* 36 (2002), 69–86.

[6] Klose, A. D., and A. H. Hielscher, "Optical tomography using the time-independent equation of radiative transfer—Part 2: Inverse model," *J. Quantitative Spectroscopy and Radiative Transfer* 72 (2002), 715–732.

[7] Abdoulaev, G. S., K. Ren, and A. H. Hielscher, "Optical tomography as a PDE-constrained optimisation problem," *Inverse Problems* 21 (2005), 1507–1530.

[8] Tarvainen, T., M. Vauhkonen, V. Kolehmainen, and J. P. Kaipio, "A hybrid radiative transfer-diffusion model for optical tomography," *Appl. Opt.* 44, no. 6, (2005), 876–886.

[9] Tarvainen, T., M. Vauhkonen, V. Kolehmainen, S. R. Arridge, and J. P. Kaipio, "Coupled radiative transfer equation and diffusion approximation model for photon migration in turbid medium with low-scattering and non-scattering regions," *Phys. Med. Biol.* 50 (2005), 4913–4930.

[10] Ren, K., G. Bal, and A. Hielscher, "Frequency domain optical tomography based on the equation of radiative transfer," *SIAM J. Sci. Comput.* 28, no. 4, (2006), 1463–1489.

[11] Arridge, S. R., "Optical tomography in medical imaging," *Inverse Problems* 15 (1999), no. 2, R41–R93.

[12] Kaipio, J., and E. Somersalo, *Statistical and Computational Inverse Problems*, New York: Springer, 2005.

[13] Schweiger, M., S. R. Arridge, M. Hiraoka, and D. T. Delpy, "The finite element model for the propagation of light in scattering media: boundary and source conditions," *Med. Phys.* 22, no. 11, (1995), 1779–1792.

[14] Heino, J., and E. Somersalo, "Estimation of optical absorption in anisotropic background," *Inverse Problems* 18 (2002), 559–657.

[15] Moulton, J. D., "Diffusion modelling of picosecond laser pulse propagation in turbid media," M. Eng. thesis, McMaster University, Hamilton, Ontario, 1990.

[16] Schweiger, M., and S. R. Arridge, "Optical tomography with local basis functions," *Journal of Electronic Imaging* 12, no. 4, (2003), 583–593.

[17] Schweiger, M., S. R. Arridge, and I. Nissilä, "Gauss-Newton method for image reconstruction in diffuse optical tomography," *Phys. Med. Biol.* 50 (2005), 2365–2386.

[18] Vogel, C. R., *Computational Methods for Inverse Problems*, Philadelphia, PA: SIAM, 2002.

[19] Ardekani, B. A., M. Braun, B. F. Hutton, I. Kanno, and H. Iida, "Minimum cross-entropy reconstruction of PET images using prior anatomical information," *Phys. Med. Biol.* 41 (1996), 2497–2517.

[20] Comtat, C., P. E. Kinahan, J. A. Fessler, T. Beyer, D. W. Townsend, M. Defrise, and C. Michel, "Clinically feasible reconstruction of 3D whole body PET/CT data using blurred anatomical labels," *Phys. Med. Biol.* 47 (2002), 1–20.

[21] Gindi, G., M. Lee, A. Rangarajan, and I. G. Zubal, "Bayesian reconstruction of functional images using anatomical information as priors," *IEEE Trans. Med. Im.* 12, no. 4, (1993), 670–680.

[22] Lu, H. H., C. M. Chen, and I. H. Yang, "Cross-reference weighted least squares estimates for positron emission tomography," *IEEE Trans. Med. Im.* 17 (1998), 1–8.

[23] Rangarajan, A., I. T. Hsiao, and G. Gindi, "A Bayesian joint mixture framework for the integration of anatomical information in functional image reconstruction," *J. Mat. Imag. Vision* 12 (2000), 119–217.

[24] Sastry, S., and R.E. Carson, "Multimodality Bayesian algorithm for image reconstruction in positron emission tomography: a tissue composition model," *IEEE Trans. Med. Im.* 16 (1997), 750–761.

[25] Som, S., B. H. Hutton, and M. Braun, "Properties of minimum cross-entropy reconstruction of emission tomography with anatomically based prior," *IEEE Trans. Nucl. Sci.* 46 (1998), 3014–3021.

[26] Zaidi, H., M. L. Montandon, and D. O. Slosman, "Magnetic resonance image-guided attenuation correction in 3D brain positron emission tomography," *Med. Phys.* 30 (2003), 937–948.

[27] Ahlfors, S. P., and G.V. Simpson, "Geometrical interpretation of fMRI-guided MEG/EEG inverse estimates," *Neuroimage* 22 (2004), no. 1, 323–332.

[28] Babiloni, F., F. Cincotti, C. Babiloni, F. Carducci, D. Mattia, L. Astolfi, A. Basilisco, P. M. Rossini, L. L. Ding, Y. Ni, J. Cheng, K. Christine, J. Sweeney, and B. He, "Estimation of the cortical functional connectivity with the multimodal integration of high-resolution EEG and fMRI data by directed transfer function," *Neuroimage* 24 (2005), 118–131.

[29] Baillet, S., L. Garnero, M. Gildas, and J.-P. Hugonin, "Combined MEG and EEG source imaging by minimization of mutual information," *IEEE Trans. on Biomedical Engineering* 46, no. 5, (1999), 522–534.

[30] Okada, E., and D. T. Delpy, "Near-infrared light propagation in an adult head model. i. modeling of low-level scattering in the cerebrospinal fluid layer," *Appl. Opt.* 42, no. 16, (2003), 2906–2914.

[31] Chang, J., H. L. Graber, P. C. Koo, R Aronson, S.-L. S. Barbour, and R.L. Barbour, "Optical imaging of anatomical maps derived from magnetic resonance images using time-independent optical sources," *IEEE Trans. Med. Im.* 16, no. 1, (1997), 68–77.

[32] Pogue, B. W., and K. D. Paulsen, "High-resolution near-infrared tomographic imaging simulations of the rat cranium by use of a priori magnetic resonance imaging structural information," *Opt. Lett.* 23 (1998), 1716–1718.

[33] Schweiger, M., and S. R. Arridge, "Optical tomographic reconstruction in a complex head model using a priori region boundary information," *Phys. Med. Biol.* 44 (1999), 2703–2721.

[34] Zhu, Q., "Imager that combines near-infrared diffusive light and ultrasound," *Opt. Lett.* 24, no. 15, (1999), 1050–1052.

[35] Zhu, Q., N. Chen, and S. H. Kurtzman, "Imaging tumour angiogenesis by use of combined near-infrared diffusive light and ultrasound," *Opt. Lett.* 25, no. 5, (2003), 337–339.

[36] Zhu, Q., S. H. Kurtzma, P. Hegde, S. Tannenbaum, M. Kane, M. Huang, N. G. Chen, B. Jagjivan, and K. Zarfos, "Utilizing optical tomography with ultrasound localization to image heterogeneous hemoglobin distribution in large breast cancers," *Neoplasia* 7, no. 3, (2005), 263–270.

[37] Ntziachristos, V., A. G. Yodh, M. D. Schnall, and B. Chance, "MRI-guided diffuse optical spectroscopy of malignant and benign breast lesions," *Neoplasia* 4, no. 4, (2002), 347–354.

[38] Guven, M., B. Yazici, X. Intes, and B. Chance, "Diffuse optical tomography with a priori anatomical information," *Phys. Med. Biol.* 50 (2005), 2837–2858.

[39] Intes, X., C. Maloux, M. Guven, B. Yazici, and N. Chance, "Diffuse optical tomography with physiological and spatial a priori constraints," *Phys. Med. Biol.* 49, no. 12, (2004), N155–N163.

[40] Brooksby, B. A., H. Dehghani, B. W. Pogue, and K. D. Paulsen, "Near-infrared (NIR) tomography breast image reconstruction with a priori structural information from MRI:

algorithm development for reconstructing heterogeneities," *IEEE J. Quantum Electron.* 9, no. 2, (March-April 2003), 199–209.

[41] Brooksby, B., S. Jiang, H. Dehghani, B. W. Pogue, and K. D. Paulsen, "Combining near infrared tomography and magnetic resonance imaging to study in vivo breast tissue: implementation of a Laplacian-type regularization to incorporate MR structure," *J. Biomed. Opt.* 10, no. 5, (2005), 0515041-10.

[42] Boverman, G., E. L. Miller, A. Li, Q. Zhang, T. Chaves, D. H Brooks, and D. A Boas, "Quantitative spectroscopic diffuse optical tomography of the breast guided by imperfect a priori structural information," *Phys. Med. Biol.* 50 (2005), 3941–3956.

[43] Corlu, A., T. Durduran, R. Choe, M. Schweiger, E. M. C. Hillman, S. R. Arridge, and A. G. Yodh, "Uniqueness and wavelength optimization in continuous-wave multispectral diffuse optical tomography," *Opt. Lett.* 28 (2003), 23.

[44] Corlu, A., R. Choe, T. Durduran, K. Lee, M. Schweiger, S. R. Arridge, E. M. C. Hillman, and A. G. Yodh, "Diffuse optical tomography with spectral constraints and wavelength optimisation," *Appl. Opt.* 44 (2005), no. 11, 2082–2093.

[45] Li, A., G. Boverman, Y. Zhang, D. Brooks, E. L. Miller, M. E. Kilmer, Q. Zhang, E. M. C. Hillman, and D. A. Boas, "Optimal linear inverse solution with multiple priors in diffuse optical tomography," *Appl. Opt.* 44 (2005), 1948–1956.

[46] Li, A., E. L. Miller, M. E. Kilmer, T. J. Brukilacchio, T. Chaves, J. Stott, Q. Zhang, T. Wu, M. Chorlton, R. H. Moore, D. B. Kopans, and D. A. Boas, "Tomographic optical breast imaging guided by three-dimensional mammography," *Journal of Applied Optics* 42 (2003), 5181–5190.

[47] Zhang, Q., T. J. Brukilacchio, A. Li, J. J. Stott, T. Chaves, E. Hillman, T. Wu, M. Chorlton, E. Rafferty, R. H. Moore, D. B. Kopans, and D. A. Boas, "Coregistered tomographic X-ray and optical breast imaging: initial results," *Journal of Biomedical Optics* 10, no. 2, (2005), 024033:1–9.

[48] Douiri, A., M. Schweiger, J. Riley, and S. R. Arridge, "Anisotropic diffusion regularisation methods for diffuse optical tomography using edge prior information," *Meas. Sci. Tech.* 18 (2007), 87–95.

[49] Bouman, C. A., and K. Sauer, "A generalised Gaussian image model for edge-preserving MAP estimation," *IEEE Trans. Image Processing* 2, no. 3, (1993), 296–310.

[50] Geman, S., and D. Geman, "Stochastic relaxation, Gibbs distributions, and the Bayesian restoration of images," *IEEE Trans. Patt. Anal. Mach. Intell.* 6, no. 6, (1984), 721–741.

[51] Rudin, L. I., S. Osher, and E. Fatemi, "Nonlinear total variation based noise removal algorithm," *Physica D* 60 (1992), 259–268.

[52] Vogel, C. R., and M. E. Oman, "Iterative methods for total variation denoising," *SIAM J. Sci. Comp.* 17 (1996), 227–238.

[53] Kaipio, J. P., V. Kolehmainen, M. Vauhkonen, and E. Somersalo, "Inverse problems with structural prior information," *Inverse Problems* 15 (1999), 713–729.

[54] Papoulis, A., and U. S. Pillai, *Probability, Random Variables, and Stochastic Processes*, New York: McGraw-Hill, 2001.

[55] Shannon, C. E., "A mathematical theory of communication," *The Bell Syst. Tech. J.* 27 (1948), 379–423.

[56] Cover, T. M., and J. A. Thomas, *Elements of Information Theory*, New York: Wiley-Interscience, 1991.

[57] Viola, P. A., *Alignment by Maximization of Mutual Information*, Tech. Report AITR-1548, MIT (1995).

[58] Maes, F., A. Collignon, D. Vandermeulen, G. Marchal, and P. J. Suetens, "Multimodality image registration by maximization of mutual information," *IEEE Trans. Med. Im.* 16, no. 2, (1997), 187–198.

[59] Hill, D. L. G., P. G. Batchelor, M. Holden, and D. J. Hawkes, "Medical image registration," *Phys. Med. Biol.* 46 (2001), no. 3, R1–R45.

[60] Somayajula, S., E. Asma, and R. M. Leahy, "PET image reconstruction using anatomical information through mutual information based priors," *Conf. Rec. IEEE Nucl. Sci. Symp. and Med. Imag. Conf.* (2005) 2722–2726.

[61] Somayajula, S., A. Rangarajan, and R. M. Leahy, "PET image reconstruction using anatomical information through mutual information based priors: a scale space approach," *Proceedings ISBI 2007* (2007) 165–168.

[62] Silverman, B. W., "Algorithm AS 176: Kernel density estimation using the fast Fourier transform," *Applied Statistics* 31, no. 1, (1982), 93–99.

[63] Scott, D. W., and S. J. Sheather, "Kernel density estimation with binned data," *Statistics Theory and Methods* 14 (1985), 1353–1359.

[64] Scott, D. W., *Multivariate Density Estimation: Theory, Practice, and Visualization*, New York: Wiley, 1992.

[65] Wand, M. P., "Fast computation of multivariate kernel estimators," *Comp. Graph. Stat.* 3 (1994), 433–445.

CHAPTER 6
Diffuse Optical Spectroscopy with Magnetic Resonance Imaging

Colin M. Carpenter and Brian W. Pogue

6.1 Introduction

Magnetic resonance imaging (MRI) has arguably the most potential of any medical imaging modality because it is uniquely sensitive not only to macroscopic and microscopic tissue structures but also to certain tissue functions and molecular species. Its volumetric data-capture approach allows submillimeter resolution images to be resolved in arbitrary geometries. An additional benefit is that it does not use ionizing radiation. Intrinsic properties such as proton density, spin-lattice relaxation time, spin-spin relaxation time, molecular diffusion and perfusion, magnetic susceptibility, and chemical shift can be probed by spatially and temporally adjusting magnetic fields applied to the tissue, and there has been widespread adoption and use in high-risk disease diagnosis. In terms of visualizing tissue contrast, there is no equivalent instrument in medical imaging [1], and the only major limitations for expanded use are cost and problems with patient claustrophobia.

However, because of its sensitivity to the many factors that influence the magnetic field, it is difficult to quantify certain tissue constituents obtained from MRI. MRI tissue contrast is affected not only by the molecular magnetic moment distributions quantified by some of the previously mentioned parameters but also by the heterogeneous environment. Magnetic heterogeneity is affected by the surroundings, including external radio frequency (RF) fields, nonuniformity in the MRI coils, and interactions from adjacent tissue. Additionally, data acquisition and image reconstruction from k-space can all add to unaccountable variations in the image produced by the MRI. These external influences can complicate the accurate quantification of tissue properties, which is helpful in monitoring long-term changes in the human body and comparing imaging results between cases.

Yet, the shortcomings of MRI in measuring tissue properties, especially hemodynamics, offer opportunities that may be satisfied with information provided by diffuse optical spectroscopic (DOS) imaging with near-infrared (NIR) light. DOS imaging is uniquely sensitive to tissue hemodynamics, and it offers the ability to quantify hemoglobin, water, lipid, and tissue microstructure, as well as recent advances demonstrating its ability to image fluorescent molecules. It may provide essential validation data to help determine what MRI contrast can be detected and quantified.

The rationale for considering DOS within MRI can be stated from several perspectives. MRI is an expensive modality as the high cost of continuously running a superconducting high-field magnet, as well as the cost of the expertise required to run the clinical exams, can be prohibitive for many locations. However, since the installation of an MR system is a long-term investment on the part of a hospital, there would be significant added value in plugging in additional devices to the MR that provide increased specificity of diagnosis or staging. Additionally, in many cases, subjects are not eligible for MRI, such as infants, subjects with metal embedded in their bodies, or subjects who cannot remain motionless. In these cases, MRI might be used sparingly, and these exams could be supplemented with DOS or other, less-intrusive methods. Additionally, coupling DOS with MRI may provide a way to track responses and changes in tissue longitudinally over many days and weeks since MRI costs are high, and the exams must be restricted to a limited number. Yet, DOS is comparatively less expensive and could be applied in a repeated manner if daily or weekly monitoring were important to track disease progression or response to therapy.

6.2 Anatomical Imaging

DOS imaging can be coupled with a high-resolution imaging modality to avoid the resolution problems that limit the value of NIR tomographic imaging caused by the high scattering nature of biological tissue in the near-infrared regime. High spatial-resolution modalities such as ultrasound [2, 3], X-ray computed tomography [4], and magnetic resonance imaging have all been used to increase the low-resolution limitations of NIR imaging. Although each modality has its benefits and shortcomings, MRI offers seemingly the greatest advantage in fusing with optical because of the high soft-tissue contrast and its volumetric nature. It also offers functional imaging, which has only recently begun to be added to NIR imaging to study hemodynamics.

Studies of MRI/optical integration can be roughly subdivided into two approaches: (1) coregistration studies between MR and optical imaging for validation or mutual information analysis, and (2) use of MR-derived prior information to synergistically improve the information from optical imaging. Both approaches are needed, as correlations between MRI and optical will help determine what information from MR can be used to improve optical images, and both provide noninvasive and nonionizing assessment of tissue, which can be used to study tissue physiology. In the latter approach, MR structural images have been shown to drastically improve the quantification of optical imaging when imaging deep tissue, as is discussed in the sections below.

Using MR structural data in optical imaging typically involves collecting T1-weighted spin-echo or gradient-echo MR images, which are coregistered with the optical instrument through radiological fiducial markers. The MR image may then be segmented into different tissue types. For breast imaging, adipose (fat), fibroglandular (parenchyma + stroma), and suspect lesions can be segmented from the MR scans. For brain imaging, the MR-derived domain can be segmented into skin, skull, gray and white matter, and CSF tissue volumes for more accurate recovery of measured optical signals.

Both T1- and T2-weighted MR images show contrast between vascular tissue and fatty tissue. T1 contrast depends on the dissipation of energy from the aligned protons to the surrounding lattice, whereas T2 contrast arises from the loss in transverse magnetization due to spin dephasing from random interactions with surrounding molecules. Another factor that affects the transverse relaxation is T2* contrast, which results from magnetic susceptibility differences in the tissue [5]. Since vascular tissue contains more blood than fatty tissue, it is a reasonable assumption that optical contrast of hemoglobin and water is correlated to vascular tissue identified by MR. Correlations between structural MR imaging and optical imaging are difficult at high resolution since the spatial resolution of optical imaging can be an order of magnitude lower than MRI. However, several studies have shown spatial correlation in hemoglobin [6–8] and similar trends in water content [9].

Suspicious lesions are best detected and characterized in the MR by dynamic contrast-enhanced MRI (DCE-MRI), a ubiquitous tool in clinical breast imaging. In practice, a paramagnetic contrast agent, a gadolinium chelate (Gd), is injected with an automated injector pump through an intravenous catheter during the series of MR imaging scans. The Gd collects in tumors because of the abnormal vasculature, distinguished by tortuousity and leakiness. The Gd shortens the T1 relaxation of water protons and thus provides positive contrast. Suspect lesions can be identified by either subtracting a postcontrast image from a precontrast image or by more sophisticated methods, such as examining contrast washout kinetics. Most systems utilize software that interprets the wash-in and washout contrast and estimates the malignancy potential of all voxels throughout the image. To delineate from cysts or benign fibroadenomas, a T2-weighted image is usually taken, which identifies fluid-dominated regions [10]. Fat suppression is often used to increase the contrast between fat and tumor tissue [11]. Although these methods have been shown in multicenter clinical trials to be extremely effective in the detection of abnormalities (upwards of 88%), their specificity to malignant tumors is modest (around 67%), even with expert analysis [10–12].

Because of the lack of specificity in breast MR tumor characterization, optically coupled MRI exams are being investigated to determine if optical contrasts can offer alternative information that may help in diagnosis of the lesion. Increased hemoglobin concentration and decreased oxygen saturation have been identified as statistically significant indicators of malignant breast lesions in the optical imaging community with stand-alone optical methods [3, 13–16]. Hemoglobin was found to be most significant when lesion size was beyond the approximately 6 mm resolution of NIR imaging in deep tissue [17]. It is thought that with the added resolution of MR, optical imaging would be even more useful for characterizing breast lesions. Ntziachristos et al. noted trends between increased hemoglobin and lower oxygenation in malignant tumors with higher spatial accuracy with MR-guided optical imaging [18]. Carpenter et al. noted not only increased hemoglobin and decreased oxygenation in tumor tissue but also increased water and increased average particle size and density with MR-guided optical imaging [19]. Another such case is shown in Color Plate 14. In this case, the data from a patient with a 1.1 cm tumor in the plane of the optical fibers was reconstructed. Increases in total hemoglobin and water content, as well as contrast in scatter size and number density, are observed that correlate well with the tumor location.

Studies by Gulsen et al. [20] and Xu et al. [8] recovered optical properties in small animals with MR guidance. Gulsen et al. confirmed an anticipated increase in optical properties in the tumor tissue; Xu et al. confirmed anticipated changes in optically recovered tissue oxygen saturation and hemoglobin concentration due to inspired O_2 and demonstrated correlation between DOS-estimated deoxyhemoglobin and MR-measured blood-oxygen-level-dependent (BOLD) signal.

6.3 Combining Hemodynamic Measures of MRI and Optical Imaging

There have been nearly two decades of innovation in MRI sequences that elucidate hemodynamic function in tissue, and there is a complex relationship between this and the information from NIR light. Imaging of tissue hemodynamics has provided information about tumor growth and treatment, as well as neurological response to stimuli, among other areas. DOS and MRI both provide measures related to total hemoglobin, oxygen saturation, blood volume, and blood flow, albeit with a complex set of accuracies and covariances. Since each system has a certain level of uncertainty about the true linearity of correlation to the vascular signal, comparing them can provide a critical level of validation in certain applications. Most investigations involving both DOS imaging and functional MRI (fMRI) have involved functional brain activation.

Blood-oxygen-level-dependent (BOLD) MRI imaging was one of the early functional sequences that was designed to map oxygen consumption in the brain. BOLD enhances the contrast caused by the magnetic susceptibility difference between diamagnetic oxyhemoglobin and paramagnetic deoxyhemoglobin [21, 22]. These susceptibility differences influence phase coherence of protons in the surrounding tissue. In BOLD imaging, the rate of loss of molecular phase coherence, $R2^*$ is increased, and signal drops in regions with decreased oxygen saturation. The BOLD contrast is commonly used in fMRI studies, which enable the imaging of the neurophysiological response of the brain to physical and visual stimulations, although it can also be used to study other vasculature [23]. Since optical imaging is also sensitive to these hemodynamics, it may also be used to study functional brain activation and tissue vasculature.

These two modalities are sensitive to different vascular tissue: while the BOLD signal arises from deoxygenated blood from a mix of large and small vessels, NIR contrast is derived from both the oxygenated and deoxygenated blood contained in smaller vessels that make up the capillary bed [24]. Although BOLD is intrinsically sensitive to all sizes of vessels [25], the BOLD signal is dominated by larger draining vessels [6, 26, 27], especially large venous vasculature, which has a larger percentage of deoxygenated blood than arterial vasculature, although spin-echo BOLD is more sensitive to microvasculature than gradient-echo BOLD. Optical imaging adds to hemodynamic information content because it is also sensitive to oxyhemoglobin and thus to arterial vasculature.

NIR imaging may add to BOLD in its ability to quantify oxy- and deoxyhemoglobin in an absolute sense [28–30], as BOLD models that quantify hemoglobin can be inaccurate, especially in tumor tissue [31]. Quantifying oxygenation with BOLD is more difficult because of the many parameters that contribute to the BOLD signal, including not only deoxyhemoglobin concentration but also hematocrit, blood volume, blood flow and tissue pH [31]. Therefore, in most BOLD studies, relative signal changes from baseline are measured.

Hemoglobin species are modeled in optical imaging by a linear system that maps the optical absorption coefficients at multiple wavelengths to chromophore concentrations. The transformation is given by

$$C = \sum_{i=1}^{nwv} \frac{\mu_a(\lambda_i)}{\varepsilon(\lambda_i, C)} \qquad (6.1)$$

where μ_a represents the absorption coefficients in tissue that are dependent on wavelength (λ), and ε represents well-known [32, 33] molar extinction coefficients that quantify the absorption of tissue components (C_i) per wavelength. Thus, optical imaging may provide more accurate quantification of tumor hemodynamics [34]. Indeed, DOS quantification has been verified by comparing oxygenation to an external chemical probe [28–30, 35]. However, optical imaging alone has limited spatial resolution as compared to fMRI and sacrifices accuracy with increasing depth [25]. Therefore, the combination of these modalities seems advantageous.

In order to establish the correlation between the two modalities, several studies have simultaneously examined optical imaging and fMRI in both the small-animal brain [7, 8] and human brain [6, 24, 36]. Studies showed similar trends between oxyhemoglobin measured by optical means and BOLD signal [8, 37, 38]. Siegel et al. [38] also found a temporal correlation between optically measured total hemoglobin (HbT) and MRI-measured cerebral plasma volume (CPV). Other studies, which have investigated the temporal and spatial correlations in more depth, reveal more similarities between the two modalities.

Kennerley et al. [7] examined simultaneous fMRI and optical imaging/laser Dopplar flowmetry in a rodent by measuring the hemodynamic response to stimulation of the whisker pad and to hypercapnic challenge. Four wavelengths of light in the green/yellow spectrum were measured sequentially with an optical-fiber bundle through a transparent window in the skull by a CCD camera. This surface image was projected into a volume image by Monte Carlo simulation, and hemodynamic parameters were quantified by measuring changes in optical absorption and multiplying these by the blood volume measured in the MRI via contrast injection. Good spatial correlation was found in the superficial cortex, although the correlation decreased with depth because of the depth limitations of optical imaging in the remittance geometry. In their study, the temporal response of the optical imaging system (~8 Hz) was faster in quantifying cerebral blood volume (CBV) and cerebral blood flow (CBF) than fMRI. Because of this temporal limitation in the MRI, an initial dip in deoxyhemoglobin upon functional activation was seen by optical methods but not by MR. This dip may correspond to changes in blood pressure or respiratory effects [6].

In the human brain, several studies have correlated BOLD MRI signal to optical hemodynamic measures, both spatially and temporally. Zhang et al. [36] and Toronov et al. [24] compared signal changes from BOLD MRI to changes in oxy- and deoxyhemoglobin with multiple fiber bundles that guided NIR light to the adult head. A Monte Carlo forward model was used along with a perturbative iterative inversion routine that constrained the solution to voxels that changed by more than 5%. They found good spatial and temporal correlation between the BOLD MRI and optical measures, observed 6 seconds after a visual paradigm, although oxyhemoglobin was found to temporally correlate more significantly. Outside these regions of BOLD signal increase, there was no significant correlation with optical changes.

Huppert et al. [6] examined the spatiotemporal correlation between BOLD MRI, NIR optical imaging, and arterial-spin-labeling (ASL) MRI in the human brain of 11 healthy subjects. In this study, fMRI data was transformed into optical data by incorporating the sensitivity of the optical instrumentation into the BOLD measurement. A similar method was proposed by Sassaroli et al. [39]. Figure 6.1 shows results comparing deoxyhemoglobin measured via BOLD and by optical methods. Correlations between BOLD and optical measurements agree in general with the findings of Toronov et al. [24] and Zhang et al. [36]. However, Huppert et al. found better spatial correlation with deoxyhemoglobin, whereas Toronov et al. and Zhang et al. found better spatial correlation with oxygenated hemoglobin. Sassaroli et al. found equal spatial correlations for both species of hemoglobin. All groups showed good temporal correlation between hemodynamics measured with optical and BOLD. ASL and optically measured hemodynamics correlated spatially and temporally most accurately to oxyhemoglobin.

Hemodynamics have been studied in tumor vasculature in the MR, and changes in tumor oxygenation, blood volume, and/or blood flow have been detected in small animal model [40], brain [41], and breast [42, 43] tumors. However, to date, hemodynamic studies of tumors involving both optical and MR imaging have been very limited. Xu et al. [8] found a strong correlation between R_2^* and optically mea-

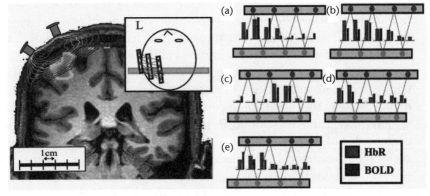

Figure 6.1 (Left) Optical sensitivity profile overlaid on an anatomical MR image. The profile is plotted in logarithmic scale, and contours indicate light-intensity changes of an order of magnitude. (Right) Temporal comparison of measured optical deoxyhemoglobin and projected BOLD response for nearest-neighbor source-detector optical probe pairs on five subjects, (a–e). (Courtesy of Huppert et al. [6]. Reproduced with permission by the SPIE, the International Society for Optical Imaging.)

sured deoxyhemoglobin. Tumor blood volume and blood flow estimates from MR and optical have yet to be compared.

Quantification of hemodynamics to study functional activation of the brain with MR has not yet been fully developed. This omission is not surprising since the source of contrast in fMRI is not sufficiently well understood to allow for accurate quantification of blood oxygen [31], although literature has been devoted to the quantification of oxygen concentration with BOLD (quantitative BOLD) [27, 44]. Absolute quantification of CBV in the human brain was successfully measured in the MR during functional activation with a Gd-DTPA contrast agent using a vascular-space-occupancy (VASO) MRI sequence [45]. Accurate quantification of oxy- and deoxyhemoglobin concentration may be improved by optical imaging, especially with the aid of spatial and or functional guidance from MRI [46–48].

6.4 MRI-Guided Optical Imaging Reconstruction Techniques

It is feasible to utilize the MR information in a manner that assists optical imaging by applying prior structural information to NIR spectral recovery. As with any multimodality technique, care must be taken regarding how much mutual information will be used in the image-reconstruction process. At the very least, MR images may be used to improve NIR image reconstruction by providing accurate tissue boundaries, which improve the accuracy of the boundary conditions [49]. Since the diffusion modeling of light often uses an assumption of an isotropic source that has propagated into the interior, proper boundary conditions can be critical to obtaining accurate solutions of the light field [50]. If it is assumed that MR T1-weighted contrast correlates well to optical contrasts, MR images may provide knowledge about internal tissue boundaries via image segmentation. Through the use of MR contrast agents, MR may also provide knowledge about suspect lesions.

Errors in segmentation of tissue types can cause errors in optically measured tissue properties, although Carpenter et al. [51] showed in simulation that the appropriate choice in image-reconstruction technique can limit errors in segmentation from 50% to less than 15%. Boverman et al. [52] showed that even using incorrectly segmented tissue will offer improvements in optical-property recovery over no structural information.

The best way to use MR-provided information is an ongoing topic of investigation. Because soft breast tissue is easily deformed when optical fibers contact the tissue, tissue boundaries cannot be perfectly modeled by any regular geometry. Using a 3D camera to create a 3D mesh of a patient breast, Dehghani et al. [53] compared reconstruction results using a conical mesh, a nondeformed patient mesh, and an accurately deformed patient mesh. They showed that a more accurate breast shape reduces artifacts in image reconstruction and provides more accurate recovery of optical properties. Even without highly deformable tissue, the MR may still provide useful information about the locations of optical probes, which is critical to minimizing model errors [54, 55]. Zhang et al. [36] improved fiber localization by using high-resolution T1-weighted images (voxel size $0.5 \times 0.5 \times 1.0$ mm), termed *probe localizers*, to ensure accurate placement of the probes.

Fibroglandular, adipose, and suspect-lesion tissue boundaries have been incorporated into image reconstruction; these algorithms essentially guide how the image is updated during the inversion process. The many different approaches that have been used to include the spatial a priori information into image reconstruction can be separated in two main categories, so-called hard and soft priors. These approaches differ in the amount of certainty in the correlation between MR and NIR contrast. Figure 6.2 demonstrates the results between using hard and soft priors to reconstruct optical images.

Hard priors constrain optical properties to update independently in each MR-defined domain. These methods enforce MR boundaries. Thus, hard prior methods assume that more correlation exists between MR and optical contrast than do soft prior methods. These algorithms have been implemented in a number of ways. Yalavarthy et al. [56], in a breast geometry, assumed that each segmented tissue type (adipose, fibroglandular, and lesion) was homogenous in the reconstruction and recovered simulated physiological properties within 3%, even with very noisy data. Brooksby et al. [57] reconstructed a homogenous adipose region but allowed unknowns to update independently on a finer-resolution-pixel basis in the fibroglandular region, which was assumed to contain the lesion. They found increased accuracy in a simulated breast domain. Schweiger and Arridge [58] used a two-step procedure in the image reconstruction of a simulated human head by first reconstructing the domain into homogeneous regions of skin, bone, gray matter, and white matter, then inserting these optical-property distributions as the initial guess for a finer-resolution reconstruction. Boas et al. [48] simulated functional brain activation and forced the optical properties to update from the initial guess only in the cortex. They found that this approach improved reconstruction accuracy, although the accuracy was limited at depth. Pogue et al. applied a similar algorithm to tissue phantoms [59] and a rat brain and recovered optical properties to within 10% [60].

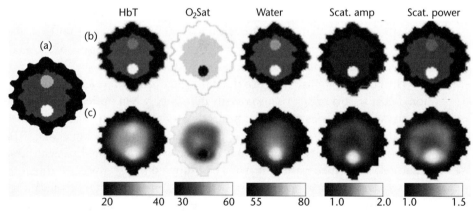

Figure 6.2 Comparison of optical-reconstruction methods that incorporate MR-derived anatomical priors. (a) Segmented tissue types as identified by MR. The upper circle is a simulated benign lesion, and the lower circle is a simulated malignant lesion. (b) Hard priors implemented in the reconstruction algorithm. Note the homogeneity of each region. (c) Soft prior reconstruction. Note the smoothing across the boundaries due to anatomical constraints implemented in the regularization of the inverse problem.

Structural MR images can alternatively be used as soft priors, which, instead of forcing optical-property boundaries to coincide with MR-defined boundaries, spatially influence the update in the optical properties from the background during the inversion. These have been implemented both approximately and statistically. Algorithms that incorporate soft priors allow changes across boundaries, reducing the error for improper segmentation [52]. Barbour et al. [61, 62] demonstrated an algorithm that assigned optical properties taken from literature to segmented adipose and fibroglandular tissues. They then simulated small lesions within the fibroglandular tissue and reconstructed the domain. They found accurate spatial and quantitative recovery, as long as the simulated lesion was a small perturbation in optical properties from the background. Brooksby et al. [54] and Yalavarthy et al. [63] incorporated smoothing operators within each tissue type in the regularization during inversion. This method was found to yield accurate recovery of hemoglobin in phantoms to within 10% [64] and was used for the group's clinical breast MR-optical studies [9, 19].

Intes et al. [47] and Guven et al. [65] incorporated structural priors in the inversion statistically through a Bayesian framework. The algorithm penalized optical-property updates across boundaries and allowed for increased contrast to be recovered in regions where a lesion was thought to exist. Optical-property recovery in simulation was accurate to within 15%, even when MR did not specify a tumor region of interest.

6.5 Other MR-Derived Contrast and Optical Imaging

It is clear that MR and optical imaging can resolve more than just hemodynamic and structural changes. MR can quantify fat and water due to the difference in the resonant frequency of the protons [66, 67]. Values of fat and water may be compared with optical imaging to compare the contrast mechanisms. This has been accomplished with high correlation in phantoms [68] but has yet to be studied in tissue. This study may be difficult in deep tissue as current state-of-the-art detection technology has limited efficiency with wavelengths most sensitive to fat and water. If the measures are found to be strongly correlated, fat and water information may aid in optical quantification in deep tissue. Assuming that they did correlate, Li et al. [69] developed a framework to incorporate water and fat priors into the optical reconstruction through a maximum a posteriori framework to recover accurate properties in simulated data.

Optical imaging is sensitive to photon scatter, which arises from changes in the index of refraction of the microscopic organelles and tissue structures. With appropriate assumptions, particle size and number density may be recovered in deep tissue [70]. The quantification of scatter may aid in tumor-tissue characterization [19, 71]. Quantification in number density may correlate to diffusion-weighted MR imaging (DWI) because DWI is highly sensitive to tissue packing density [72].

Beyond MR and optical static data, dynamic changes may aid in the characterization of tissue function and structure. Diamond et al. [46] extended the incorporation of priors in optical imaging to include dynamic changes in blood pressure and heart rate through a state-space model in simulated adult-brain images. Dynamic changes elucidated by optical [73] and MR imaging will be an important next step in tissue imaging.

6.6 Hardware Challenges to Merging Optical and MRI

Operation of high-precision optical devices in a high magnetic field creates complications in instrumentation, space constraints, and uniformity of the magnetic field.

Typically, optical instrumentation operates in the control room outside the MRI, and long optical fibers enter the room through a magnetically shielded conduit. Thus, fibers can be expensive and are more prone to damage. Limitations in space from the size of the bore and the size of the MR coil prevent ideal optical interfaces. Because metal components create artifacts and potential safety hazards in the MRI, positioning equipment for optical components must be constructed from nonmagnetic materials, such as plastic. Even diamagnetic metals such as brass will distort the magnetic field due to eddy currents in the material. However, metal is superior to plastic in resistance to wear and precision in manufacturing. If these materials are to be used, they should be kept well away from the imaging domain. Care also must be taken in the design of optical-fiber interfaces, which may create imaging artifacts because of the magnetic susceptibility difference between the interface and the subject. Time constraints also pose challenges of simultaneously operating these two modalities, especially in humans, as some of the limited available clinical imaging time must be devoted to accurate optical positioning. Figure 6.3

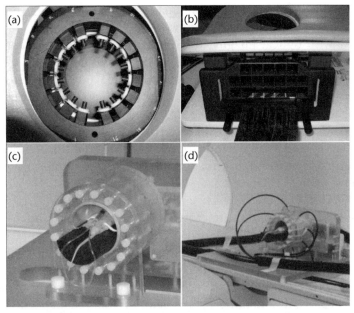

Figure 6.3 Optical/MR multimodality instruments. (a, b) Commercial MR breast coil integrated with (a) circular fiber interface for breast imaging with simulated object overlaid, or (b) slab geometry fiber interface for transmission and remission breast imaging. (c) Customized small-animal MR/optical coil, and (d) experimental setup in a full-body MR bore [75].

shows several different implementations of optical imaging systems that operate concurrently in the MR.

6.7 Optical/MR Contrast Agents

In addition to the intrinsic contrast that may be examined with optical imaging, contrast agents are realizing greater use in the biomedical optics community because of the increased contrast possible. Furthermore, contrast washout dynamics may yield information about the function and pathology of tissue. Since fluorescent agents can be selectively excited and subsequently identified by their spectral signature, they may offer increased flexibility, sensitivity, and specificity compared to MRI contrast agents, where crosstalk in magnetic contrast is more severe. Also, the field of fluorescent agents is massive compared to MRI contrast agents. However, lack of resolution in deep tissue will still limit the localization and quantification of fluorescent agents unless they are combined with a high-resolution modality such as MRI [74, 75]. This resolution limitation and the desire to correlate contrast agents with several modalities has led to investigations that inject both optical and MR contrast agents, as well as to the development of joint optical/MR agents, which are generally in preclinical use [76–78].

Optical and MR contrast agents may be injected sequentially or bound and injected simultaneously. Optical contrast agents are either nonspecific and gather in tumors, similar to Gd-DTPA, or are tagged to pathological or functional markers and injected into the vasculature. Contrast enhancement was shown to be spatially similar between indocyanine green (ICG) optical and Gd-DTPA MR contrast in breast tumors. Corlu et al. [79] demonstrated similar spatial localization in breast tissue between Gd-DTPA MR contrast and ICG fluorescence, and Ntziachristos et al. [55] showed spatial correlation from simultaneous imaging of MR Gd-DTPA and ICG absorption. Cuccia et al. [80] compared the pharmacokinetics of two optical contrast agents, ICG and methylene blue, in rat tumors and showed spatial correlation to Gd MR enhancement. Because of the similar spatial localization between MR and optical contrasts, a preliminary study by Davis et al. [75] used MR structural information to better quantify fluorescence yield in an epithelial growth-factor-receptor-targeted fluorescent probe in U-251 brain tumor models in mice.

Bimodality agents that bind to receptors that are overexpressed in tumors have been studied both in vitro and in vivo. Larson et al. [81] bound nanoparticles to epidermal growth factor receptors that were specific to breast cancer cells (MDA-MB-468) in vitro. Xu et al. [76] found specificity to ovarian tumors in mice in vivo with a fluorescently labeled avadin bound to a biotin-gadolinium(III) dendrimer molecule. Melancon et al. [77] found higher sensitivity with optical contrast agents than with MR contrast agents by binding a Gd-DTPA molecule to poly-L-glutamic acid and an NIR813 dye used for tagging cancerous lymph nodes in mice bearing human oral squamous-cell carcinomas (DM14). Color Plate 15 shows a comparison of the two modalities. This study found that at a dose of 0.002 mmol of Gd/kg, brachial lymph nodes were not detected by MR but were reliably visualized with optical fluorescence. By combining high spatial localization of MR contrast agents with the advantages of optical contrast, abundant opportunities exist to identify potential biomarkers.

6.8 Outlook for MR-Optical Imaging

Intrinsic optical imaging combined with MR has two main potential uses: as a clinical tool to help determine function or pathology and as a research tool to further the understanding of MR contrast. Its future depends on the extent to which MR contrasts can be accurately quantified. The field of MR is growing at a fast rate, and advances in the understanding of its contrast will continue. If BOLD contrast is able to quantify hemodynamics in tumors, optical imaging of hemodynamics in deep tissue may be short-lived. However, the future of optical contrast agents seems to be much more promising. Using MR to provide a map onto which fluorescent markers may be imaged has the potential to be a revolutionary multimodality tool, both in research and in the clinic.

References

[1] Liang, Z., and P. Lauterbur, *Principles of magnetic resonance imaging: A signal processing perspective.* IEEE Press Series in Biomedical Engineering. New York: IEEE Press, 2000.

[2] Zhu, Q., N. Chen, and S. H. Kurtzman, "Imaging tumor angiogenesis by use of combined near-infrared diffusive light and ultrasound." *Opt. Lett.* 28(5) (2003): 337–339.

[3] Zhu, Q., et al., "Benign versus malignant breast masses: Optical differentiation with US-guided optical imaging reconstruction." *Radiology* 237(1) (2005): 57–66.

[4] Zhang, Q., et al., "Coregistered tomographic X-ray and optical breast imaging: Initial results." *J. Biomed. Opt.* 10(2) (2005): 024033.

[5] Bushberg, J., et al., *The essential physics of medical imaging.* 2nd ed. Philadelphia: Lippincott Williams & Wilkins, 2002.

[6] Huppert, T., et al., "Quantitative spatial comparison of diffuse optical imaging with blood oxygen level–dependent and arterial spin labeling–based functional magnetic resonance imaging." *J. Biomed. Opt.* 11(6) (2006): 064018.

[7] Kennerley, A., et al., "Concurrent fMRI and optical measures for the investigation of the hemodynamic response function." *Mag. Res. Med.* 54 (2005): 354–365.

[8] Xu, H., et al., "Magnetic resonance imaging–coupled broadband near-infrared tomography system for small animal brain studies." *Appl. Opt.* 44(10) (2005): 2177–2188.

[9] Brooksby, B., et al., "Imaging breast adipose and fibroglandular tissue molecular signatures using hybrid MRI-guided near-infrared spectral tomography." *Proc. Natl. Acad. Sci. USA* 103 (2006): 8828–8833.

[10] Kuhl, C., "The current status of breast MR imaging Part I: Choice of technique, image interpretation, diagnostic accuracy, and transfer to clinical practice." *Radiology* 244(2) (2007): 672–691.

[11] Orel, S. G., and M. Schnall, "MR imaging of the breast for detection, diagnosis, and staging of breast cancer." *Radiology* 220 (2001): 13–30.

[12] Bluemke, D., et al., "Magnetic resonance imaging of the breast prior to biopsy." *JAMA* 292(22) (2004): 2735–2742.

[13] Chance, B., et al., "Breast cancer detection based on incremental biochemical and physiological properties of breast cancers: A six-year, two-site study." *Acad. Radiol.* 12(8) (2005): 925–933.

[14] Intes, X., "Time-domain optical mammography SoftScan initial results." *Acad. Radiol.* 12(8) (2005): 934–947.

[15] Fantini, S., et al., "Spatial and spectral information in optical mammography." *Technol. Canc. Res. Treat.* 4(5) (2005): 471–482.

[16] Cerussi, A., et al., "In vivo absorption, scattering, and physiologic properties of 58 malignant breast tumors determined by broadband diffuse optical spectroscopy." *J. Biomed. Opt.* 11(4) (2006): 044005.

[17] Poplack, S. P., et al., "Electromagnetic breast imaging: Results of a pilot study in women with abnormal mammograms." *Radiology* 243(2) (2007): 350–359.

[18] Ntziachristos, V., et al., "MRI-guided diffuse optical spectroscopy of malignant and benign breast lesions." *Neoplasia* 4(4) (2002): 347–354.

[19] Carpenter, C. M., et al., "Image-guided spectroscopy provides molecular-specific information in vivo: MRI-guided spectroscopy of breast cancer hemoglobin, water, and scatterer size." *Opt. Lett.* 32(8) (2007): 933–935.

[20] Gulsen, G., et al., "Combined diffuse optical tomography (DOT) and MRI system for cancer imaging in small animals." *Technol. Canc. Res. Treat.* 5(4) (2006): 351–363.

[21] Ogawa, S., et al., "Brain magnetic resonance imaging with contrast dependent on blood oxygenation." *PNAS* 87 (1990): 9868–9872.

[22] Frahm, J., et al., "Dynamic imaging of human brain oxygenation during rest and photic-stimulation." *JMRI* 2(5) (1992): 501–505.

[23] Howe, F., et al., "Issues in flow and oxygenation dependent contrast (FLOOD) imaging of tumors." *NMR Biomed.* 14 (2001): 497–506.

[24] Toronov, V., X. Zhang, and A. Webb, "A spatial and temporal comparison of hemodynamic signals measured using optical and functional magnetic resonance imaging during activation in the human primary visual cortex." *NeuroImage* 34(3) (2007): 1136–1148.

[25] Dunn, J. F., et al., "BOLD MRI vs. NIR spectrophotometry: Will the best technique come forward?" *Adv. Exper. Med. Biol.* 454 (1998): 103–113.

[26] Boxerman, J., et al., "The intravascular contributions of fMRI signal change: Monte Carlo modeling and diffusion-weighted studies." *Mag. Res. Med.* 34 (1995): 4–10.

[27] He, X., and D. Yablonskiy, "Quantitative BOLD: Mapping of human cerebral deoxygenated blood volume and oxygen extraction fraction: Default state." *Mag. Res. Med.* 57 (2007): 115–126.

[28] Kurth, C. D., et al., "A dynamic phantom brain model for near-infrared spectroscopy." *Phys. Med. Biol.* 40(12) (1995): 2079–2092.

[29] Holzschuh, M., et al., "Dynamic changes of cerebral oxygenation measured by brain tissue oxygen pressure and near infrared spectroscopy." *Neurolog. Res.* 19 (1997).

[30] Quaresima, V., et al., "Oxidation and reduction of cytochrome oxidase in the neonatal brain observed by in vivo near-infrared spectroscopy." *Biochim. Biophys. Acta* 1366(3) (1998): 291–300.

[31] Baudelet, C., and B. Gallez, "Current issues in the utility of blood oxygen level–dependent MRI for the assessment of modulations in tumor oxygenation." *Curr. Med. Imag. Rev.* 1(3) (2005).

[32] Prahl, S. A., Oregon Medical Laser Center Web site.

[33] Eker, C., *Optical characterization of tissue for medical diagnosis.* PhD thesis, Department of Physics, Lund Institute of Technology, 1999.

[34] Srinivasan, S., et al., "Developments in quantitative oxygen saturation imaging of breast tissue in vivo using multispectral near-infrared tomography." *Antiox. Redox Signal.* 9(8) (2007): 1–14.

[35] Srinivasan, S., et al., "Spectrally constrained chromophore and scattering NIR tomography improves quantification and robustness of reconstruction." *Appl. Opt.* 44(10) (2004): 1858–1869.

[36] Zhang, X., V. Toronov, and A. Webb, "Simultaneous integrated diffuse optical tomography and functional magnetic resonance imaging of the human brain." *Opt. Exp.* 13(14) (2005): 5513–5521.

[37] Chen, Y., et al., "Correlation between near-infrared spectroscopy and magnetic resonance imaging of rat brain oxygenation modulation." *Phys. Med. Biol.* 48 (2003): 417–427.

[38] Siegel, A., et al., "Temporal comparison of functional brain imaging with diffuse optical tomography and fMRI during rat forepaw stimulations." *Phys. Med. Biol.* 48 (2003): 1391–1403.

[39] Sassaroli, A., et al., "Spatially weighted BOLD signal for comparison of functional magnetic resonance imaging and near-infrared imaging of the brain." *NeuroImage* 33 (2006): 505–514.

[40] Karczmar, G., et al., "Effects of hyperoxia on T2* and resonance frequency weighted magnetic resonance images of rodent tumors." *NMR Biomed.* 7(1994): 3–11.

[41] Provenzale, J. M., et al., "Diffusion-weighted and perfusion MR imaging for brain tumor characterization and assessment of treatment response." *Radiology* 239(3) (2006): 632–649.

[42] Kuhl, C. K., et al., "Breast neoplasms: T_2^* susceptibility-contrast, first-pass perfusion MR imaging." *Radiology* 202(1) (1997): 95–97.

[43] Deliffe, J. P., et al., "Breast cancer: Regional blood flow and blood volume with magnetic-susceptibility-based MR imaging: Initial results." *Radiology* 223 (2002): 558–565.

[44] van Zijl, P., et al., "Quantitative assessment of blood flow, blood volume and blood oxygenation effects in functional magnetic resonance imaging." *Nat. Med.* 4(2) (1998): 159–167.

[45] Lu, H., et al., "Novel approach to the measurement of absolute cerebral blood volume using vascular-space-occupancy magnetic resonance imaging." *Mag. Res. Med.* 54 (2005): 1403–1411.

[46] Diamond, S., et al., "Dynamic physiological modeling for functional diffuse optical tomography." *NeuroImage* 30 (2006): 88–101.

[47] Intes, X., et al., "Diffuse optical tomography with physiological and spatial a priori constraints." *Phys. Med. Biol.* 49 (2004): N155–N163.

[48] Boas, D., and A. Dale, "Simulation study of magnetic resonance imaging–guided cortically constrained diffuse optical tomography of the human brain function." *Appl. Opt.* 44(10) (2005): 1957–1968.

[49] Li, C., et al., "Using a priori structural information from magnetic resonance imaging to investigate the feasibility of prostate diffuse optical tomography and spectroscopy: A simulation study." *Med. Phys.* 34(1) (2007): 266–274.

[50] Schweiger, M., et al., "Image reconstruction in optical tomography in the presence of coupling errors." *Appl. Opt.* 46(14) (2007): 2743–2746.

[51] Carpenter, C. M., et al., "A comparison of edge constrained optical reconstruction methods incorporating spectral and MR-derived spatial information." *Proc. SPIE* (2007): 6431.

[52] Boverman, G., et al., "Quantitative spectroscopic diffuse optical tomography of the breast guided by imperfect a priori structural information." *Phys. Med. Biol.* 50 (2005): 3941–3956.

[53] Dehghani, H., et al., "Breast deformation modeling for image reconstruction in near-infrared tomography." *Phys. Med. Biol.* 49 (2004): 1131–1145.

[54] Brooksby, B., et al., "Combining near infrared tomography and magnetic resonance imaging to study in vivo breast tissue: Implementation of a Laplacian-type regularization to incorporate MR structure." *J. Biomed. Opt.* 10(5) (2005): 050504.

[55] Ntziachristos, V., et al., "Concurrent MRI and diffuse optical tomography of breast after indocyanine green enhancement." *Proc. Natl. Acad. Sci. USA* 97(6) (2000): 2767–2772.

[56] Yalavarthy, P. K., et al., "Weight-matrix structured regularization provides optimal generalized least-squares estimate in diffuse optical tomography." *Med. Phys.* 34(6) (2007): 2085–2098.

[57] Brooksby, B., et al., "Near infrared (NIR) tomography breast image reconstruction with a priori structural information from MRI: Algorithm development for reconstructing heterogeneities." *IEEE J. STQE* 9(2) (2003): 199–209.

[58] Schweiger, M., and S. R. Arridge, "Optical tomographic reconstruction in a complex head model using a priori region boundary information." *Phys. Med. Biol.* 44(11) (1999): 2703–2721.

[59] Pogue, B. W., H. Zhu, C. Nwaigwe, T. O. McBride, U. L. Osterberg, K. D. Paulsen, and J. F. Dunn, "Hemoglobin imaging with hybrid magnetic resonance and near-infrared diffuse tomography." *Adv. Expt. Med. Biol.* 530 (2003): 215–224.

[60] Pogue, B. W., and K. D. Paulsen, "High-resolution near-infrared tomographic imaging simulations of the rat cranium by use of a priori magnetic resonance imaging structural information." *Opt. Lett.* 23(21) (1998): 1716.

[61] Barbour, R. L., et al., "MRI-guided optical tomography: Prospects and computation for a new imaging method." *IEEE Comp. Sci. Eng.* 2 (1995): 63–77.

[62] Chang, J., H. L. Graber, P. C. Koo, R. Aronson, S. S. Barbour, and R. L. Barbour, "Optical imaging of anatomical maps derived from magnetic resonance images using time-independent optical sources." *IEEE Trans. Med. Imag.* 16 (1997): 68–77.

[63] Yalavarthy, P. K., et al., "Structural information within regularization matrices improves near infrared diffuse optical tomography." *Opt. Exp.* 15(13) (2007): 8043–8058.

[64] Brooksby, B., et al., "Spectral-prior information improves near-infrared diffuse tomography more than spatial-prior." *Opt. Lett.* 30(15) (2005): 1968–1970.

[65] Guven, M., et al., "Diffuse optical tomography with a priori anatomical information." *Phys. Med. Biol.* 12 (2005): 2837–2858.

[66] Glover, G. H., and E. Schneider, "Three-point Dixon technique for true water/fat decomposition with B_0 inhomogeneity correction." *Mag. Res. Med.* 18 (1991): 371–383.

[67] Reeder, S., et al., "Multi-coil Dixon chemical species separation with an iterative least squares method." *Mag. Res. Med.* 51 (2004): 35–45.

[68] Merritt, S., et al., "Comparison of water and lipid content measurements using diffuse optical spectroscopy and MRI in emulsion phantoms." *Technol. Canc. Res. Treat.* 2(6) (2003): 563–569.

[69] Li, A., et al., "Optical linear inverse solution with multiple priors in diffuse optical tomography." *Appl. Opt.* 44(10) (2005): 1948–1956.

[70] Wang, X., et al., "Image reconstruction of effective Mie scattering parameters of breast tissue in vivo with near-infrared tomography." *J. Biomed. Opt.* 11(4) (2006): 041106.

[71] Bigio, I. R., et al., "Diagnosis of breast cancer using elastic-scattering spectroscopy: Preliminary clinical results." *J. Biomed. Opt.* 5(2) (2000): 221–228.

[72] Neil, J., "Diffusion imaging concepts for clinicians." *J. Mag. Res. Imag.* 27 (2007): 1–7.

[73] Piao, D., et al., "Instrumentation for video-rate near-infrared diffuse optical tomography." *Rev. Sci. Instr.* 76 (2005): 124301.

[74] Davis, S. C., et al., "Magnetic resonance–coupled fluorescence tomography scanner for molecular imaging." *Rev. Sci. Instr.* 79(6) (2008): 064302.

[75] Davis, S. C., et al., "Image-guided diffuse optical fluorescence tomography implemented with Laplacian-type regularization." *Opt. Exp.* 15(7) (2007): 4066–4082.

[76] Xu, H., et al., "Preparation and preliminary evaluation of a biotin-targeted, lectin-targeted, dendrimer-based probe for dual-modality magnetic resonance and fluorescence imaging." *Bioconj. Chem.* 18 (5) (2007): 1474–1482.

[77] Melancon, M., et al., "Development of a macromolecular dual-modality MR-optical imaging for sentinel lymph node mapping." *Invest. Radiol.* 42(8) (2007): 569–578.

[78] Lisy, M., et al., "Fluorescent bacterial magnetic nanoparticles as bimodal contrast agents." *Invest. Radiol.* 42(4) (2007): 235–241.

[79] Corlu, A., et al., "Three-dimensional in vivo fluorescence diffuse optical tomography of breast cancer in humans." *Opt. Exp.* 15(11) (2007): 6696–6716.

[80] Cuccia, D. J., et al., "In vivo quantification of optical contrast agent dynamics in rat tumors by use of diffuse optical spectroscopy with magnetic resonance imaging coregistration." *Appl. Opt.* 42(16) (2003): 2940–2950.

[81] Larson, T., et al., "Hybrid plasmonic magnetic resonance nanoparticles as molecular specific agents for MRI/optical imaging and photothermal therapy of cancer cells." *Nanotechnology* 18 (2007): 325101.

CHAPTER 7
Software Platforms for Integration of Diffuse Optical Imaging and Other Modalities

Fred S. Azar

7.1 Introduction

7.1.1 A Platform for Diffuse Optical Tomography

Near-infrared (NIR) diffuse optical tomography (DOT) relies on functional processes and provides unique measurable parameters with potential to enhance breast-tumor-detection sensitivity and specificity. For example, several groups have demonstrated the feasibility of breast tumor characterization based on total hemoglobin concentration, blood oxygen saturation, water and lipid concentration, and scattering [1–17].

The functional information derived with DOT is complementary to structural and functional information available to conventional imaging modalities, such as magnetic resonance imaging (MRI), X-ray mammography, and ultrasound. Thus, the combination of functional data from DOT with structural/anatomical data from other imaging modalities holds potential for enhancing tumor-detection sensitivity and specificity. In order to achieve this goal of data fusion, two general approaches can be employed. The first, concurrent imaging, physically integrates the DOT system into the conventional imaging instrument; this approach derives images in the same geometry and at the same time. The second approach, nonconcurrent imaging, employs optimized stand-alone DOT devices to produce 3D images that must then be combined with those of the conventional imaging modalities via software techniques; in this case, the images are obtained at different times and often in different geometries.

Thus far, a few DOT systems have been physically integrated into conventional imaging modalities such as MRI [18–22], X-ray mammography [4], and ultrasound [8] for concurrent measurements; however, these DOT systems are often limited by the requirements of the "other" imaging modality, for example, restrictions on metallic instrumentation for MRI, hard breast compression for X-ray mammography, limited optode combinations for ultrasound (as well as MRI and X-ray), and time constraints. On the other hand, among the stand-alone DOT systems available today, only a few attempts have been made to quantitatively compare DOT images of the same breast cancer patient to those of other imaging modalities [9, 22] obtained at different times because the nonconcurrent coregistration problem presents many challenges. It is therefore desirable to develop quantitative and systematic methods for data fusion that utilize the high-quality data and versatility of the stand-alone imaging systems.

In this chapter, we describe the techniques in a novel software imaging platform required for combining nonconcurrent MRI and DOT: the Optical and Multimodal Imaging Platform for Research Assessment and Diagnosis (OMIRAD) [23–28]. The OMIRAD platform enables multimodal 3D image visualization and manipulation of data sets based on a variety of 3D-rendering techniques, and through its ability to simultaneously control multiple fields of view, OMIRAD can streamline quantitative analyses of structural and functional data. OMIRAD is the result of 4 years of work to develop and test a prototype platform specifically designed for multimodal optical-data visualization, fusion, and analysis, including the ability to share data and analysis results across several institutions. Our preliminary study takes an important step toward improved diagnosis and treatment of breast cancer patients with DOT and MRI. Coregistration combines structural and functional data from multiple modalities. Segmentation and fusion will also enable a priori structural information derived from MRI to be incorporated into the DOT reconstruction algorithms. The combined MRI/DOT data set provides information in a more useful format than the sum of the individual data sets, and we expect the platform to have a substantial impact on the standardization of diffuse optical imaging systems and, therefore, on the translation of optical imaging research prototypes into viable clinical systems. In this section, we describe the results of experiments performed in collaboration with the team of Professor Arjun G. Yodh at the University of Pennsylvania (Philadelphia, Pennsylvania) [29].

7.1.2 A Platform for Diffuse Optical Spectroscopy

Near-infrared (NIR) diffuse optical spectroscopy (DOS) may provide accurate monitoring of neoadjuvant chemotherapy of breast cancer. DOS characterizes tissue function (e.g., water, lipid, or hemoglobin concentration) and is a noninvasive and low-cost technique that may enable regular and accurate monitoring of the efficiency of drug treatments [30]. We present a 3D visualization and guidance system (HANDHELD) for handheld optical imaging devices such as DOS. The system provides a patientcentric approach, which enables more accurate longitudinal studies, 3D reconstruction of optical handheld measurements, joint analysis with other imaging modalities, and easier validation and translation into the clinic. The combined guidance system/DOS instrument becomes particularly useful for monitoring neoadjuvant chemotherapy in breast cancer patients and for longitudinal studies where measurement reproducibility is critical. The custom-built visualization and guidance system comprises a magnetic tracking device and a software platform optimized for a well-defined workflow. The use of magnetic trackers in medical imaging has become quite popular, especially in the 3D ultrasound community [31], where the objective is to provide the missing third axis of conventional 2D probes, biopsy needle tracking [31–33], or virtual clinical environments [34–37] to coregister tools with anatomical data for guiding procedures.

DOS is a noninvasive, bedside technique that quantitatively measures NIR (650 to 1,000 nm) absorption and reduced-scattering spectra [38]. Absorption spectra are used to calculate the tissue concentrations of oxygenated and reduced hemoglobin, water, and bulk lipid. DOS rapidly (e.g., in a few seconds) provides quantitative, functional information about tumor biochemical composition with a handheld probe, making it potentially desirable from a patient perspective. Measurements are acquired while the patient lies prone. The handheld DOS probe is placed on the breast and translated by hand across a region of interest (ROI). Currently, spatial locations are marked on the breast with a surgical pen. However, the best reproducibility comes when the patient positioning, ROI, and probe orientation are maintained between measurement sessions. The HANDHELD guidance system stores the ROI and probe orientation with respect to a 3D breast anatomical map. Measurement repeatability in longitudinal studies is further improved by correcting for patient movement and breathing. The system will also provide tools for coregistration of DOS results with other imaging modalities. The visualization and guidance system uses a magnetic tracking device (pciBIRD, Ascension Technology, Burlington, Vermont). In this section, we describe the results of experiments performed in collaboration with the team of Professor Bruce J. Tromberg at the Beckman Laser Institute (Irvine, California) [39].

7.2 Imaging Platform Technologies

7.2.1 Multimodal Imaging Workflow for DOT Applications

The OMIRAD platform enables multimodal integration and visualization of data from DOT and MRI. Figure 7.1 describes a typical workflow that a user may follow.

1. *Input*: The software platform accepts two types of data formats:
   - *For MRI data sets:* Digital Imaging and Communications in Medicine (DICOM), the widely accepted format [25];
   - *For DOT data sets:* Time-Resolved Optical Absorption and Scattering Tomography (TOAST), developed at University College London [40], and Near-Infrared Frequency-Domain Absorption and Scatter Tomography (NIRFAST), developed at Dartmouth College (Hanover, New Hampshire) [41], two formats used in the DOT image-reconstruction community.

   Data sets are converted into a common binary format through a user-friendly interface. Then a Patient Browser (in the Import Module shown in Figure 7.1) allows the user to select any two 3D data sets for visualization and/or registration.
2. *Visualization:* The visualization stage permits the user to inspect each data set, both through volume rendering and multiplanar reformatting (MPR) visualization, and to define the volume of interest (VOI) through morphological operations such as punching. Punching involves determining a 3D region of an object from the 2D region specified on the orthographic

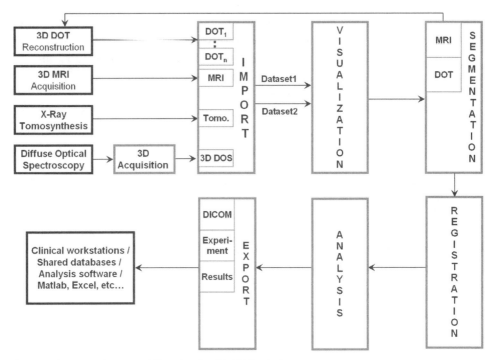

Figure 7.1 Typical user workflow for the OMIRAD platform.

projection of the same object. This 3D region can then be removed or retained. This type of operation enables easy editing of 3D structures. This is a particularly important stage, as the user removes parts of the data that should not be used in the registration process.

3. *Segmentation:* The breast MR image-segmentation technique enables a priori structural information derived from MRI to be incorporated into the reconstruction of DOT data (details are given in Section 7.2.3).

4. *Registration:* The user may decide to roughly align one volume to the other before starting the automatic registration procedure (details are given in Section 7.2.2).

5. *Analysis:* Once the registration is complete, several tools are available to the user for assessment of the results, including fused synchronized MPR and volume manipulation.

Color Plate 16 exhibits the visualization platform showing same-patient MRI and DOT (blood volume) data sets before registration. After the appropriate color-transfer functions are applied, one can clearly observe the location of the invasive ductal carcinoma diagnosed in this patient breast.

7.2.2 3D-DOT/3D-MRI Image-Registration Algorithm

3D-DOT/3D-MRI image registration presents several new challenges. Because registration of DOT to MR acquired nonconcurrently has not been extensively studied, no standard approach has been established for this problem. We present here a new approach specifically devised to address the challenges of DOT/MR image registration. DOT images have much lower anatomical resolution and contrast than MRI, and the optical-reconstruction process typically uses a geometric model of the breast. In the case of Professor Yodh's DOT device at the University of Pennsylvania, the constraining geometric model of the breast is a semiellipsoid. Also, the patient breast is compressed axially in the DOT imaging device and sagittally in the MRI machine, and, of course, the breast is a highly deformable organ. We note that this case may be considered as a "worst-case" scenario in terms of the difference in breast compression. The same registration technique may be used or extended for other breast-compression configurations.

For this task, we require that registration be automatic with little prior user interaction and robust enough to handle the majority of patient cases. In addition, the process should be computationally efficient for applicability in practice and yield results useful for combined MRI/DOT analysis.

At this time, automatic image registration is an essential component in medical imaging systems. The basic goal of intensity-based image-registration techniques is to align anatomical structures in different modalities. This is done through an optimization process, which assesses image similarity and iteratively changes the transformation of one image with respect to the other until an optimal alignment is found [42]. Computation speed is a critical issue and dictates applicability of the technology in practice. Although feature-based methods are computationally more efficient, they are notoriously dependant on the quality of the extracted features from the images [43].

In intensity-based registration, volumes are directly aligned by iteratively computing a volumetric similarity measure based on the voxel intensities. Since the number of computations per iteration is high, the overall registration process is very slow. In cases where mutual information (MI) is used, sparse sampling of volume intensity could reduce the computational complexity while compromising the accuracy [44, 45]. In [46], a projection-based method for 2D-2D image registration is proposed. In this method, the projections along the two axes of the image are computed. Horizontal and vertical components of the shift are then computed using a one-dimensional cross-correlation-based estimator. This technique is robust in the presence of temporal and spatial noise and computationally efficient compared to the 2D-correlation-based shift estimator. In [47], the authors formulate 3D-3D registration cost function as the summation of three 2D-3D optimization cost functions. The optimization is then done concurrently on the sum of the cost functions, which are identically parameterized. Furthermore, images are preprocessed to extract a binary segmentation. Projection images from the binary segmentation are used to compute similarity measures. The key is to choose a well-behaved similarity measure that can robustly characterize a metric for the volumes [48]. In order to make such an algorithm practical, the computational time must also be reduced. In [48], researchers suggest random sampling of the volume data sets and computation performance based only on these random samples in order to decrease the computational load. In [49], the authors propose a hybrid technique, which selects a set of high-interest points (i.e., landmarks) within the volume and tries to do registration based on those points only.

Let us consider two data sets to be registered to each other. One data set is considered the reference and is commonly referred to as the "fixed" data set. The other data set is the one onto which the registration transformation is applied. This data set is commonly referred to as the "moving" data set. Registration of volumetric data sets (i.e., fixed and moving) involves three steps: (1) computation of the similarity measure quantifying a metric for comparing volumes; (2) an optimization scheme, which searches through the parameter space (e.g., six-dimensional rigid body motion) in order to maximize the similarity measure; and (3) a volume-warping method, which applies the latest computed set of parameters to the original moving volume to bring it a step closer to the fixed volume.

Our proposed approach is a novel combination of the methods described in [50] and [51]: we compute 2D *projection images* from the two volumes for various *projection geometries* and set up a *similarity measure* with an optimization scheme that searches through the *parameter space*. These images are registered within a 2D space, which is a subset of the 3D space of the original registration transformations. Finally, we perform these registrations successively and iteratively in order to estimate all the registration parameters of the original problem.

We further optimize the performance of projection and 2D-2D registration similarity computation through the use of graphics processing units (GPUs). Details and general validation of this novel approach have been recently presented [52]. Multiple two-dimensional signatures (or projections) can represent the volume robustly depending on the way the signatures are generated. An easy way to understand the idea is to derive the motion of an object by looking at three perpendicular shadows of the object (see Figure 7.2).

Figure 7.3 provides an illustration of different transformation models used in medical image registration: rigid, affine, and free-form transformations. Nonrigid registration, depending on complexity, can be classified in two ways: (1) affine transformations [see Figure 7.4(c)], which include nonhomogeneous scaling and/or shearing; and (2) free-form transformations [see Figure 7.3(d)], which include arbitrary deformations at the voxel level. These transformations can be based on intensity, shape, or material properties. The dominant transformation observed across the MR and DOT data sets is due to the difference in compression axis (lateral compression for MR versus axial compression for DOT); this transformation can be modeled using affine parameters. DOT images do not possess enough local structure information for computation of a free-form deformation mapping to register a DOT to an MR data set.

Given the above challenges, we used the following parameters in the nonrigid registration algorithm:

- *Projection images:* We use maximum-intensity-projection (MIP) techniques. MIP is a computer-visualization method for 3D data that projects in the visualization plane the voxels with maximum intensity that fall in the way of parallel rays traced from the viewpoint to the plane of projection.
- *Projection geometries:* We use three mutually orthogonal 2D MIPs in order to achieve greater robustness in the registration algorithm.
- *Similarity measure:* We use normalized mutual information [48]. Mutual information measures the information that two random variables A and B

7.2 Imaging Platform Technologies

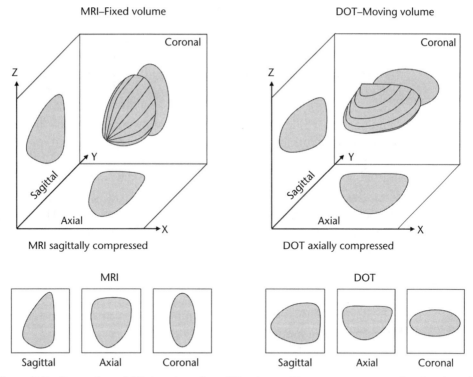

Figure 7.2 Generation of 2D signatures from 3D volumes. The arrows represent the direction of 2D projections in the three mutually orthogonal directions. (*From:* [29]. © 2007 SPIE. Reprinted with permission.)

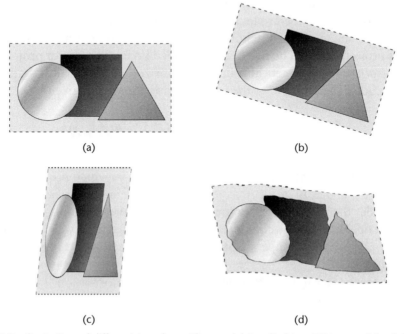

Figure 7.3 Illustration of different transformation models applied to a 2D image: (a) original image, (b) rigid transformation, (c) affine transformation, and (d) free-form transformation. (*From:* [29]. © 2007 SPIE. Reprinted with permission.)

share. It measures how knowledge of one variable reduces the uncertainty of the other. For example, if A and B are independent, then knowing A does not give any information about B and vice versa, so their normalized mutual information is zero. On the other hand, if A and B are identical, then all information given by A is shared with B; therefore, knowing A determines the value of B and vice versa, and the normalized mutual information is equal to its maximum possible value of 1. Mutual information quantifies the distance between the joint distribution of A and B from what it would be if A and B were independent. In our case, the moving data set is deformed until the normalized mutual information between it and the fixed data set is maximized.

- *Parameter space:* We use rigid body motion (translation and rotation) and independent linear scaling in all three dimensions. This results in a nine-dimensional parameter space enabling nonrigid registration: three parameters for translation in x, y, and z; three parameters for rotations about three axes; and three parameters for linear scaling in each of the x-, y-, and z-directions.

Mathematically, the estimate of the nine degrees of freedom (DOF) homogeneous transformation matrix T^9 is initially given by

$$T^9 = \arg \max_{T^9} S^3 \left(I_f, \Gamma^3_{T^9}(I_m) \right) \tag{7.1}$$

where $\Gamma^3_{T^9}$ is the six DOF mapping operator, S^3 estimates the similarity metric between two volumes, and I_f and I_m are the fixed and moving volumetric data, respectively. Both $\Gamma^3_{T^9}$ and S^3 have a superscript of three to indicate that the operations are over three dimensions. We can reformulate the registration-optimization process so it can be applied to each of the two-dimensional signatures, or projections, using the five DOF homogeneous transformation matrix defined in the plane of projection, T^5_P. The five degrees of freedom in the plane of projection correspond to horizontal and vertical translation, horizontal and vertical scaling, and in-plane rotation. The estimate of the transformation matrix is given by

$$T^5_P = \arg \max_{T^5_P} S^2 \left(\Phi_P(I_f), \Gamma^2_{T^5_P}(\Phi_P(I_m)) \right) \tag{7.2}$$

where Φ_P is an orthographic projection operator, which projects the volume points onto an image plane; P is a 4×4 homogeneous transformation matrix, which encodes the principal axis of the orthographic projection; $\Gamma^2_{T^5_P}$ is a three DOF mapping operator; and S^2 computes the similarity metric between 2D projections. Here, $\Gamma^2_{T^5_P}$ and S^2 have a superscript of two to indicate that the operations are over two dimensions.

Since the similarity metric here is mutual information [i.e., $S^2 \equiv h(A) + h(B) - h(A, B)$], (7.2) can be rewritten as

$$T^5_P = \arg \max_{T^5_P} \left[h(A) + h(B) - h(A, B) \right] \tag{7.3}$$

where $A = \Phi_P(I_f)$, $B = \Gamma^2_{T_P^S}(\Phi_P(I_m))$, $h(x)$, is the entropy of a random variable x, and $h(x, y)$ is the joint entropy of two random variables x and y.

Entropy is a measure of variability and is defined as $h(x) \equiv -\int p(x)\ln p(x)dx$, and $h(x,y) \equiv -\int \ln(p(x,y))dxdy$ [48], where $p(x)$ is the probability density function (PDF) of variable x, and $p(x,y)$ is the joint PDF of variables x and y. The entropy h is discretely computed as

$$H(I_I) = -\sum_{I=L}^{H} p_{I_I}(I)\log p_{I_I}(I) \text{ and } H(I_I, I_J) = -\sum_{I=L}^{H}\sum_{J=L}^{H} p_{I_I,I_J}(I,J)\log p_{I_I,I_J}(I,J) \quad (7.4)$$

where I_I and I_J are two given images; I and J are the intensities ranging from lower limit L (e.g., 0) to higher limit H (e.g., 255) for I_I and I_J, respectively. $p_{I_I}(I)$ is the PDF of image I_I, and $p_{I_I I_J}(I, J)$ is the joint PDF of images I_I and I_J. Here, a PDF is represented by a normalized image histogram.

Figure 7.4 shows the algorithm flowchart. Figure 7.4(a) shows the global registration flowchart. For a number of iterations n (typically $n = 3$), the three mutually orthogonal 2D signatures are generated (sagittal, coronal, and axial) for both the fixed and moving volumes. After each 2D signature generation, the moving 2D signature is registered to the fixed 2D signature. This process is shown schematically in Figure 7.4(b) and explained in detail next.

1. First, the Δ variables are initialized:
   $\Delta scale = \Delta scale\_initial; \Delta trans = \Delta trans\_initial; \Delta rot = \Delta rot\_initial$
2. Then, for step $k = 1$ to m
   a. Compute the deformation steps:

   $$\Delta scale = \frac{\Delta scale}{Divider}; \Delta trans = \frac{\Delta trans}{Divider}; \Delta rot = \frac{\Delta rot}{Divider};$$

   b. Compute the initial similarity measure $S^2_{initial}$ between the two 2D signatures.
   c. Scale moving volume vertically by $\pm\Delta scale$, then estimate $S^2_{scale-vert}$. If an improvement has been made (i.e., $S^2_{scale-vert} > S^2_{initial}$), then go to the next step; otherwise, do not apply this scaling operation.
   d. Scale moving volume horizontally by $\pm\Delta scale$, then estimate $S^2_{scale-horiz}$. If an improvement has been made (i.e., $S^2_{scale-horiz} > S^2_{scale-vert}$), then go to the next step; otherwise, do not apply this scaling operation.
   e. Translate moving volume vertically by $\pm\Delta trans$, then estimate $S^2_{transvert}$. If an improvement has been made (i.e., $S^2_{transvert} > S^2_{scale-vert}$), then go to the next step; otherwise, do not apply this translation operation.
   f. Translate moving volume horizontally by $\pm\Delta trans$, then estimate $S^2_{transhoriz}$. If an improvement has been made (i.e., $S^2_{transhoriz} > S^2_{transvert}$), then go to the next step; otherwise, do not apply this translation operation.

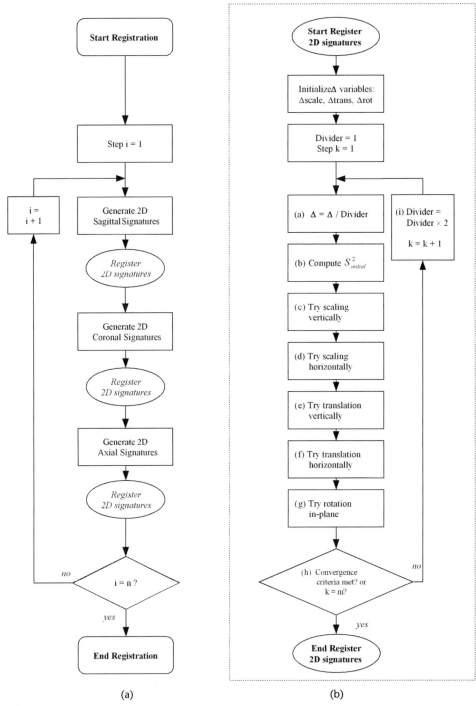

Figure 7.4 Flowcharts for the registration process: (a) global registration flowchart, and (b) 2D-signatures registration flowchart. (*From:* [29]. © 2007 SPIE. Reprinted with permission.)

g. Rotate moving volume in-plane by $\pm\Delta rot$, then estimate S^2_{rot}. If an improvement has been made (i.e., $S^2_{rot} > S^2_{transhoriz}$), then go to the next step; otherwise, do not apply this rotation operation.

h. Convergence criteria:

If $0 < |S_{rot}^2 - S_{inital}^2| \leq \Delta S^2$ or $Divider > Divider\_threshold,$ then end k-loop.

i. If no improvements have been made (i.e., $S^2_{rot} = S^2_{initial}$), then decrease the deformation steps (i.e., $Divider = Divider \times 2$).

The variables are initialized at the beginning of the registration process and are typically set to the following: $n = 3$, $m = 40$, $\Delta scale\_initial = 4$ mm, $\Delta trans\_initial = 4$ mm, $\Delta rot\_initial = 4°$, $Divider\_threshold = 40$.

7.2.3 Breast MRI Image Segmentation

Our proposed segmentation approach is based on the random walker algorithm. In this case, the segmentation technique requires little user interaction and is computationally efficient for practical applications.

This algorithm, originally developed in [53] and extended in [54] to incorporate intensity priors, can perform multilabel, semiautomated image segmentation: given a small number of pixels with user-defined labels, one can analytically (and quickly) determine the probability that a random walker starting at each unlabeled pixel will first reach one of the prelabeled pixels. By assigning each pixel to the label for which the greatest probability is calculated, high-quality image segmentation may be obtained (Figure 7.5). This algorithm is formulated in discrete space (i.e., on a graph) using combinatorial analogs of standard operators and principles from continuous potential theory, allowing it to be applied in arbitrary dimensions.

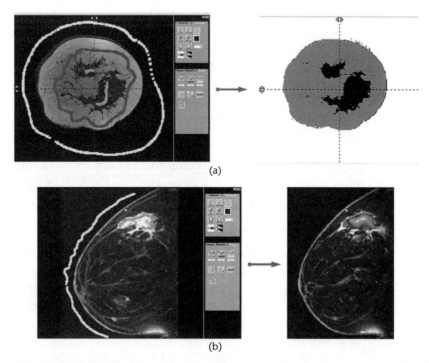

Figure 7.5 Breast MRI 3D image segmentation based on random walkers: (a) segmenting fatty from nonfatty tissue, and (b) segmenting tumor from nontumor tissue. (*From:* [29]. © 2007 SPIE. Reprinted with permission.)

Usually, T1-weighted MR imaging is performed: images show lipid as bright and parenchyma as dark. Tumor also tends to be dark. Minimal user initialization is required. We have developed a workflow customized for this type of breast MRI segmentation:

1. Using a custom-made interactive visual interface, the user scrolls through axial, sagittal, and coronal views of the MRI data set. In each view, the user selects one or two slices that best incorporate all tissue types.
2. The user draws three types of seed points using a virtual "brush" on each of the selected slices in order to indicate different tissue types: fatty tissue, nonfatty tissue (parenchyma and/or tumor), and tissue outside the breast.
3. The algorithm generates a mask file representing the result of the segmentation. Each voxel in the generated mask is assigned a value ("fatty," "nonfatty," or "outside") indicating the type of tissue.
4. The segmented mask file can finally be incorporated into a more accurate reconstruction of physiological quantities (such as THC) to generate the DOT data set.

This algorithm can be used to distinguish fatty from nonfatty tissue and tumor from nontumor tissue, as shown in Figure 7.5. Since the objective of this initial study is to show how nonconcurrent data may be registered and jointly analyzed, we should note that we did not use here the results of MRI segmentation to improve the DOT reconstructions. Rather, we used the MRI segmentation to isolate the tumor tissue in the image.

One significant advantage of spatially registering DOT to MRI data is the ability to treat anatomical information from MRI data as prior information in the DOT chromophore-concentration and scattering-variables reconstruction process. By segmenting fatty from nonfatty tissue in an MR data set, for example, we can provide a priori data about the tissue that interacts with light in a DOT imaging device. This information can further be incorporated in solving the inverse problem associated with the photon-diffusion equation and lead to a more precise reconstruction of physiological quantities (such as hemoglobin concentration).

7.2.4 Image-Based Guidance Workflow and System for DOS Applications

HANDHELD is an easy-to-use and highly interactive image-based guidance platform. We define two workflows:

1. *Reference session:* A baseline reference scan of the breast surface is performed. The shape of the surface and the position of the measurements are stored according to the following steps: (1) calibrate the magnetic sensors if necessary, (2) scan the surface of the breast (i.e., generate the reference surface), (3) acquire new measurements, and (4) store data.
2. *Current session:* The patient comes back for a follow-up scan. In order to complete measurements at the same locations as in the reference session, the physician performs the following steps: (1) calibrate sensors if necessary, (2) load reference surface and measurements, (3) scan the patient's breast again (i.e., generate the current surface), (4) align the current surface to the

reference surface and then project the reference measurements onto the current surface (these become the guiding locations for the new measurements), (5) acquire the new measurements based on the location and orientation of the reference measurements, and (6) store data.

To enable these scenarios, HANDHELD uses three magnetic sensors: (1) one sensor attached to a pointer used to scan the breast surface, (2) one sensor rigidly attached to the DOS probe used to locate measurements, and (3) one sensor securely taped to the patient chest for tracking respiration and other body movements.

- *Generation of a patient coordinate system:* Using the first sensor, a patient coordinate system is built from some easily identifiable landmarks [Color Plate 17(a)]: nipple N, sternal extremities of the left clavicle S_L and right clavicle S_R, and the xyphoid process P_X. The last three points define the orientation of the axis of the new coordinate system:

$$\vec{k} = \pm \frac{\overline{S_L P_X} \otimes \overline{S_R P_X}}{\left\| \overline{S_L P_X} \otimes \overline{S_R P_X} \right\|} \text{ and } \vec{k} \cdot \overline{P_X N} \geq 0 \quad \vec{j} = \frac{\overline{P_X S_L} + \overline{P_X S_R}}{\left\| \overline{P_X S_L} + \overline{P_X S_R} \right\|} \quad \vec{i} = \vec{j} \otimes \vec{k} \quad (7.5)$$

- *Scanning of the breast surface and mesh reconstruction:* As shown in Color Plate 17(b), the operator draws, using the tracked pointer, a number of curves on the breast, which produce a point cloud [Color Plate 17(c)]. Sampling of curves is achieved by selecting a minimum distance $d_{min}^{acquistion}$ between two consecutive data points. In order to reconstruct a surface mesh using triangular elements [Color Plate 17(d)], we perform an advanced tridimensional sculpture of Delaunay-based triangulation (3DDT) using an implicit function [55]. A 3DDT of a point cloud (P_i) is a subdivision of the convex hull of (P_i) into tetrahedra, where the circumsphere of each tetrahedron contains none of (P_i). We construct a table T with corresponding facets of the 3DDT and generate a surface mesh from all facets, belonging to only one tetrahedron (i.e., select in T the facets without any correspondent).
- *Reference/current surface alignment:* When comparing the current surface to the reference surface, the patient coordinate systems are not the same, and the breast is probably in a different position and orientation from one time point to another. In order to guide measurements on the current surface, it is important to align the current and reference surfaces. First, we match the two patient coordinate systems and then refine the alignment by finding the best rigid transformation using an iterative closest point (ICP)–based algorithm involving a least-square fitting [56].

7.3 Computing the Accuracy of a Guidance and Tracking System

7.3.1 Global Accuracy of the System

This experiment measures the global accuracy of the system on a deformable breast self-examination simulator. The breast on the simulator is soft and deformable.

Four physical points were drawn on the breast. A reference session was completed on all four marked locations. Then, five current sessions with different positions of the breast simulator were also performed. We used the system guidance to locate the position of each of the four marks, and we measured the physical distance between the sensor extremity and the corresponding mark. We also measured the repeatability of the orientation of the sensor by comparing the current local orientation of the probe to the reference. This experiment took into account all sources of error. The results are shown in Figure 7.6: average positional error = 1.9 mm, and angular error = 2.6°, which are well within the system design criteria of 5 mm and 5°, respectively.

7.3.2 Motion Tracking

Another experiment on a patient shows how the third magnetic sensor compensates for patient breathing and movements during a measurement session. The third magnetic sensor is securely taped to the top of the left chest [position 2 in Figure 7.7(a)]. The tracking sensor was placed on the breast near the nipple [position 1 in Figure 7.7(a)]. The volunteer was asked to perform five types of movements during 10 second periods: (1) normal breathing, (2) deep breathing, (3) lying up and down in the

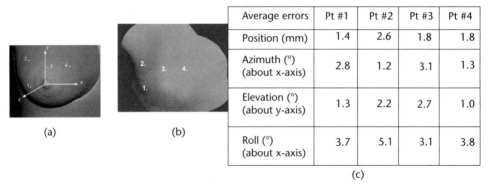

Average errors	Pt #1	Pt #2	Pt #3	Pt #4
Position (mm)	1.4	2.6	1.8	1.8
Azimuth (°) (about x-axis)	2.8	1.2	3.1	1.3
Elevation (°) (about y-axis)	1.3	2.2	2.7	1.0
Roll (°) (about x-axis)	3.7	5.1	3.1	3.8

(a)   (b)   (c)

Figure 7.6 Experiment 1: Marked points (a) on the breast and (b) in the application. (c) Results table: average current measurement errors (errors in position are physically measured); errors in angle measured in the current patient coordinate system.

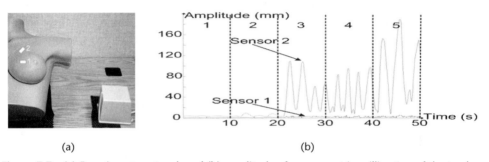

(a)   (b)

Figure 7.7 (a) Experiment protocol, and (b) amplitude of movement in millimeters of the tracking sensor in the patient coordinate system and of patient-taped sensor in the global coordinate system. The point sampling rate is 15 Hz.

chair, (4) lateral movements (rotation around the spine), and (5) a combination of 1, 3, and 4. The results in Figure 7.7(b) show that this setup compensates for patient breathing and movement (with an average amplitude error of 1.6 mm) and strengthens translational efforts. The errors are mainly due to the dynamic behavior of the magnetic tracker when a certain movement speed is reached.

7.4 Application to Nonconcurrent MRI and DOT Data of Human Subjects

A study involving three patients was performed. This study provides an initial answer to a vital question regarding MRI/DOT data analysis: how can functional information on a tumor obtained from DOT data be combined with the anatomical information about the tumor derived from MRI data?

Three MRI and three DOT [displaying total hemoglobin concentration (THC)] data sets are used in this experiment:

1. *Patient 1:* MRI ($256 \times 256 \times 22$ with $0.63 \times 0.63 \times 4.0$ mm pixel size) and mastectomy show an invasive ductal carcinoma of the left breast. The size of the tumor was 2.1 cm, as measured from pathology.
2. *Patient 2:* MRI ($256 \times 256 \times 60$ with $0.7 \times 0.7 \times 1.5$ mm pixel size) and biopsy show an invasive ductal carcinoma of the left breast. The size of the tumor was 5.3 cm, as measured from the MRI (Patient 2 was a neoadjuvant chemo patient and did not have surgery until later).
3. *Patient 3:* MRI ($512 \times 512 \times 56$ with $0.35 \times 0.35 \times 3.93$ mm pixel size) and mastectomy show an invasive in situ ductal carcinoma in the right breast. The size of the tumor was 2.0 cm, as measured from pathology.

All DOT image acquisitions are similar and show the patient total hemoglobin concentration (THC). The procedure described in the typical workflow (Figure 7.1) was used for visualizing, editing, and registering the MRI and DOT data sets. However, since the objective of this initial study is to show how nonconcurrent data may be registered and jointly analyzed, we did not use the results of MRI segmentation to improve the DOT reconstructions.

A quantitative analysis of the resulting data is not trivial. We propose a simple analysis method that provides valuable functional information about the carcinoma. Using the MRI/DOT registered data, we calculate the differences in THC between the volumes inside and outside the segmented tumor as follows:

1. Segment tumor from nontumor tissue in the breast MRI data set using our segmentation approach.
2. Calculate the following statistical quantities from the DOT data set within the resulting segmented tumor and nontumor volumes (this is a trivial task since the DOT and MRI data sets are now registered):
    - a. Average THC value over the entire breast: α;
    - b. Average THC value within the tumor volume defined by the MRI segmentation: β;

- c. Standard deviation of THC for the entire breast: σ.
3. Calculate a new difference measure defined as the distance from α to β in terms of σ.

The computed quantities are described in Figure 7.8(a). Figure 7.8(b) shows the computed statistical quantities as well as the difference measures. As expected, all DOT data sets show average tumor THC values, one to three standard deviations higher than the average breast THC values. The results also show large variability in average breast THC values from one patient to another (varying from 21 to 31 μM). This justifies the use of our difference measure μ, which defines a normalized quantity allowing interpatient comparisons. These results confirm that the tumor areas in the patient breasts exhibit significantly higher THC than their surroundings. Color Plate 18 shows the visual results of the registration algorithm when applied to real patient data sets. We show superimposed MRI and DOT images (3D renderings and 2D fused images) before and after registration. As can be qualitatively ascertained from the figures, registration has greatly improved the alignment of the DOT and MRI data sets. The images also show a significant overlap between the location of the tumors in the MRI and DOT data sets. Patient 3 shows particularly good correlation between the two modalities. The combination of DOT and MR image resolution, the registration technique, and the segmentation accuracy in MR all affect the final outcome. Can registration errors significantly affect the quantification of the results? Certainly this is possible, but a larger-scale study is required to better characterize the effect of the registration error. Indeed, this issue is significant when automatic segmentation is employed and when quantitative values are derived, especially in the case of small pathologies. Variations in the target registration error (TRE) cause variations in the overlap of the MR segmentation to the THC in the DOT data set, which in turn cause variations in the quantification of the computed difference measure μ. However, because the THC is a slowly varying quantity in the DOT data set, we expect small variations in μ.

In order to test this hypothesis, we simulated variations in the TRE by translating incrementally the MR segmentation area in the direction of maximum THC gra-

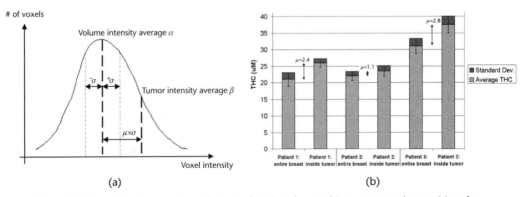

Figure 7.8 (a) THC distribution in a DOT data set showing the resulting computed quantities after DOT-MRI image registration. (b) Statistical values computed in the registered DOT data sets: the segment middle points are the average THC values (α inside the breast, β inside the tumor); the segment endpoints represent one standard deviation spread σ; and μ is the difference measure (distance from α to β in terms of σ). (*From:* [29]. © 2007 SPIE. Reprinted with permission.)

dient in the DOT data set. This enabled us to assess the upper bound of the quantification error due to TRE variations. The MR segmentation area was translated 1, 2, 3, 4, and 5 mm. Then, the different statistics were computed again, and variations in the difference measure μ are shown in Color Plate 18(d).

As Color Plate 18(d) shows, in all cases the difference measure decreases in amplitude as the translation distance is increased. This shows that the MR segmentation area is translated away from the THC "hotspot" in the DOT data sets. The variations of μ from the baseline (translation = 0 mm) in all cases are less than 15%, and μ remains equal to or larger than 1 (i.e., the average THC inside the segmentation area remains more than one standard deviation away from the overall data set average THC). Even though these results are limited to only three patients, they exhibit a relative robustness of the registration-segmentation-quantification approach to errors in automatic registration and segmentation. It is also worth noting that these results may apply more generally to patients with breast cancer tumors of sizes within the range tested, between 2 and 5 cm, which is typical for chemotherapy monitoring.

The most efficient way to improve the coregistration technique in the near future will be to provide additional structural information on the DOT data set. One way to achieve this goal is to provide a more accurate surface map of the patient's breast as it is scanned in the DOT device, using stereo cameras for example. A more precise surface map may enable us in a near future to use more complex voxel-based and/or physics-based nonrigid registration techniques and to achieve better MR- DOT data set alignment, especially for patients whose cancer tumors are smaller than 1 cm in size.

7.5 Conclusion

A new software platform was developed and tested for multimodal integration and visualization of DOT and MRI data sets. The platform enables qualitative and quantitative analysis of DOT and MRI breast data sets and combines the functional and structural data extracted from both types of images. The methods integrate advanced multimodal registration and segmentation algorithms along with a straightforward and well-defined workflow. The methods require little prior user interaction and are robust enough to handle a majority of patient cases, are computationally efficient for practical applications, and yield results useful for combined MRI/DOT analysis. The techniques presented in this chapter offer additional advantages:

- More flexibility than integrated MRI/DOT imaging systems in system design and patient positioning;
- The ability to independently develop a stand-alone DOT system without the stringent limitations imposed by the MRI device environment;
- Combined analysis of structural and functional data derived simultaneously from both modalities;
- Enhancement of DOT data reconstruction through the use of MRI-derived a priori structural information.

The development of a multimodal imaging platform contributes to the important long-term goal of enabling a standardized direct comparison of the two modalities (MRI and DOT), and we anticipate that it will have a positive impact on the standardization of optical imaging technology by establishing common data formats and processes for sharing data and software, which in turn will allow direct comparison of different modalities, validation of new versus established methods in clinical studies, development of commonly accepted standards in postprocessing methods, creation of a standardized MR-DOT technology platform, and, eventually, translation of research prototypes into clinical imaging systems.

We also presented a 3D visualization and guidance system for handheld optical imaging devices and, more specifically, for diffuse optical spectroscopy (DOS). The system provides a patientcentric approach, which enables more accurate longitudinal studies (especially important in chemotherapy monitoring), 3D reconstruction of optical handheld measurements, joint analysis and fusion with other imaging modalities, and easier validation and translation into the clinic. The combined guidance system/DOS instrument becomes particularly useful for monitoring neoadjuvant chemotherapy in breast cancer patients and for longitudinal studies in which measurement reproducibility is critical. A custom-built visualization and guidance system, combined with a well-defined workflow, provides the means for precise image-guided measurements, breast-surface reconstruction, 3D reconstruction of optical properties, and serial data registration. We presented experiments that confirmed the stability and accuracy of the system as well as improvements that will enable translation of DOS technology into the clinical environment.

Acknowledgments

We would like to acknowledge the contributions of University of Pennsylvania collaborators Arjun G. Yodh, Regine Choe, Alper Corlu, Soren Konecky, and Kijoon Lee; Beckman Laser Institute collaborators Bruce J. Tromberg and Albert Cerussi; and Siemens collaborators Ali Khamene and Leo Grady. We would also like to acknowledge the work of Benoit de Roquemaurel and Mazen el-Bawab for key implementations in OMIRAD and in HANDHELD. This work was sponsored in part by the National Institutes of Health and the National Cancer Institute (U54 CA105480).

References

[1] Colak, S. B., M. B. van der Mark, G. W. Hooft, J. H. Hoogenraad, E. S. van der Linden, and F. A. Kuijpers, "Clinical optical tomography and NIR spectroscopy for breast cancer detection," *IEEE J. Quant. Electron.* 5 (1999): 1143–1158.

[2] Pogue, B. W., S. P. Poplack, T. O. McBride, W. A. Wells, K. S. Osterman, U. L. Osterberg, and K. D. Paulsen, "Quantitative hemoglobin tomography with diffuse near-infrared spectroscopy: Pilot results in the breast," *Radiology* 218 (2001): 261–266.

[3] Jiang, H. B., N. V. Iftimia, Y. Xu, J. A. Eggert, L. L. Fajardo, and K. L. Klove, "Near-infrared optical imaging of the breast with model-based reconstruction," *Acad. Radiol.* 9 (2002): 186–194.

[4] Li, A., et al., "Tomographic optical breast imaging guided by three-dimensional mammography," *Appl. Opt.* 42 (2003): 5181–5190.

[5] Torricelli, A., L. Spinelli, A. Pifferi, P. Taroni, R. Cubeddu, and G. M. Danesini, "Use of a nonlinear perturbation approach for in vivo breast lesion characterization by multi-wavelength time-resolved optical mammography," *Opt. Exp.* 11 (2003): 853–867.

[6] Pera, V. E., E. L. Heffer, H. Siebold, O. Schutz, S. Heywang-Kobrunner, L. Gotz, A. Heinig, and S. Fantini, "Spatial second-derivative image processing: An application to optical mammography to enhance the detection of breast tumors," *J. Biomed. Opt.* 8 (2003): 517–524.

[7] Jakubowski, D. B., A. E. Cerussi, F. Bevilacqua, N. Shah, D. Hsiang, J. Butler, and B. J. Tromberg, "Monitoring neoadjuvant chemotherapy in breast cancer using quantitative diffuse optical spectroscopy: A case study," *J. Biomed. Opt.* 9 (2004): 230–238.

[8] Zhu, Q., S. H. Kurtzma, P. Hegde, S. Tannenbaum, M. Kane, M. Huang, N. G. Chen, B. Jagjivan, and K. Zarfos, "Utilizing optical tomography with ultrasound localization to image heterogeneous hemoglobin distribution in large breast cancers," *Neoplasia* 7 (2005): 263–270.

[9] Choe, R., et al., "Diffuse optical tomography of breast cancer during neoadjuvant chemotherapy: A case study with comparison to MRI," *Med. Phys.* 32 (2005): 1128–1139.

[10] Chance, B., S. Nioka, J. Zhang, E. F. Conant, E. Hwang, S. Briest, S. G. Orel, M. D. Schnall, and B. J. Czerniecki, "Breast cancer detection based on incremental biochemical and physiological properties of breast cancers: A six-year, two-site study," *Acad. Radiol.* 12 (2005): 925–933.

[11] Grosenick, D., K. T. Moesta, M. Möller, J. Mucke, H. Wabnitz, B. Gebauer, C. Stroszczynski, B. Wassermann, P. M. Schlag, and H. Rinneberg, "Time-domain scanning optical mammography: I. Recording and assessment of mammograms of 154 patients," *Phys. Med. Biol.* 50 (2005): 2429–2450.

[12] Grosenick, D., H. Wabnitz, K. T. Moesta, J. Mucke, P. M. Schlag, and H. Rinneberg, "Time-domain scanning optical mammography: II. Optical properties and tissue parameters of 87 carcinomas," *Phys. Med. Biol.* 50 (2005): 2451–2468.

[13] Taroni, P., A. Torricelli, L. Spinelli, A. Pifferi, F. Arpaia, G. Danesini, and R. Cubeddu, "Time-resolved optical mammography between 637 and 985 nm: Clinical study on the detection and identification of breast lesions," *Phys. Med. Biol.* 50 (2005): 2469–2488.

[14] Schmitz, C. H., et al., "Design and implementation of dynamic near-infrared optical tomographic imaging instrumentation for simultaneous dual-breast measurements," *Appl. Opt.* 44 (2005): 2140–2153.

[15] Yates, T., J. C. Hebden, A. Gibson, N. Everdell, S. R. Arridge, and M. Douek, "Optical tomography of the breast using a multi-channel time-resolved imager," *Phys. Med. Biol.* 50 (2005): 2503–2518.

[16] Intes, X., "Time-domain optical mammography SoftScan: Initial results," *Acad. Radiol.* 12 (2005): 934–947.

[17] Cerussi, A., N. Shah, D. Hsiang, A. Durkin, J. Butler, and B. J. Tromberg, "In vivo absorption, scattering, and physiologic properties of 58 malignant breast tumors determined by broadband diffuse optical spectroscopy," *J. Biomed. Opt.* 11 (2006): 044005.

[18] Ntziachristos, V., A. G. Yodh, M. Schnall, and B. Chance, "Concurrent MRI and diffuse optical tomography of breast after indocyanine green enhancement," *Proc. Natl. Acad. Sci. USA* 97 (2000): 2767–2772.

[19] Brooksby, B., B. W. Pogue, S. Jiang, H. Dehghani, S. Srinivasan, C. Kogel, T. D. Tosteson, J. Weaver, S. P. Poplack, and K. D. Paulsen, "Imaging breast adipose and fibroglandular tissue molecular signatures by using hybrid MRI-guided near-infrared spectral tomography," *Proc. Natl. Acad. Sci. USA* 103 (2006): 8828–8833.

[20] Li, D., P. M. Meaney, T. D. Tosteson, S. Jiang, T. Kerner, T. O. McBrice, B. W. Pogue, A. Hartov, and K. D. Paulsen, "Comparisons of three alternative breast modalities in a common phantom imaging experiment," *Med. Phys.* 30(8) (2003): 2194–2205.

[21] Brooksby, B., H. Dehghani, B. W. Pogue, and K. D. Paulsen, "Near infrared (NIR) tomography breast image reconstruction with a priori structural information from MRI: Algorithm development for reconstructing heterogeneities," *IEEE J. Sel. Top. Quant. Electron.* (special issue on lasers in biology and medicine) 9(2) (2003).

[22] Shah, N., J. Gibbs, D. Wolverton, A. Cerussi, N. Hylton, and B. J. Tromberg, "Combined diffuse optical spectroscopy and contrast-enhanced magnetic resonance imaging for monitoring breast cancer neoadjuvant chemotherapy: A case study," *J. Biomed. Opt.* 10(5) (2005): 051503.

[23] Azar, F. S., K. Lee, R. Choe, A. Corlu, J. Pearson, F. Sauer, and A. G. Yodh, "A software platform for multi-modal information integration and visualization: Diffuse optical tomography and MRI of breast cancer" (proffered talk), *Third Annual Meeting of the International Society for Molecular Imaging, Symposium X: Methods of Multimodality Imaging: Fusion Instruments and Software Solutions*, Abstract #069, St. Louis, MO, September 9–12, 2004, 96.

[24] Azar, F. S., M. ElBawab, A. Khamene, K. Lee, R. Choe, A. Corlu, S. D. Konecky, A. G. Yodh, and F. Sauer, "Multimodal 3D registration of non-concurrent diffuse optical tomography with MRI of breast cancer," *Fourth Annual Meeting of the International Society for Molecular Imaging, Multimodal Imaging Instrumentation*, Abstract #186, 4(3) (2005): 264.

[25] Florin, C., M. ElBawab, and F. S. Azar, "A new method for increasing the flexibility of DICOM tags management in application-specific integration," *DICOM 2005 International Conference—Digital Imaging and Communications in Medicine*, Abstract #B402, Budapest, Hungary, 2005.

[26] Azar, F. S., K. Lee, R. Choe, A. Corlu, S. D. Konecky, A. G. Yodh, and F. Sauer, "A novel approach for joint analysis of non-concurrent magnetic resonance imaging and diffuse optical tomography of breast cancer," *Fifth Annual Meeting of the International Society for Molecular Imaging, Advances in Multimodality Imaging*, Abstract #324, 5(3) (2006): 275.

[27] Konecky, S. D., R. Wiener, N. Hajjioui, R. Choe, A. Corlu, K. Lee, S. M. Srinivas, J. R. Saffer, R. Freifelder, F. S. Azar, J. S. Karp, and A. G. Yodh, "Characterization of breast lesions using diffuse optical tomography and positron emission tomography," *SPIE Photonics West—Multimodal Biomedical Imaging II*, Conference 6431, Session 4, Abstract #6431-20, San Jose, CA, January 20–25, 2007.

[28] Azar, F. S., K. Lee, R. Choe, A. Corlu, S. D. Konecky, and A. G. Yodh, "Joint analysis of non-concurrent magnetic resonance imaging and diffuse optical tomography of breast cancer," *SPIE Photonics West—Optical Tomography and Spectroscopy of Tissue*, Conference 6434, Session 10, Abstract #6434-45, San Jose, CA, January 20–25, 2007.

[29] Azar, F. S., K. Lee, A. Khamene, R. Choe, A. Corlu, S. D. Konecky, F. Sauer, and A. G. Yodh, "Standardized platform for coregistration of non-concurrent diffuse optical and magnetic resonance breast images obtained in different geometries," *J. Biomed. Opt.* (special section on optical diagnostic imaging from bench to bedside) 12(5) (2007): 051902.

[30] Cerussi, A., et al., "Predicting response to breast cancer neoadjuvant chemotherapy using Diffuse Optical Spectroscopy," *Proc. Natl. Acad. Sci. USA* 104(10) (2007): 4014–4019.

[31] Ellsmere, J., et al., "A new visualization technique for laparoscopic ultrasonography," *Surgery* 136(1) (2004): 84–92.

[32] Leotta, D. F., "An efficient calibration method for freehand 3-D ultrasound imaging systems," *Ultrasound Med. Biol.* 30(7) (2004): 999–1008.

[33] Khamene, A., et al., "An augmented reality system for MRI-guided needle biopsies," *Proc. Med. Meets Virt. Real.* 11 (2003): 151–157.

[34] Barratt, D. C., et al., "Optimisation and evaluation of an electromagnetic tracking device for high-accuracy three-dimensional ultrasound imaging of the carotid arteries," *Ultrasound Med. Biol.* 27(7) (2001): 957–968.

[35] Sauer, F., et al., "A head-mounted display system for augmented reality image guidance: Towards clinical evaluation for iMRI-guided neurosurgery," *Proc. Med. Comput. Comput.-Assist. Intervent.*, Utrecht, the Netherlands, 2001, 701–716.

[36] Khamene, A., et al., "Local 3D reconstruction and augmented reality visualization of free-hand ultrasound for needle biopsy procedures," *Proc. Med. Image Comput. Comput.-Assist. Intervent.* (MICCAI '03), Montreal, Canada, 2003, 344–355.

[37] Sauer, F., et al., "Augmented reality visualization of ultrasound images: System description, calibration, and features," *Proc. 4th Int. Symp. Augment. Real.* (ISAR 2001), New York, 2001, 30–39.

[38] Cerussi, A., et al., "In vivo absorption, scattering, and physiologic properties of 58 malignant breast tumors determined by broadband diffuse optical spectroscopy," *J. Biomed. Opt.* 11(4) (2006): 044005.

[39] Azar, F. S., A. Cerussi, B. deRoquemaurel, E. Flannery, S. H. Chung, J. Ruth, and B. J. Tromberg, "A 3D image-based guidance system for handheld optical imaging devices," *Optical Society of America, BIOMED Meeting*, St. Petersburg, FL, March 16–19, 2008.

[40] Schweiger, M., "Application of the finite element method in infrared image reconstruction of scattering media," PhD thesis, University of London, 1994.

[41] See www-nml.dartmouth.edu/nir/downloads.html.

[42] Maintz, J., and M. Viergever, "A survey of medical image registration," *Med. Image Anal.* 2 (1998): 1–36.

[43] Hill, D. L. G., et al., "Registration of MR and CT images for skull base surgery using pointlike anatomical features," *Br. J. Radiol.* 64 (767) (1991): 1030–1035.

[44] Colignon, A., et al., "Automated multi-modality image registration based on information theory," *IPMI* (1995): 263–274.

[45] Wells, W., et al., "Multi-modal volume registration by maximization of mutual information," *Med. Image Anal.* 1 (1996): 32–52.

[46] Cain, S. C., M. M. Hayat, and E. E. Armstrong, "Projection-based image registration in the presence of fixed-pattern noise," *IEEE Trans. Image Process.* 10 (2001): 1860–1872.

[47] Chan, H., and A. C. S. Chung, "Efficient 3D-3D vascular registration based on multiple orthogonal 2D projections," *2nd Int. Work. Biomed. Image Regist.* (WBIR) 2717 (2003): 301–310.

[48] Wells, M., et al., "Multi-modal volume registration by maximization of mutual information," *Med. Image Anal.* 1(1) (1996): 35–51.

[49] Huesman, R. H., et al., "Deformable registration of multi-modal data including rigid structures," *IEEE Trans. Nucl. Sci.* 50(3) (2003): 1879–1882.

[50] Cain, S. C., M. M. Hayat, and E. E. Armstrong, "Projection-based image registration in the presence of fixed-pattern noise," *IEEE Trans. Image Process.* 10 (2001): 1860–1872.

[51] Chan, H., and A. C. S. Chung, "Efficient 3D-3D vascular registration based on multiple orthogonal 2D projections," *2nd Int. Work. Biomed. Image Regist.* (WBIR) (2003): 301–310.

[52] Khamene, A., R. Chisu, W. Wein, N. Navab, and F. Sauer, "A novel projection-based approach for medical image registration," *Third International Workshop on Biomedical Image Registration*, Utrecht, the Netherlands, July 9–11, 2006.

[53] Grady, L., and G. Funka-Lea, "Multi-label image segmentation for medical applications based on graph-theoretic electrical potentials," *8th ECCV04, Workshop on Computer Vision Approaches to Medical Image Analysis and Mathematical Methods in Biomedical Image Analysis*, Prague, Czech Republic, May 15, 2004.

[54] Grady, L., "Multilabel Random Walker image segmentation using prior models," *Proc. IEEE Comput. Soc. Int. Conf. Comput. Vis. Pattern Recog.* 1 (June 2005): 763–770.

[55] Boissonnat, J.-D., and F. Cazals, "Smooth surface reconstruction via natural neighbor interpolation of distance functions," *Proc. 16th ACM Symp. Computation. Geom.* (2000): 223-232.

[56] Besl, P., and N. McKay, "A method for registration of 3-D shapes," *Pattern Anal. Mach. Intellig.* 14(2) (1992): 239–256.

Selected Bibliography

Azar, F. S., D. N. Metaxas, and M. D. Schnall, "Methods for modeling and predicting mechanical deformations of the breast under external perturbations," *Med. Image Anal.* 6(1) (2002): 1–27.

Choe, R., A. Corlu, K. Lee, T. Durduran, S. D. Konecky, M. Grosicka-Koptyra, S. R. Arridge, G. J. Czerniecki, D. L. Fraker, A. DeMichele, B. Chance, M. A. Rosen, and A. G. Yodh, "Diffuse optical tomography of breast cancer during neoadjuvant chemotherapy: A case study with comparison to MRI," *Med. Phys.* 32(4) (2005): 1128–1139.

Corlu, A., R. Choe, T. Durduran, K. Lee, M. Schweiger, E. M. C. Hillman, S. R. Arridge, and A. G. Yodh, "Diffuse optical tomography with spectral constraints and wavelength optimization," *Appl. Opt.* 44 (2005): 2082–2093.

Culver, J. P., R. Choe, M. J. Holboke, L. Zubkov, T. Durduran, A. Slemp, V. Ntziachristos, B. Chance, and A. G. Yodh, "Three-dimensional diffuse optical tomography in the parallel plane transmission geometry: Evaluation of a hybrid frequency domain/continuous wave clinical system for breast imaging," *Med. Phys.* 30 (2003): 235–247.

CHAPTER 8
Diffuse Optical Spectroscopy in Breast Cancer: Coregistration with MRI and Predicting Response to Neoadjuvant Chemotherapy

Bruce J. Tromberg, Natasha Shah, Catherine Klifa, Albert E. Cerussi, Nola M. Hylton, and Ang Li

8.1 Introduction

Near-infrared (NIR) diffuse optical methods that employ a direct quantitative approach to measuring tissue physiology may be a beneficial adjunct to current imaging methods for breast cancer detection, particularly in challenging cases of younger women, subjects with high mammographic density, and individuals undergoing presurgical neoadjuvant chemotherapy. The technique presented in this chapter, broadband diffuse optical spectroscopy (DOS) employs near-infrared light (650 to 1,000 nm) to provide noninvasive quantitative assessment of the tissue concentration of oxyhemoglobin (ctO_2Hb), deoxyhemoglobin (ctHHb), water (ctH_2O), and lipid, as well as the bulk-tissue scattering parameter (μ'_s). These tissue biomarkers convey information on fundamental biologic processes, such as angiogenesis, necrosis, edema, cellular metabolism, and matrix composition. Several studies have shown that there is high optical and physiological contrast between tumors and normal tissues in the NIR [1–7] and that DOS is acutely sensitive to the biology of healthy breast [8–12]. Because DOS methods focus on tissue function rather than structure, DOS may be suitable for younger women with dense breasts. In addition, DOS is relatively inexpensive, does not employ ionizing radiation, and can be used for frequent screening or monitoring of high-risk women and individuals undergoing chemo- or radiation therapies [13].

This chapter devotes a section each to two promising features of DOS: (1) coregistration with MRI, and (2) monitoring and predicting neoadjuvant-chemotherapy response. The first section explains how DOS can be validated with an established imaging technique (MRI) and highlights the complementary nature of these methods. The second section focuses on the application of DOS to a specific clinical problem: monitoring and predicting breast tumor response to presurgical neoadjuvant chemotherapy.

8.2 Coregistration with MRI

Overall validation of DOS techniques by established imaging methods is necessary for its development as a clinical technique. Due to the diffusive nature of NIR light propagation in tissue, the main disadvantage to DOS is inherently low spatial resolution. Contrast-enhanced magnetic resonance imaging (cMRI) is ideal for direct comparison with DOS because it provides detailed anatomical images as a context for understanding the origin of DOS signals. Water and lipid spectral signatures from DOS can be compared to T2- and T1-weighted images, respectively [14], while vascular information provided by cMRI can be directly correlated to DOS hemoglobin signals [15].

This section directly compares DOS-derived quantitative physiological data with MRI in healthy, benign, and malignant breast-tissue types in vivo. In addition, a case study of DOS/cMRI is presented that highlights the complementary sensitivity of both methods to presurgical neoadjuvant-chemotherapy response. The purpose of this section is to report studies that validate the accuracy and sensitivity of broadband DOS and to evaluate its potential as a possible adjunct to MRI.

8.2.1 Materials and Methods

8.2.1.1 Subjects

Six healthy, "normal" volunteers and three patients with known or suspected breast lesions were examined using MRI and DOS. All subjects provided informed, written consent and HIPPA compliance under protocols approved by the institution's Committee on Human Research.

Normal volunteers were recruited by internal university advertisement and selected if they had no prior or suspected breast disease. The six healthy subjects ranged from 22 to 54 years of age (mean age 33 ± 13 years). The three lesion patients presented in this paper were concurrently enrolled in an MRI research protocol and recruited for the DOS study. Patient 1 is a 54-year-old postmenopausal woman diagnosed with an invasive ductal carcinoma, and Patient 2 is a 45-year-old woman with a fibroadenoma. Patient 3, who was in the chemotherapy study, is a 54-year-old postmenopausal female undergoing neoadjuvant chemotherapy for invasive ductal carcinoma of the right breast. All studies were performed at the University of California, San Francisco, Magnetic Resonance Science Center.

8.2.1.2 DOS Instrumentation and Measurements

A detailed description of the instrumentation and theory employed in DOS measurements (Figure 8.1) is presented elsewhere [16, 17], but a brief explanation is provided here. The DOS system [Figure 8.1(a)] employs two integrated techniques to determine the complete tissue NIR absorption (μ_a) and scattering (μ'_s) spectra. The frequency-domain photon-migration (FDPM) component employs six fiber-coupled laser diodes (λ = 658, 682, 785, 810, 830, and 850 nm) that are intensity-modulated at frequencies ranging from 50 to 600 MHz. The average optical power launched into the tissue by the FDPM lasers is about 10 to 20 mW. A steady-state (SS) compo-

8.2 Coregistration with MRI

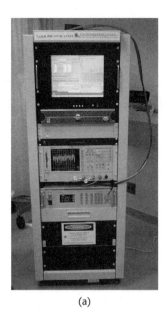
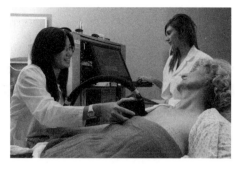

Figure 8.1 (a) Photograph of the laser breast-scanner instrument, and (b) bedside measurement.

nent consists of a high-intensity tungsten-halogen source (Micropak HL2000-HP, Ocean Optics, Dunedin, Florida) and a 16 bit spectrometer (Oriel MS1271i, Intraspec IV CCD, Newport Oriel Instruments, Stratford, Connecticut). DOS measurements are made with the subject in the supine position using a handheld probe [Figure 8.2(b)] equipped with an FDPM laser fiber bundle, avalanche photodiode detector (module C5658 with S6045-03 silicon APD, Hamamatsu, San Diego, California), and SS source and detector fibers. The source-detector separation distance was fixed in these studies at 28 mm, from which we estimate a mean sampling depth of approximately 10 mm in the tissue. The actual tissue volume interrogated, which is determined by multiple light scattering and absorption, extends above and below the mean sampling depth and is estimated to approximately 8 to 10 cm^3. Figure 8.2(a) shows a schematic of the handheld probe and light penetration.

Resulting FDPM and SS data are fit to a mathematical model of diffusive light transport to determine μ_a and μ'_s spectra in the NIR [18]. From the spectral information, tissue concentrations of ctHHb, ctO$_2$Hb, lipid, and ctH$_2$O are calculated using their wavelength-dependent molar extinction coefficients [18, 19]. From these parameters, total hemoglobin concentration (ctTHb = ctHHb + ctO$_2$Hb) and tissue hemoglobin oxygenation saturation (S$_t$O$_2$ = ctO$_2$Hb/ctTHb) × 100%) are calculated. A contrast function, the tissue optical index (TOI), has been defined to indicate tissue metabolism where TOI = (ctHHbctH$_2$O)/[lipid].

DOS measurement positions are marked on the skin using a surgical skin pen. The handheld probe is placed on one of the marked locations for the duration of a measurement then moved to the next discrete position. The total time for one DOS measurement is currently approximately 6 seconds (earlier versions of our instrument with approximately 30 second acquisition were used in some of the reported studies). Two DOS measurements are made at each location.

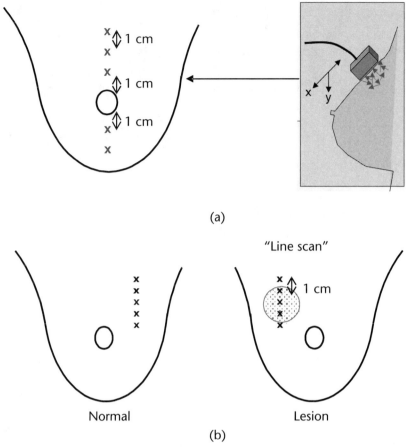

Figure 8.2 (a) Measurement scheme for normal volunteers and cartoon of handheld probe orientation on breast: of five measurements performed in a vertical line centered at the nipple, three started 1 cm above the areolar border spaced 1 cm apart, and two started 1 cm below the areola spaced 1 cm apart. (b) Measurement scheme for lesion patients: DOS measurements were spaced 1 cm apart in a line ("linescan") centered across the lesion. A linescan in the identical location on the contralateral breast was performed for comparison.

DOS measurements were correlated to MR images by using vitamin A tablets, which enhance on MRI, as fiducial markers. The fiducials were placed on each of the premarked DOS positions and affixed to the skin with tape. For lesion measurements DOS measurements were spaced 1 cm apart in a line ("linescan") centered across the lesion [Figure 8.2(b)]. To sample different regions of breast tissue in normal volunteers, five DOS measurements were made in a vertical line centered at the nipple, and three measurements were made above and two below the areola at 1 cm intervals [Figure 8.2(a)].

8.2.1.3 MRI Measurements

All MRIs were performed on a 1.5T Signa system (GE Medical Systems, Milwaukee, Wisconsin) using a bilateral phased-array breast coil with the subject in the prone position.

- *Healthy volunteers:* Unilateral, fat-suppressed, T1-weighted images were acquired using a 3D fast-gradient recalled-echo (3DFGRE) sequence, with the following imaging parameters: repetition time (TR) = 8.4 ms, echo time (TE) = 4.2 ms, number of excitations (NEX) = 2, 256 × 256 matrix, field of view (FOV) = 180, and slice thickness = 2 mm with no gap between slices. Non-fat-suppressed images were acquired with TR = 7.9; other imaging parameters remained the same.

- *Patient 1:* Unilateral, fat-suppressed, T1-weighted images were acquired using a 3DFGRE sequence with the same imaging parameters used for the volunteer scans. In addition, a T2-weighted fast-spin-echo (FSE) sequence was acquired with TR = 5,500 ms, TE = 90.664 ms, NEX = 2,256 × 256 matrix, FOV = 180, and slice thickness = 3.3 mm slice thickness with 0.5 mm gap between slices.

- *Patient 2:* A bilateral scan was performed using a fat-suppressed 3DFGRE sequence and the following imaging parameters: TR = 8.90 ms, TE = 4.2 ms, NEX = 1,512 × 512 matrix, slice thickness = 2.3 mm with no gap between slices. In addition, a bilateral T2 FSE sequence was acquired with TR = 5,200 ms, TE = 89.096 ms, NEX = 2,512 × 512 matrix, FOV = 320, and slice thickness = 3.2 mm with 0.5 mm gap between slices. Both Patients 1 and 2 received intravenous gadolinium at a dose of 0.1 mmol/kg using an indwelling catheter. Images were acquired at 0, 2.5, and 7.5 minutes after contrast injection.

- *Patient 3:* Unilateral, fat-suppressed, T1-weighted cMRI of the breast was performed using a 3D fast-gradient recalled-echo (3DFGRE) sequence using the following imaging parameters: TR = 8.4 ms, TE = 4.2 ms, NEX = 2, 256 × 192 matrix, FOV = 180, and slice thickness = 2 mm. Contrast agent gadolinium-diethylenetriaminepentaacetic acid (Gd-DTPA) was administered at a dose of 0.1 mmol/kg using an indwelling catheter. Three high-resolution images were acquired in succession, one preceding and two following Gd-DTPA injection. Each image required 5 minutes for a complete scan. Central-phase encoding lines of each data set were acquired midway through the scan, yielding effective contrast sample times of 0, 2.5, and 7.5 minutes for the precontrast (S_0), early postcontrast (S_1), and late postcontrast (S_2) images, respectively. In addition to cMRI, T2-weighted images were acquired using a 2D fast-spin-echo sequence with the following parameters: TR = 5,500 ms, TE = 90 ms, NEX = 2, 256 × 192 matrix, FOV = 180, and slice thickness = 3 mm with a 0.5 mm gap between slices.

8.2.2 Results

Combined DOS and MRI measurements were performed in a total of nine women, six healthy, premenopausal volunteers, two case studies with known lesions, and one patient with locally advanced breast cancer undergoing neoadjuvant chemotherapy.

8.2.2.1 Normal Volunteers

Figure 8.3 shows a T1-weighted, nonfat-suppressed sagittal MRI with five DOS positions clearly indicated by fiducial markers. One MR fat and one MR tissue-thickness value was determined at each marker by measuring the length of rays perpendicular to the skin going through fatty (dark gray lines) and glandular tissue (light gray lines), respectively. Seven breasts in six healthy subjects (22 to 56 years old) were measured for a total of 35 points. DOS physiological values were calculated for each position and correlated to MRI-determined glandular and fatty tissue thickness. Figure 8.4(a) shows DOS-derived water content and lipid concentration versus glandular tissue thickness. Water content is positively correlated with glandular tissue thickness ($r = 0.85$), while lipid content is inversely correlated ($r = -0.79$). Subjects who appear to have either purely fatty or glandular tissue in the optically probed region have measurable water and lipid content. For example, the subject with approximately 0 cm fatty tissue (by MRI) displays 30% to 40% lipid and 45% to 49% ctH_2O, while the subject with approximately 0 cm glandular tissue has 11% ctH_2O. Figure 8.4(b) shows that the hemoglobin parameters ctO_2Hb and $ctHHb$ also correlate with glandular tissue thickness. $ctHHb$ shows a stronger positive relationship ($r = 0.81$) and is primarily indicative of tissue oxygen utilization. Interestingly, the subject with approximately 0 cm glandular tissue has approximately 12 μM total hemoglobin (ctTHb).

Each measurement position was segregated into dominantly fatty or glandular categories by using a ratio of glandular tissue (GT) thickness to fat tissue (FT) thickness, where GT/FT > 1 is glandular and GT/FT < 1 is fatty. Table 8.1 compares the average values for each parameter based on the tissue type ($n = 9$, fatty; $n = 24$, glandular). The results correlate the optically measured composition with the two dominant tissue types determined by MRI. Although the S_tO_2 is comparable in both tissues, glandular tissue has 70% greater ctO_2Hb, 60% greater $ctHHb$, twofold greater ctH_2O, and 20% less lipid. The TOI is 4.5 times greater for glandular versus fatty tissue for all subjects. However, the mean TOI contrast (coefficient of variation $= (\sigma/x) \times 100\%$) within individuals for glandular/fatty was 33%.

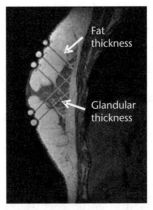

Figure 8.3 T1-weighted sagittal MR image of a healthy, premenopausal breast acquired using a nonfat-suppressed 3D fast-gradient recalled-echo sequence (8.4/4.2). The five vitamin A fiducials correspond to five DOS measurement positions. Fat thickness (dark gray lines) and glandular tissue thickness (light gray lines) were calculated at each fiducial location by measuring the length of rays perpendicular to the skin from the breast surface.

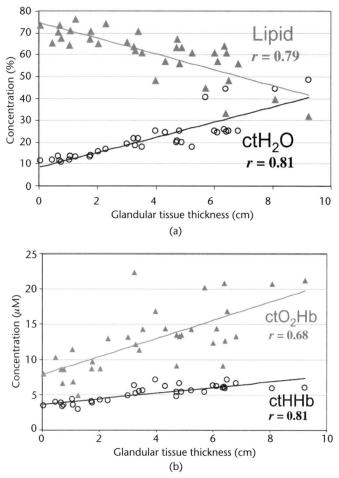

Figure 8.4 Scatter plots show the correlation of DOS-derived parameters to MRI morphology: (a) DOS-derived lipid concentration (triangles) and ctH$_2$O (circles) versus MRI-derived glandular tissue thickness at 35 measurement positions on six premenopausal volunteers with healthy breast tissue. (b) DOS-derived ctO$_2$Hb (triangles) and ctHHb (circles) versus MRI-derived glandular tissue thickness. The linear correlation coefficient, r, is provided.

8.2.2.2 Case Studies of Three Lesions

We present three case studies to illustrate how the presence of a lesion perturbs background normal physiological properties. The results demonstrate that regions of increased enhancement on contrast-enhanced T1-weighted and T2-weighted images correlate with DOS-derived hemoglobin and ctH$_2$O, respectively.

Table 8.1 Average DOS Physiological Parameters for Dominantly Fatty ($n = 9$) or Dominantly Glandular ($n = 24$) Tissue (Error Bars Represent Standard Deviation to the Mean)

	Lipid (%)	Water (%)	ctHHb (μM)	ctO$_2$Hb (μM)	S$_t$O$_2$ (%)	TOI
Glandular ($n = 24$)	57.6 ± 4	25.0 ± 9.4	5.7 ± 0.8	14.1 ± 4	70.7 ± 5	2.92 ± 2.2
Fatty ($n = 9$)	70.2 ± 4	12.5 ± 1.1	3.7 ± 0.4	8.3 ± 2	68.5 ± 3	0.65 ± 0.1

Case 1: Invasive Ductal Carcinoma

A sagittal, T1-weighted, Gd-DTPA-enhanced, fat-suppressed MRI of a 54-year-old postmenopausal woman reveals a $3.7 \times 3.9 \times 3.9$ cm tumor with a strongly enhancing periphery and large central nonenhancing area of necrosis in the lateral right breast (Figure 8.5), confirmed to be an invasive ductal carcinoma on pathology. The lesion is superficial with skin involvement, and the surrounding parenchyma is predominantly fatty. The central enhancement on the corresponding T2-weighted sagittal image indicates a fluid-filled necrotic core. The DOS linescan consisted of 11 points superior to inferior across the lesion and the surrounding normal tissue. The lesion is situated between DOS positions 5 to 9. The lesion in positions 6 to 7 is superficial and samples largely tumor tissue with little or no contribution of normal tissue to the signal. Positions 1 to 4 and 10 to 11 represent surrounding normal tissue. Corresponding DOS results [Figure 8.6(a, b)] exhibit a three- to fourfold increase in ctH_2O at the lesion center ($81.4 \pm 0.3\%$) compared to the surrounding normal parenchyma ($25.1 \pm 4\%$) and a concomitant drop in the lipid ($15.5 \pm 3\%$ versus $77 \pm 2\%$). The ctHHb and ctO_2Hb curves [Figure 8.6(b)] show a peak at positions 5 and 6, corresponding to the lesion rim: ctO_2Hb is approximately twofold greater at the lesion peak compared to the normal tissue periphery ($43.9 \pm 5 \mu M$ versus $23.7 \pm 6 \mu M$), and ctHHb is threefold greater ($18.9 \pm 2 \mu M$ versus $6.6 \pm 2 \mu M$). The relative increase of ctHHb to ctO_2Hb at the lesion center reflects a 20% decrease in S_tO_2 at the necrotic core (61% versus 81%). The TOI shows a 46-fold contrast at the lesion peak compared to the surrounding tissue (102 ± 31.4 versus 2.2 ± 1).

Case 2: Fibroadenoma

A bilateral, Gd-DTPA-enhanced, fat-suppressed MRI of a 45-year-old premenopausal woman reveals a $2.2 \times 2.2 \times 2.1$ cm mass with T2-weighted and T1-weighted Gd-DTPA enhancement with nonenhancing septations consistent with known fibroadenoma; the surrounding parenchyma is heterogeneously dense. The DOS linescan consisted of five points superior to inferior across the lesion and surrounding normal tissue. The tumor is situated in DOS positions 2 to 4; positions 1

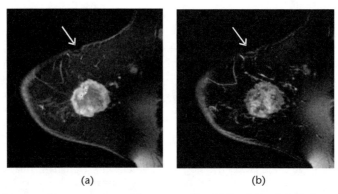

(a)   (b)

Figure 8.5 A 54-year-old postmenopausal woman with a $3.7 \times 3.9 \times 3.9$ cm invasive ductal carcinoma: (a) T1-weighted, contrast-enhanced sagittal MR image acquired using a fat-suppressed 3D fast-gradient recalled-echo sequence (8.4/4.2), and (b) corresponding T2-weighted sagittal image acquired using a fast-spin-echo sequence (5500/90.664). Arrows indicate vitamin A fiducials.

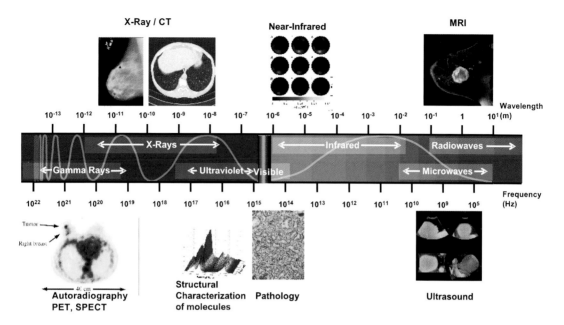

Color Plate 1 Electromagnetic spectrum and associated imaging modalities.

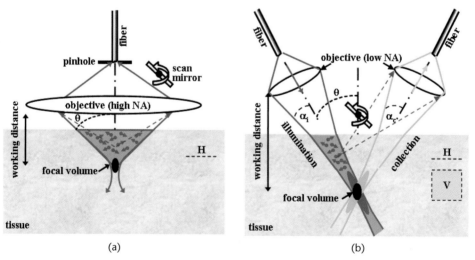

Color Plate 2 Confocal microscopy architectures. (a) In the single-axis configuration, the fiber (pinhole) is aligned with the optical axis and uses a high-numerical-aperture (NA) objective to achieve subcellular resolution. Geometry often limits the working distance; thus, the scanning mechanism (mirror) is placed in the preobjective position. (b) In the dual-axes architecture, separate low-NA objectives create a long working distance, and the overlap of the two beams (black oval) achieves subcellular resolution. Postobjective scanning is now allowed and provides a large field of view and scalability of the optics to millimeter dimensions. Off-axis light collection reduces the effects of tissue scattering (dashed lines) and allows for the collection of both vertical (V) and horizontal (H) cross-sectional images.

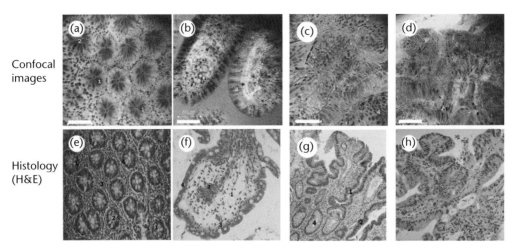

Color Plate 3 In vivo confocal images collected with Pentax EC-3870K: (a) normal colonic mucosa, (b) terminal ileum, (c) intraepithelial neoplasia, and (d) adenocarcinoma following intravenous administration of fluorescein. Corresponding histology is shown below in (e–h); scale bar = 80 μm. (© 2004 Elsevier. Reprinted with permission.)

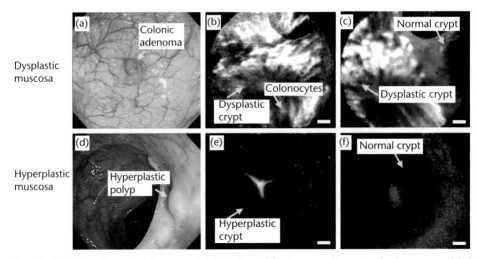

Color Plate 4 Binding of targeted fluorescent-labeled peptides to premalignant colonic mucosa. (a) Conventional white-light image of a colonic adenoma is shown. (b) In vivo confocal fluorescence image of colonic adenoma following topical administration reveals peptide binding to dysplastic colonocytes. (c) Confocal image at adenoma: normal border shows preferential binding of peptides to dysplastic rather than normal crypt with an average target-to-background ratio of 5. (d) White-light image of hyperplastic polyp is shown. (e, f) No binding of target peptide to hyperplastic or normal crypts was seen. Scale bars = 20 μm.

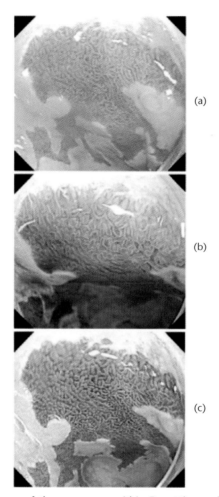

Color Plate 5 Endoscopic images of the same area within Barrett's esophagus using (a) high-resolution endoscopy with optical magnification, (b) chromoendoscopy with indigo carmine, and (c) narrow-band imaging (NBI) (Chapter 3, [70] Reprinted with permission).

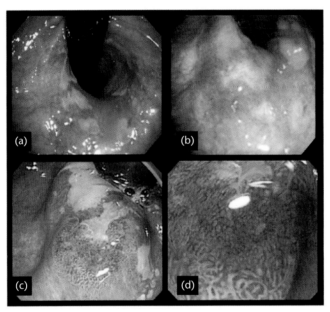

Color Plate 6 Images of a Barrett's esophagus lesion with high-grade intraepithelial neoplasia (HGIN) detected with autofluorescence imaging (AFI) and narrowband imaging (NBI). (a) During inspection with white light, this area was not judged as suspicious. (b) The area around the small squamous island in the middle of the image showed a blue-violet autofluorescence imaging color. (c, d) With NBI, irregular and disrupted mucosal patterns were found. The histopathology confirmed the presence of HGIN (Chapter 3, [89] Reprinted with permission).

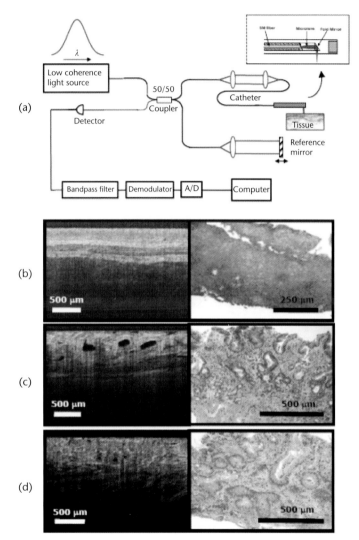

Color Plate 7 (a) The schematic diagram of time-domain endoscopic OCT system with inset showing the schematic of OCT imaging catheter. The optical beam from the catheter can be scanned either linearly or circularly to generate cross-sectional images. (b–d) In vivo ultrahigh resolution endoscopic OCT image (left) and corresponding histology (right) from: (b) normal esophagus, (c) Barrett's esophagus, and (d) high-grade dysplasia (Chapter 3, [99] Reprinted with permission).

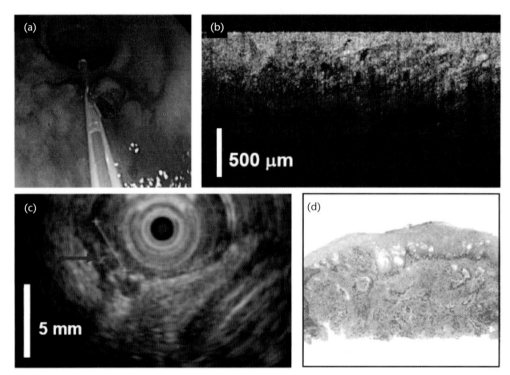

Color Plate 8 Ultrahigh-resolution endoscopic OCT image of adenocarcinoma beneath squamous mucosa: (a) white light endoscopic view; (b) endoscopic OCT image; (c) endoscopic ultrasound images of the same nodule (indicated by the red arrow); and (d) corresponding histology (Chapter 3, [99] Reprinted with permission).

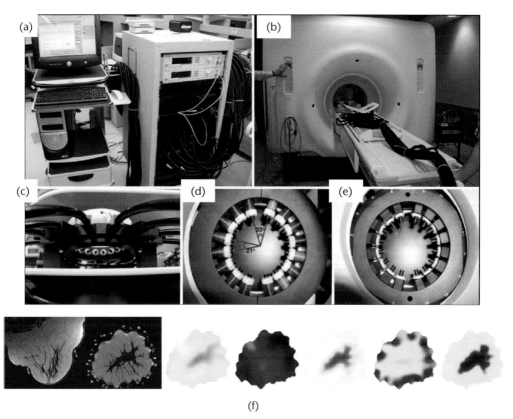

Color Plate 9 The Dartmouth NIR/MRI systems. (a) Photograph of the portable NIR instrumentation and control console is shown. (b) Optical fibers extend from the system into the MRI. (c) Open architecture breast array coil houses the optical fiber positioning system. (d) The first and (e) second generation MR-compatible fiber-positioning mechanisms are shown. (f) One set of breast MRI/NIR images is shown. (*From:* Chapter 4, [74]. © 2006 National Academy of the Sciences of the USA. Reprinted with permission.)

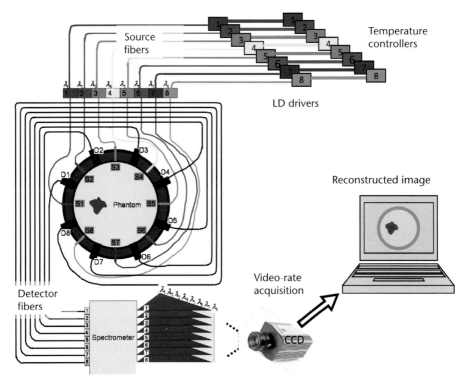

Color Plate 10 The spectral-encoding NIR tomography system developed by Dartmouth NIR imaging group: system schematic diagram.

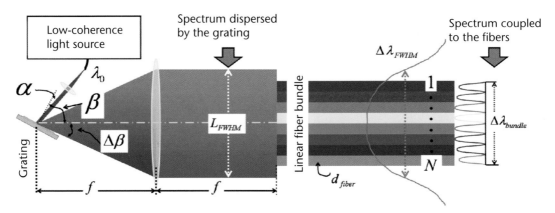

Color Plate 11 The principle of spread spectral encoding based on a wideband (low-coherence) light source. The dispersion of the wideband light can be coupled to a linear fiber bundle within which each channel has a small wavelength offset from neighboring ones to form a spread spectral encoding among the source channels.

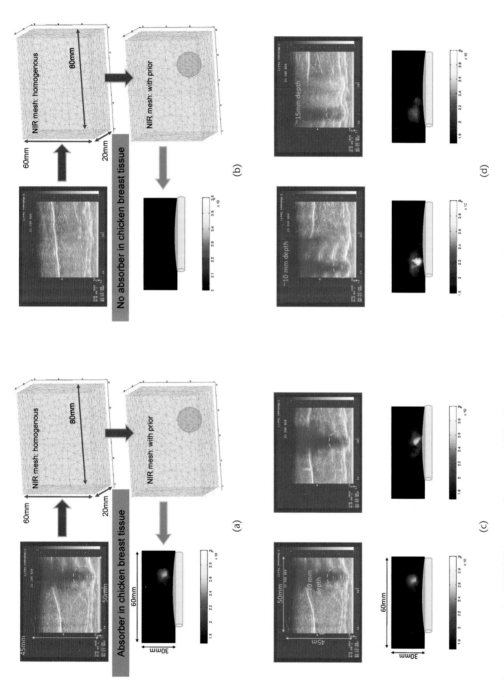

Color Plate 12 Concurrent sagittal HIR/US images taken from chicken breast tissue using the trans-redal HIR/US probe: (a) with an absorbing target at approximately 1 cm depth, (b) with no absorbing target, (c) with the absorbing target displaced longitudinally, and (d) with the absorbing target displaced about 5 mm deeper.

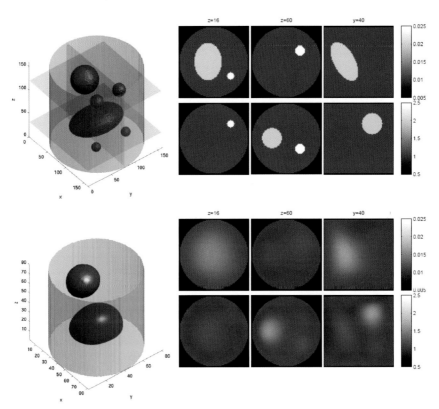

Color Plate 13 Top: target object. Left: cylinder with location of the embedded absorption (red) and scattering inclusions (blue). The position of the cross-sectional planes used for displaying the reconstruction results is indicated in gray. Right: cross sections $z = 16$, $z = 60$, and $y = 40$ through the absorption and scattering target. Bottom: TV prior with flat weighting. Reconstructions, displayed as iso-surfaces (left) and cross sections (right).

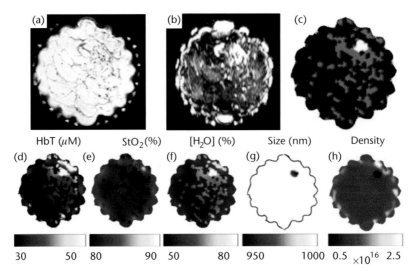

Color Plate 14 (a) T1-weighted and (b) Gd-enhanced T1 weighted MR coronal slice of the breast near the fiber plane. (c) MR image coarsely segmented into adipose, fibroglandular, and suspect lesion; (d–h) functional optical images consisting of (d) total hemoglobin, (e) oxygen saturation, (f) water percent, (g) scatter particle size, and (h) scatter particle number density.

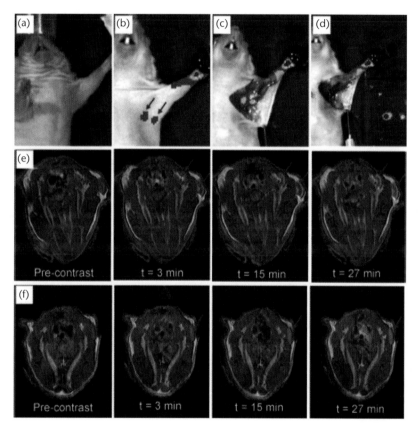

Color Plate 15 Optical/MR images of the axial and brachial lymph nodes in male nude mice. (a–d) Optical fluorescence images of (a) precontrast overlay of white light and fluorescence, (b) overlay of white light and fluorescence images 1 hour after contrast injection, (c) fluorescence image without skin, and (d) fluorescence image after surgical resection. (e, f) T1-weighted MR images obtained during contrast injection of (e) 0.02 mmol Gd/kg, and (f) 0.002 mmol/kg, with arrows indicating lymph nodes. (Chapter 6, Courtesy of Melancon et al. [77].)

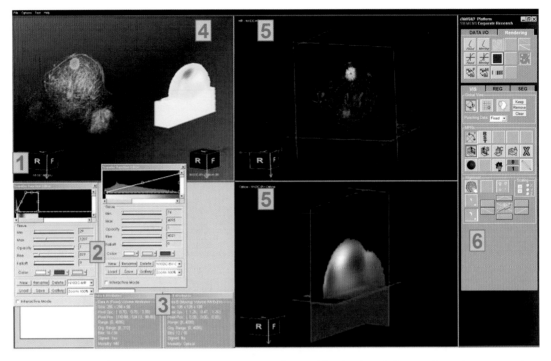

Color Plate 16 Visualization platform showing MRI and DOT (blood volume) datasets from the same patient before registration. After the appropriate transfer functions are applied, one can clearly observe the location of the invasive ductal carcinoma diagnosed in this patient breast. The following components are shown from left to right: (1) orientation cube, (2) transfer function editors, (3) data attribute windows, (4) volume rendering window, (5) MPR windows, and (6) command tabs [29]. (Reprinted with permission.)

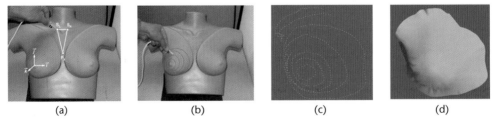

Color Plate 17 Handheld imaging system: (a) patient coordinate system; (b) scanning of the breast surface; (c) 3D point cloud; and (d) textured surface mesh.

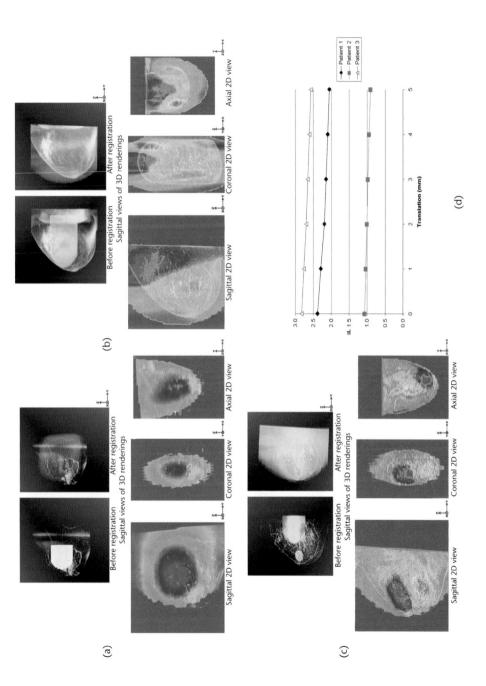

Color Plate 18 Superimposed MRI and DOT images (3D renderings, and 2D fused images) of Patients (a) 1, (b) 2, and (c) 3 before and after registration. The 2D fused images show the cross-sections going through the center of the tumor. (d) Variations in μ for each patient, due to translations of the MR segmentation area inside the THC DOT dataset.

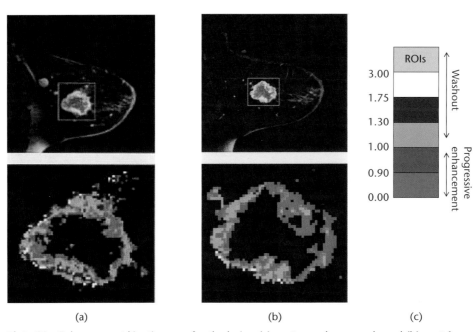

Color Plate 19 Enhancement kinetic maps for the lesion (a) post one chemo cycle and (b) post four chemo cycles. Blue (dark gray) pixels represent progressive enhancement and yellow (light gray) pixels correspond to contrast agent washout.

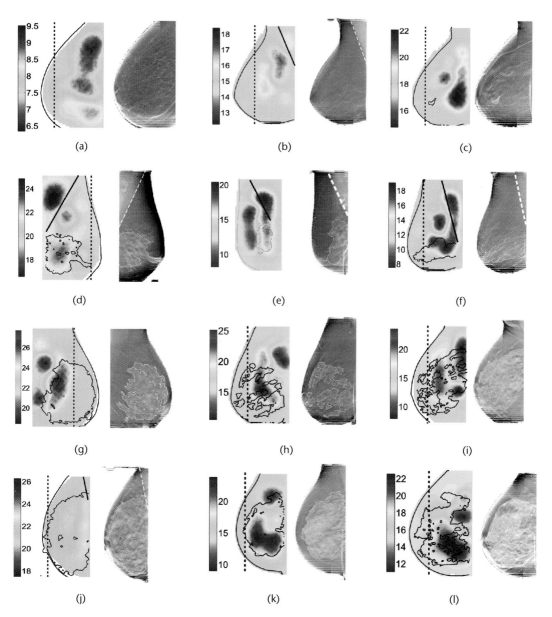

Color Plate 20 Reconstructed total hemoglobin concentration ([HbT]) and DBT images for various subjects. (a–c) The images in the first row are examples of fatty breast reconstructions, (d–f) show scattered density breasts, (g–i) show heterogeneously dense breasts, and (j–l) show extremely dense breasts. All images are slices extracted along a horizontal plane from the reconstructed 3D [HbT] maps. The black dashed line denotes the edge of optical source/detector coverage. The white dashed line on the DBT slice and the black solid line on the [HbT] images denote the boundaries of the chest-wall muscle regions. (Use permitted by the IEEE.)

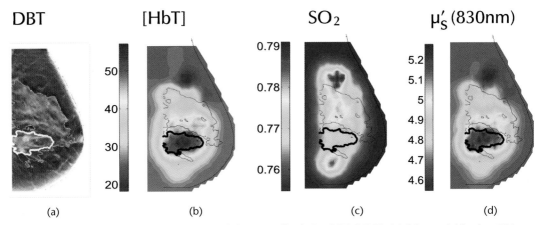

Color Plate 21 (a) The DBT image slice and the optically derived (b) [HbT], (c) SO_2, and (d) μ'_s at 830 nm (cm^{-1}) images for breast with a 3-cm invasive ductal carcinoma (IDC) collocating with a ductal carcinoma in situ (DCIS). (Use permitted by the Radiological Society of North America.)

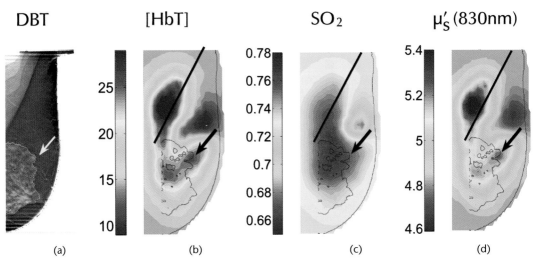

Color Plate 22 (a) The DBT image slice and the optically derived (b) [HbT], (c) SO_2, and (d) μ'_s at 830 nm (cm^{-1}) images for breast with a 1-cm invasive ductal carcinoma (IDC). An arrow points to the location of the tumor on each image. (Use permitted by the Radiological Society of North America.)

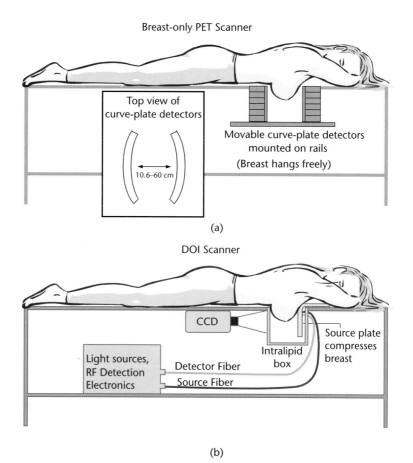

Color Plate 23 (a) Breast-only PET scanner. The breast hangs freely between the two movable detector units. (b) DOI breast scanner. The breast is mildly compressed to 5.5–7.5 cm.

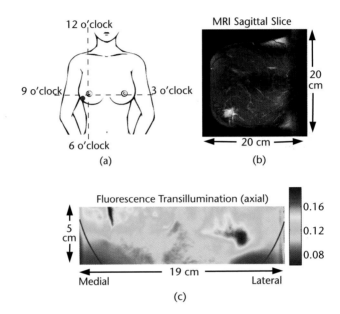
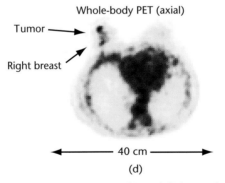

Color Plate 24 (a) Illustration of the tumor location. (b) Gadolinium-enhanced sagittal MR image slice showing the tumor in the lower left corner. (c) Fluorescent transillumination image (explained in text). (d) Axial slice from ^{18}F-FDG whole-body PET image. The view is from the patient's feet (i.e., the right breast appears on the left side). [Figures (a–c) from Chapter 10, [63]. © 2007 Optical Society of America. Reprinted with permission.]

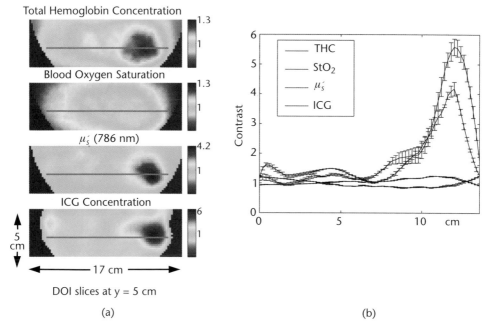

Color Plate 25 Images of total hemoglobin, blood oxygen saturation, μ'_s, and ICG concentration. (a) Axial slices through the plane containing the tumor are shown. (b) Graphs of the values in the images along a horizontal line passing through the center of the tumor. (*From:* Chapter 10, [63]. © 2007 Optical Society of America. Reprinted with permission.)

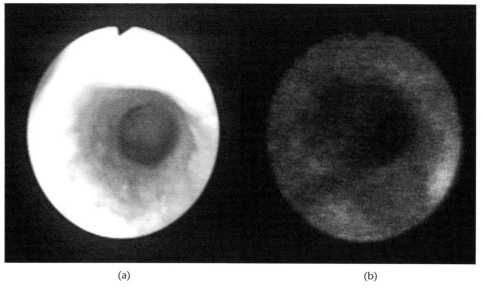

Color Plate 26 Barrett's esophagus imaged with (a) white light and (b) broadband blue light 3 hours post oral ALA at 2 mgkg^{-1}. (Photos courtesy of Dr. Ralph DaCosta, Toronto, Ontario, Canada.)

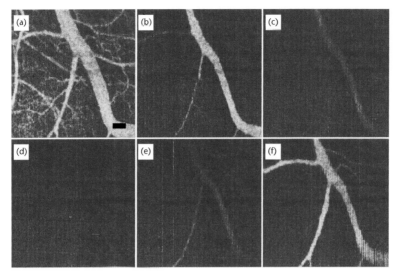

Color Plate 27 Speckle variance OCT imaging of Visodyne-mediated PDT within a 1×1 mm region of the dorsal skin-fold window chamber mouse model (fluence rate =167 mWcm^{-2}, total fluence =100 Jcm^{-2}). This series of images show complete shutdown of vessels and subsequent reperfusion of major vessels post PDT. (a) $T = 0$ minute (start irradiation with 690 nm laser). (b) $T = 2$ minutes. (c) $T = 7$ minutes. (d) $T = 10$ minutes (stop irradiation). (e) $T = 12$ minutes. (f) $T = 20$ minutes. Scale bar: 100 μm. (Courtesy of A. Mariampillai, V. Yang, and A. Vitkin.)

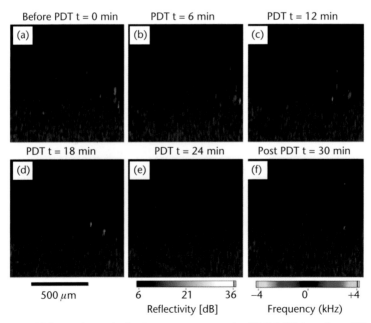

Color Plate 28 Interstitial Doppler optical coherence tomography (IS-DOCT) imaging of Photofrin-mediated PDT (fluence rate = 15 mWcm^{-2}, fluence = 22 Jcm^{-2}) in the IS-DOCT region of interest in a rat Dunning prostate xenograft model. (a–f) IS-DOCT imaging sequence of color-Doppler blood detection overlaid onto structural IS-DOCT images for PDT treatment. Complete vascular shutdown occurred with reprofusion of vessels post PDT treatment. (Photo courtesy of Beau Standish.)

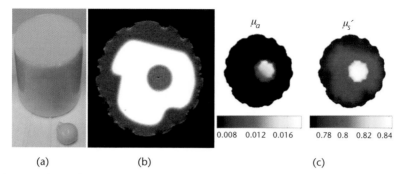

(a) (b) (c)

Color Plate 29 A gelatin phantom is shown in (a) a photograph and (b) a T1-weighted MRI image of the structure in cross-section. The inner layer (light region) contains Gadolinium for MR contrast (1% by volume). The inner inclusion is a 2 cm diameter sphere. (c) The NIR images were reconstructed by using the interior structural information of the MRI. (Chapter 12, [84].)

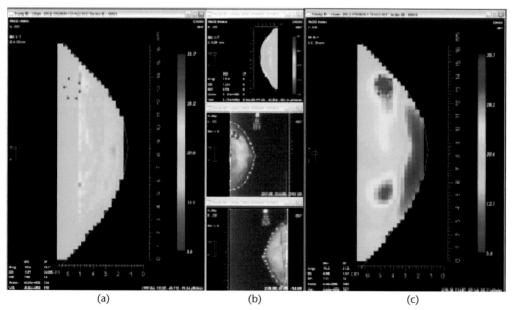

(a) (b) (c)

Color Plate 30 (a) Mammogram with cranio-caudal (CC) view of left breast, (b) CC view of first slice of left breast's 3D oxyhemoglobin image, and (c) third slice of CC view of the oxyhemoglobin image displayed on the review workstation. The lesion is defined by the clinician on the 2D mammogram (blue dotted circle). Through the colocalization software, the ROI is automatically remapped onto the optical image and automatically positioned on every slice.

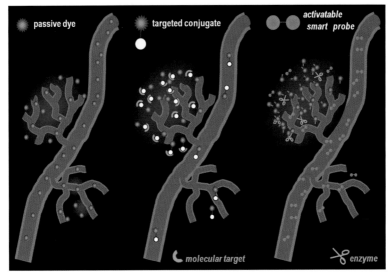
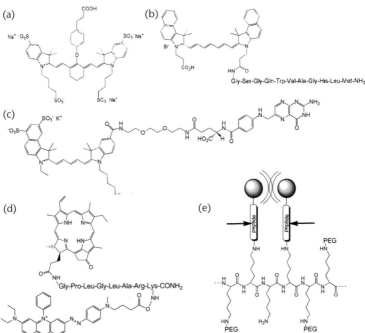

Color Plate 31 Illustration of the general routes to optical contrast including passive, targeted, and activatable agents shown in a tumor vasculature model. Examples representing chemical structures of fluorescent imaging probes are depicted: (a) nonspecific dye IRDye78 (Chapter 16, [12]), (b) cyanine dye-peptide conjugate Cybesin (Chapter 16, [13]), (c) Cy5.5-conjugate with folate (Chapter 16, [14]), (d) pyropheophorbide a construct with MMP-7 peptide substrate and BHQ-3 quencher (Chapter 16, [15]), and (e) activatable graft polymer with enzymatically cleavable peptide-Cy5.5 units (Chapter 16, [16]).

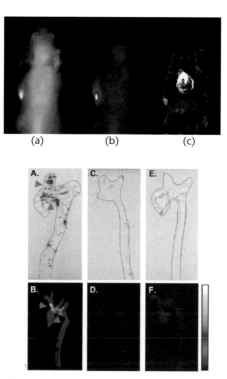

Color Plate 32 Examples of biological imaging performance of MRI/optical probes comparing MRI with fluorescence imaging. Upper row: imaging of lymph nodes using a PAMAM dendrimer covalently loaded with Gd-DTPA and Cy5.5 (Chapter 16, [86]): (a) white light/fluorescence, (b) fluorescence false color, and (c) intensity projection MRI from 3D gradient echo sequence. Lower row: Imaging of atherosclerotic plaques using a VCAM-1 targeting peptide conjugated to a fluorescent iron oxide nanoparticle [see illustration of Figure 16.2(a)]; ex vivo MRI and fluorescence of ApoE−/− mouse (A, B) showing uptake, controls (wild type mouse in C, D and nontargeted particle E, F) without probe accumulation (Chapter 16, [74]).

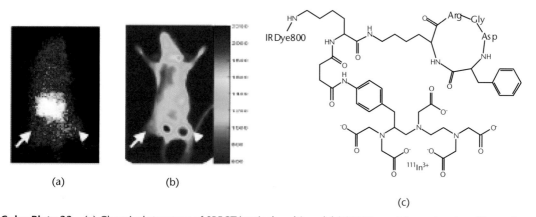

Color Plate 33 (a) Chemical structure of SPECT/optical multimodal (K)RGD-peptide conjugate with cyanine dye IRDye800 (LiCOR) and DTPA labeled with indium-111: comparative in vivo imaging of $\alpha\beta_3$-positive human melanoma tumors in mice using (b) scintigraphy and (c) fluorescence reflectance imaging (Chapter 16, [97, 98]).

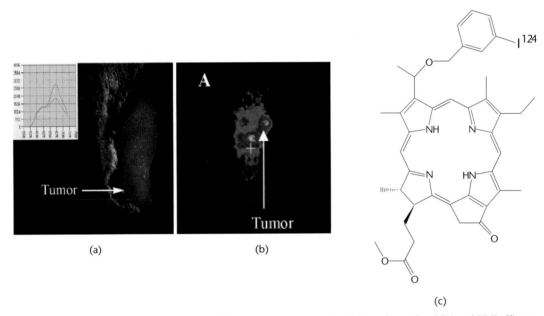

Color Plate 34 (a) Chemical structure of PET/optical pyropheophorbide probe with additional PDT efficacy, (b) in vivo tumor imaging (24 hours) with "cold" compound after spectral unmixing procedure, and (c) parallel PET imaging experiment using the "hot" derivative carrying iodine-124 radionuclide (Chapter 16, [101]).

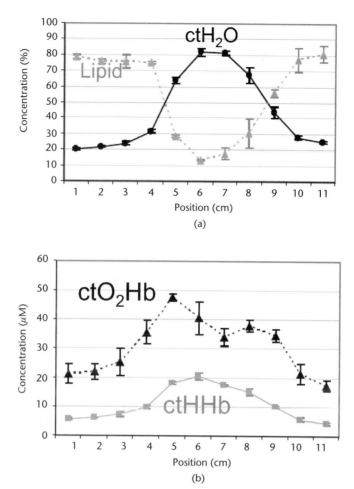

Figure 8.6 Corresponding DOS-derived physiological properties for Patient 1: (a) ctH$_2$O and lipid and (b) ctO$_2$Hb and ctHHb concentrations were determined at 11 positions at 1.0 cm intervals over the lesion and surrounding tissue. Error bars represent the standard deviation of repeat measurements [10].

and 5 probe normal tissue with the presence of glandular tissue at positions 4 and 5. DOS results (Figure 8.7) display a 50% increase in ctO$_2$Hb in the tumor compared to the surrounding normal tissue (22.4 ± 2 μM versus 14.6 ± 2 μM) and a 70% increase at the tumor center (24.9 μM), 30% greater ctHHb (5.0 ± 0.8 μM versus 3.8 ± 0.2 μM), 64% greater ctH$_2$O (36.2 ± 2% versus 22.1 ± 2%), and a 15% decrease in adipose content (68.4 ± 3% versus 80.3 ± 3%). The TOI is approximately 2.5 times greater for the fibroadenoma at the tumor center (2.64 ± 0.07 versus 1.06 ± 0.10).

Case 3: Monitoring Chemotherapy in Conjunction with cMRI
These data were reported by Shah et al. [14] in 2005 and correspond to the patient described in Case 1. Fat-suppressed, T1-weighted sagittal cMRI of the right breast taken 14 days after the initial Adriamycin/Cytoxan (AC) chemotherapy cycle revealed a 3.7 × 3.9 × 3.9 cm invasive ductal carcinoma with a central area of

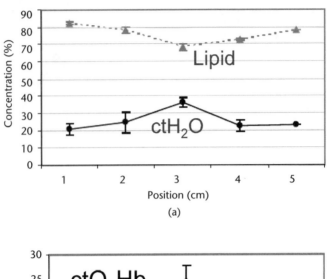

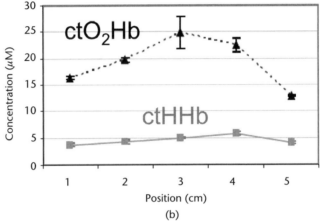

Figure 8.7 Corresponding DOS-derived results for Patient 2: (a) ctH_2O (circles) and lipid (triangles) and (b) ctO_2Hb (triangles) and ctHHb (squares) concentrations were determined at five positions at 1 cm intervals over the lesion and surrounding tissue. Error bars represent standard deviation of repeat measurements.

necrosis and strong peripheral rim enhancement in the upper lateral right breast [Figure 8.8(a)]. The composition of the surrounding breast tissue is mostly fatty, as indicated by the dark T1 regions. The T2-wieghted sagittal image of the same breast shows increased intensity in the central area of the tumor mass, indicating high water content in the necrotic core. The calculated tumor volume was 21.9 cc.

DOS-derived parameters of the right breast show that there were significant differences between tissue at the lesion center compared to the periphery. There was a 3- to 4-fold increase in water content ($81.4 \pm 1\%$ versus $24 \pm 3\%$, respectively), and a 2- to 2.5-fold increase in ctTHB ($56 \pm 7\,\mu M$ versus $27 \pm 4\,\mu M$). Concurrently, there were large reductions in lipid content (13% to 30% versus $78 \pm 2\%$) and S_tO_2 ($66 \pm 0.2\%$ versus $78 \pm 1\%$). The scatter power increased from 0.3 to 0.7 in normal tissue to 1.1 ± 0.1 at the center of the lesion, and the scattering is 0.86 ± 0.05 mm^{-1} at 658 nm for all positions.

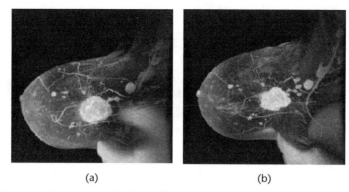

Figure 8.8 Maximum intensity projections of the lesion (a) after one cycle of chemotherapy, and (b) after four cycles of chemotherapy. The lesion measures 3.7 × 3.9 × 3.9 cm in (a) versus 3.1 × 3.5 × 2.8 in (b).

MRI examination 14 days after the fourth cycle of AC revealed a 3.1 × 3.5 × 2.8 cm lesion and a 5 to 10 mm reduction in each dimension from the previous MRI, with a reduced tumor volume of 13.7 cc (Figure 8.8). Changes in enhancement kinetics were determined by segmenting the lesion into regions with different enhancement kinetics. Color Plate 19 shows enhancement kinetic maps of a sagittal slice through the lesion obtained from cMRIs at both time points. Image regions where contrast enhancement at the late postcontrast time point (S_2) is greater than the early postcontrast time point (S_1) represent progressive enhancement and are colored blue (dark gray). Pixels where $S_1 = S_2$ correspond to regions that enhance quickly and wash out; these regions are colored yellow (light gray). After one cycle of AC, 51.3% of the tumor displays contrast-agent washout; after the fourth cycle, 26.1% of the tumor displays contrast-agent washout. Peak enhancement also decreased; after one cycle of AC, the mean percentage-enhancement (PE) value for the top 5% of enhancing voxels in the digitized MRI is 271.8% above background. After the fourth cycle of chemotherapy, the corresponding mean PE was 163.9%. These changes indicate that a reduction in contrast-enhancement and signal wash-out has occurred in the lesion in conjunction with a drop in tumor size.

Figure 8.9 shows DOS results for both time points. The shapes of the linescans indicate that all measured parameters are sensitive to the decrease in tumor size. Full-width, half-maximum scans of water, ctTHB, and lipid reveal an approximately 1 cm drop in tumor size [Figure 8.9(a, b, d)], while S_tO_2 values change over a region corresponding to approximately 2 cm [Figure 8.9(c)]. There is a 43.7% overall reduction in total hemoglobin concentration (41.6 μM versus 23.4 μM), and the peak water concentration is similar at both time points (81% versus 75%). However, there is a 17.1% reduction in the overall water content of the lesion (44.4% versus 36.8%), as well as a 7% decrease in S_tO_2, and the lipid content has increased by approximately two- to threefold in all positions across the tumor.

Table 8.2 compares changes in cMRI anatomic and kinetic parameters with DOS calculations. The 39.7% decrease in peak enhancement indicates vascular-perfusion changes and agrees well with the 38.7% drop in total hemoglobin content determined by DOS. The 37.6% reduction in tumor volume is commensurate with optical measurements that show a 33% increase in lipid.

Table 8.2 Comparison of Changes in Kinetic MRI Contrast Parameters and DOS Parameters at Two Time Points in Chemotherapy

	Tumor Volume (cc)	Peak Enhancement (Top 5% of Voxels, Percentage above t_0)	Percentage of Tumor Volume with SER ≥ 1.30	ctTHB (Peak Values, μM)	S_tO_2 (Peak Values, %)	ctTHB Average Values (μM)	Water-Content Average Values (%)	Lipid-Content Average Values (%)
Post chemo 1	21.7	271.8	14.54	56.02	74.9	41.6	44.4	48.6
Post chemo 4	13.8	163.9	4.48	34.3	68.1	23.4	36.8	71.9
Difference (%)	−36.4	−39.7	−69.0	−38.7	−9.1	−43.7	−17.1	+33.0

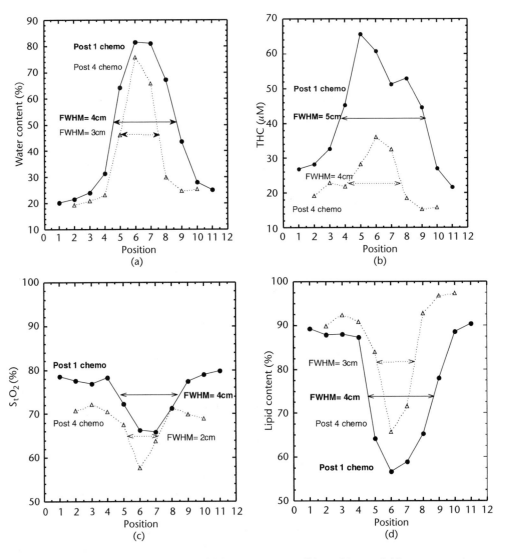

Figure 8.9 Comparison of DOS-derived (a) water content, (b) total hemoglobin concentration, (c) tissue oxygen saturation, and (d) lipids for the lesion after one cycle of chemotherapy and four cycles of chemotherapy. The full-width, half-maximum (FWHM) is indicated on each linescan.

8.2.3 Discussion

The results presented in this section help establish the accuracy and reliability of DOS-derived physiological properties by validation with high-resolution MRI in normal, benign, and malignant breast tissue in vivo. The strong quantitative relationship between DOS lipid and water measurements and MRI morphology in the six premenopausal women support the sensitivity of DOS to compositional differences between glandular- and fatty-tissue compartments across a range of ages. Correlations between ctO_2Hb, $ctHHb$, and cMRI demonstrate DOS sensitivity to subtle changes in metabolism and vascularity present in more active glandular tissues. $ctHHb$ correlates more strongly to tissue composition and may be a better indicator of tissue metabolism than ctO_2Hb. Thus, DOS measurements report both structural and functional properties in distinct regions in the breast. This is summarized in the TOI, a combination of anatomical and functional parameters, which shows a 4.5-fold difference in regions of dominant fatty tissue versus dominant glandular tissue.

Hemoglobin concentration is related to blood-volume fraction in a discrete region of tissue. The total hemoglobin concentration is a measure of tissue vascularity and, in malignant cases, angiogenesis. Gd-DTPA-enhancement patterns of three lesions correspond to regions of elevated tissue hemoglobin measured by DOS. This correlation is anticipated because contrast-agent delivery to the tumor occurs via blood perfusion. Thus, MRI contrast-enhancement intensity and kinetics are employed as indicators of increased vascularity and/or angiogenic factors.

DOS provides complementary vascular information to MRI since the DOS hemoglobin signal is heavily weighted toward microvascular components. MRI structural resolution limits its sensitivity to comparatively larger vessels. Furthermore, DOS directly measures the presence of absolute hemoglobin concentration and hemoglobin oxygen saturation by spectral features of the heme group, whereas MR enhancement is reported in relative terms and dependent upon complex vascular variables for contrast-agent delivery [20].

For example, in the necrotic core of the invasive ductal carcinoma, there is a lack of Gd-DTPA enhancement, whereas DOS measures elevated hemoglobin. In this region of the tumor, DOS may be detecting the presence of nonvascular hemoglobin or hemoglobin breakdown products not accessible to Gd-DTPA. Thus, the 20% decrease in S_tO_2 observed in the invasive ductal carcinoma is likely associated with necrotic tissue. This value is consistent with previously reported data in an animal model, which showed an 18% decrease in S_tO_2 in necrotic versus viable, well-perfused tissue [21].

One source of error in this study is the patient geometry between the two modalities. DOS measurements were made in the supine position, whereas MRI measurements were made in the prone position. This produces an error in depth and tissue-thickness measurements, especially in the tangential measurements made in the premenopausal studies. Despite this design limit, a strong correlation was observed. Coregistration methods that explicitly address this limitation are described in Chapter 7.

The effects of chemotherapy further support MRI/DOS anatomic and functional correlations. Reduction in tumor size determined by DOS line scan FWHM changes (approximately 1 cm for water, lipid, and ctTHb linescans) generally agree with changes in dimension established by MRI (0.4 to 1.4 cm, Figure 8.8). It is also important to note that DOS measurements were made at 1.0 cm intervals, thus the coarseness of resolution of DOS may also play a role in determining lesion size.

Changes in quantitative parameters derived from cMRI also correlate with DOS-derived physiological parameters. The decrease in tumor volume (37.6%) corresponds to an increase in tumor lipid over all position (33%) between the two time points. The increase in lipid content reflects the greater contribution of normal (fatty) breast tissue to the weighted average of the DOS signal which occurs with a decrease in tumor volume. Peak water content levels are similar at both time points (81% versus 75%), reflecting the absence of significant alterations in the fluid-filled necrotic center of the lesion. Further support that peak water signals primarily reflect a fluid-filled structure is provided by a concomitant decrease in scattering. The overall water content (determined from all positions) decreased approximately 17% following chemotherapy, probably due to changes in tumor edema and cellularity.

Note that the size of the lesion did not change dramatically, but overall total hemoglobin decreased considerably (41.6 versus 23.4 μM) which is validated by an approximately 40% decrease in peak enhancement and an overall reduction in signal washout in cMRI (Color Plate 19 and Table 8.2). These observations confirm that significant functional response to AC therapy can occur in diseased tissue that cannot be assessed by changes in lesion size alone [18, 19, 22]. They provide additional support for the idea that DOS and cMRI have complementary sensitivity to similar hemodynamic processes.

8.3 Monitoring and Predicting Response to Breast Cancer Neoadjuvant Chemotherapy

In the previous section, we compared DOS with cMRI in order to validate the functional and structural origins of optical signals. DOS-derived physiological data were shown to correlate with cMRI measurements of necrosis, vasculature, and lesion size. Changes in kinetic parameters correlate with changes in DOS-derived physiological parameters during chemotherapy. In this section, we demonstrate that DOS measurements alone can predict final, postsurgical pathological response in 11 breast cancer patients undergoing a 3 month Adriamycin/Cytoxan (AC) neoadjuvant-chemotherapy treatment. Our goal is to provide oncologists with quantitative information that could be used to optimize therapy for individual patients, evaluate the efficacy of novel dosing regimens, and assist in the development and characterization of experimental therapeutics. The results of this study have been previously presented in a more detailed report [23].

8.3.1 Materials and Methods

This study uses the same DOS instrument and similar measurement procedures as described in the previous section.

8.3 Monitoring and Predicting Response to Breast Cancer Neoadjuvant Chemotherapy

8.3.1.1 Patient Characteristics

We studied 11 cancer patients receiving neoadjuvant chemotherapy. All subjects provided informed, written consent according to an institution-approved protocol (University of California Irvine 02-2306). The average subject age was 47.4 ± 11.4 years with a range of 30 to 65, and the average body mass index was 28.8 ± 5.6 with a range of 21.6 to 41.2. Before treatment, the average tumor maximum-length axis was 37 ± 23 mm, with a median of 30 mm and a range of 18 to 95 mm. Two subjects were premenopausal, and the remaining nine were postmenopausal. Final pathological response was determined from standard pathology. Initial lesion sizes were determined by ultrasound. Pathological response was stratified into "responders" ($n = 6$) and "nonresponders" ($n = 5$). Consistently with radiological definitions, responders were defined as subjects with greater than 50% change in the maximum-tumor axis in final pathology dimensions relative to the initial maximum-axis dimension. The remaining subjects were considered nonresponders.

8.3.1.2 Chemotherapy Treatment Sequence

Nine of the 11 patients were treated with three to four cycles of A/C therapy, followed by three to four cycles of taxanes. The remaining two subjects received three cycles of A/C therapy without the taxanes. Each chemotherapy cycle lasted 3 weeks.

8.3.1.3 Measurement Sequence

Linescans were performed within 1 week before and 1 week after the initial A/C treatment. Initial DOS measurements were performed 2 to 4 weeks after the diagnostic biopsy. At each location, broadband optical absorption and reduced-scattering spectra were obtained (Figure 8.10). On average, measurements were performed 1.8 ± 4.5 days before and 6.5 ± 1.4 after the initial A/C therapy. Baseline measurements were performed within 1 week of therapy. We removed intersubject variations by analyzing the ratio of pretherapy and posttherapy tumor measurements; thus, no change has the value of unity. Measurements were also performed on the contralateral normal breast to serve as a measure of normal physiological variations, although the effects of chemotherapy are not localized. Thus, patients served as their own controls.

8.3.2 Results

8.3.2.1 DOS Sensitivity: Binary Classification

Table 8.3 summarizes the observed changes in all five measured DOS base parameters for a simple binary response classification of "responder" versus "nonresponder" (see Section 8.3.1). The best predictor of therapeutic response was ctHHb. The average ctHHb relative value was 1.02 ± 0.05 in the nonresponder group, compared to a 27% drop (0.73 ± 0.17) in the responder group, which was a statistically significant difference ($Z = 0.008$, 2 tailed, 95% confidence). ctO_2Hb also decreased significantly after therapy ($Z = 0.02$). Unlike ctHHb, both responders and nonresponders dropped in ctO_2Hb: nonresponders by 18% (0.82 ± 0.10)

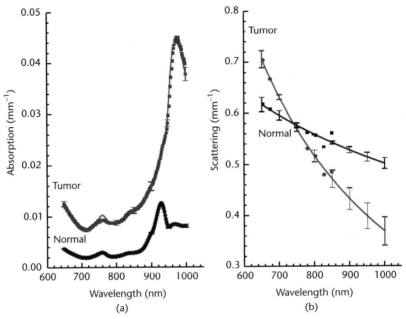

Figure 8.10 Near-infrared (a) absorption and (b) reduced-scattering spectra obtained noninvasively from a 30 mm diameter tumor in the breast of a neoadjuvant-chemotherapy subject. The heightened absorption results from a combination of increased hemoglobin and water relative to normal breast tissue (left panel). The sharp spectral decrease in scattering, as reflected in the scatter-power measurement, is likely due to increases in both vessel density and fibrous tissue in tumor tissue relative to normal breast tissue (right panel). These tumor spectra were obtained from the +10 mm position, whereas the normal spectra were taken from the corresponding location on the contralateral normal side.

Table 8.3 Single-Parameter Predictors: Summary of the Observed Relative Changes in All Five Measured DOS Base Parameters for a Simple Binary Response Classification of "Responder" Versus "Nonresponder"

Parameter	Responder (N = 6)	Nonresponder (N = 5)	Z
ctHHb (μm)	0.73 ± 0.17	1.02 ± 0.05	0.008*
ctO$_2$Hb (μm)	0.67 ± 0.06	0.82 ± 0.10	0.03*
ctH$_2$O (%)	0.89 ± 0.2	0.96 ± 0.03	0.41
ctH$_2$O (relative)	0.80 ± 0.08	0.96 ± 0.03	0.008*
Lipid (%)	1.30 ± 0.3	1.11 ± 0.14	0.41
SP	0.88 ± 0.20	0.97 ± 0.20	0.93

* = significant result; 1 = no change

and responders by 33% (0.67 ± 0.06). These findings confirm our previous single-subject report of chemotherapy-induced anemia that affects systemic oxygen delivery, causing a drop in ctO$_2$Hb. In contrast, ctHHb, a sensitive index of local oxygen consumption, is unaffected by systematic changes [13].

ctH$_2$O also changed in response to neoadjuvant chemotherapy (Table 8.3). For the nonresponder group, ctH$_2$O values remained nearly constant (0.96 ± 0.03), whereas for the responder group, ctH$_2$O decreased (0.89 ± 0.2). The difference between these changes, however, was not statistically significant ($Z = 0.4$). The reason for this lack of significance is that in some cases, ctH$_2$O increased after therapy (an initial effect we have seen previously [13]). In other patients, ctH$_2$O arrived at a peak value a few days after therapy and then decreased below the baseline on average 1 week later. If we consider the absolute value of the change from baseline, the relative ctH$_2$O changes (20%) are significant ($Z = 0.008$). The dynamics of this ctH$_2$O increase and subsequent decrease is likely due to individual variations in tumor drug response, edema, and necrosis.

8.3.2.2 DOS Predictive Value

Calculations of sensitivity and specificity for predicting the known final pathological response were performed using discriminant analysis. The results of single-parameter analysis show that ctHHb is the best predictor of response (83% sensitivity, 100% specificity), followed by relative changes in ctH$_2$O (80% sensitivity, 100% specificity). One patient of the 11 was misclassified when only ctHHb was used as a predictor. ctO$_2$Hb also performed well in this limited sample (83% sensitivity, 80% specificity). Parameters that report more on the structural nature of tissue (i.e., lipids and SP) were not good single predictors, presumably because more time is needed before significant changes in tumor size can be detected. If we use a second parameter in the discrimination analysis (e.g., relative water changes and ctHHb), we find that perfect classification can be achieved (i.e., 100% sensitivity and 100% sensitivity).

The scatter plot in Figure 8.11 shows ctH$_2$O versus ctHHb for both pathological responders (■) and nonresponders (▲). The error bars represent the differences between subsequent linescans on the same date (generally about 5% variation). There is clear separation of responders from nonresponders on the basis of tumor biochemical activity. All of the five nonresponders are essentially near unity on both axes, while the responders display a more pronounced change response in both ctHHb and ctH$_2$O. Note that ctH$_2$O change plotted here is not the absolute value as described earlier.

8.3.2.3 DOS Sensitivity: Tertiary Classification

All subjects can be reclassified according to a more clinically relevant scheme. Figure 8.12 provides the same information as previously but using more rigorous complete (cpR), partial (ppR), and nonpathologic response (npR) criteria. Error bars are not presented for the cpR group since only one subject achieved cpR. Also note that meaningful statistical comparisons are not possible given the heavy imbalance of subjects between categories. Nevertheless, a clear trend suggests that the extent of pathologic response is proportional to the degree of change in DOS-measured parameters. It does not appear that there are significant differences between the lipid signals of ppR and npR. Yet, it does appear that there may be meaningful differences between the ppR and npR groups for both ctHHb and ctH$_2$O. Although

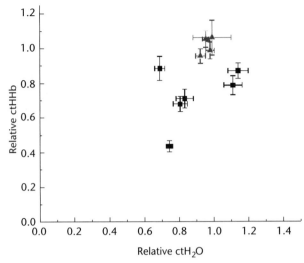

Figure 8.11 Scatter plot of noninvasively measured ctHHb and ctH_2O responses for both pathological responders (■) and nonresponders (▲). A relatively tight pattern is observed for the nonresponders on both axes, whereas responders display significantly higher changes in both ctHHb and ctH_2O. Note that the ctH_2O values are not the delta-ctH_2O values described in the text. Error bars represent the standard deviation of two linescans over the same tissue region.

this may also be true of the SP, the high degree of variation within the ppR group obscures this result.

8.3.3 Discussion

Anthracycline derivatives, such as the doxorubicin used in this trial, have been found to induce both an early increase in apoptotic activity and a decrease in proliferation [24]. A key question is whether these early apoptotic and proliferative changes in tumors can produce macroscopically detectable light-scattering signals that are predictive of pathological response and are consistent with known mechanisms. DOS, which relies solely on endogenous contrast in this study, does not directly measure proliferation or apoptosis. However, DOS-measured tissue hemoglobin [25] is representative of tumor microvasculature [26], which, in turn, is sensitive to cellular metabolism.

The overall decrease in ctTHb during chemotherapy is a consequence of alterations in tumor cell metabolism, blood vessel density, and systemic effects. These processes can be separated, in part, by considering ctO_2Hb and ctHHb independently. As was previously described, a portion of the ctO_2Hb decrease can be attributed to the impact of anemia, while ctHHb is representative of tumor-tissue oxygen consumption. As tumor cells undergo apoptosis and reduced proliferation rates, oxygen delivery and consumption diminish. DOS measurements are sensitive to these events, as indicated by the drop in ctO_2Hb and ctHHb levels, respectively. With increased cell death, the loss of oxygen-consuming sources (i.e., cells) causes tumor ctHHb levels to drop even further.

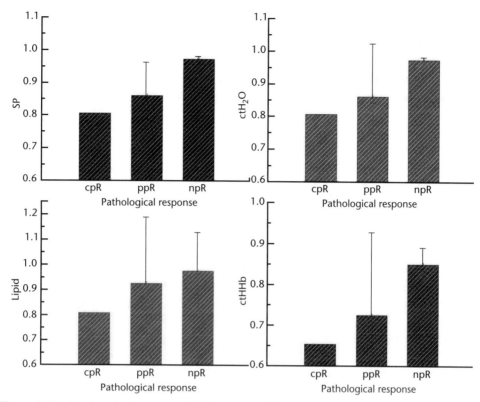

Figure 8.12 Noninvasively measured DOS responses for complete pathological responders (cpR), pathological partial responders (ppR), and pathological nonresponders (npR). Each panel represents one DOS basis parameter. The proper trends are observed, but small numbers prevent any appropriate statistical analysis. Nonresponders are clearly separated from the complete responder; however, there is high variance within the partial-response category. Error bars represent the standard deviation of the subjects within each category.

8.4 Summary and Conclusions

The validation of DOS by high-resolution cMRI provides a necessary step in the development of the technique as a new modality in breast clinical management. Combining high-resolution functional information from cMRI with DOS measurements provides better accuracy in interpreting DOS signals. Understanding the optical signature of different tissue types can lead to the development of more accurate diagnostic indices involving several optical parameters. In addition, optical methods can be used to understand the origin of complex vascular factors involved in cMRI enhancement kinetics since tissue-component concentrations are measured directly and not inferred [27]. Ultimately, combining DOS with MRI can lead to a more accurate classification of tissue types and enhance lesion diagnostic and prognostic capabilities in vivo.

An important clinical application of DOS is monitoring and predicting neoadjuvant chemotherapy, which is increasingly prescribed for patients with locally advanced disease in order to reduce primary tumor size, minimize metastasis impact, and improve breast-tissue conservation during surgery. DOS provides endogenous in vivo biomarkers that report on tissue biochemical status, which may predict the degree of pathological response in treated tumors. Thus, using DOS measurements may become a practical bedside approach for monitoring and predicting chemotherapy response in individual patients.

Acknowledgments

This work was made possible by the National Institutes of Health (NIH) National Center for Research Resources (NCRR), the Laser Microbeam and Medical Program (LAMMP, P41RR01192), the California Breast Cancer Research Program, and the National Cancer Institute's (NCI) Network for Translational Research: Optical Imaging (NTROI) program (U54CA105480) and NIH ROM CA 069587. Beckman Laser Institute programmatic support is provided by the Air Force Office of Scientific Research (AFOSR) and the Beckman Foundation. We wish to thank Amanda Durkin for her contributions in constructing and shipping the laser breast scanner (LBS) instrument to the University of California, San Francisco (UCSF); Jessica Gibbs, the clinical coordinator for the study; and Evelyn Proctor from the UCSF Magnetic Resonance Science Center. We would also like to thank Dr. David Hsiang, Dr. John Butler, and Dr. Rita Mehta. Finally, we wish to thank the subjects who generously volunteered for this study.

References

[1] Srinivasan, S., et al. "Near-infrared characterization of breast tumors in vivo using spectrally constrained reconstruction." *Technol. Canc. Res. Treat.* 4(5) (2005): 513–526.

[2] Nioka, S., and B. Chance. "NIR spectroscopic detection of breast cancer." *Technol. Canc. Res. Treat.* 4(5) (2005): 497–512.

[3] Chance, B., et al. "Breast cancer detection based on incremental biochemical and physiological properties of breast cancers: A six-year, two-site study." *Acad. Radiol.* 12(8) (2005): 925–933.

[4] Grosenick, D., H. Wabnitz, K. T. Moesta, J. Mucke, P. M. Schlag, and H. Rinneberg. "Time-domain scanning optical mammography: II. Optical properties and tissue parameters of 87 carcinomas." *Phys. Med. Biol.* 50(11) (2005): 2451–2468.

[5] Gu, X., Q. Zhang, M. Bartlett, L. Schutz, L. L. Fajardo, and H. Jiang. "Differentiation of cysts from solid tumors in the breast with diffuse optical tomography." *Acad. Radiol.* 11(1) (2004): 53–60.

[6] Zhu, Q., et al. "Ultrasound-guided optical tomographic imaging of malignant and benign breast lesions: Initial clinical results of 19 cases." *Neoplasia* 5(5) (2003): 379–388.

[7] Pogue, B. W., et al. "Quantitative hemoglobin tomography with diffuse near-infrared spectroscopy: Pilot results in the breast." *Radiology* 218(1) (2001): 261–266.

[8] Shah, N., et al. "Noninvasive functional optical spectroscopy of human breast tissue." *Proc. Natl. Acad. Sci. USA* 98(8) (2001): 4420–4425.

[9] Srinivasan, S., et al. "Interpreting hemoglobin and water concentration, oxygen saturation, and scattering measured in vivo by near-infrared breast tomography." *Proc. Natl. Acad. Sci. USA* 100(21) (2003): 12349–12354.

[10] Cerussi, A. E., et al. "Sources of absorption and scattering contrast for near-infrared optical mammography." *Acad. Radiol.* 8(3) (2001): 211–218.

[11] Cubeddu, R., C. D'Andrea, A. Pifferi, P. Taroni, A. Torricelli, and G. Valentini. "Effects of the menstrual cycle on the red and near-infrared optical properties of the human breast." *Photochem. Photobiol.* 72(3) (2000): 383–391.

[12] Pogue, B. W., et al. "Characterization of hemoglobin, water, and NIR scattering in breast tissue: Analysis of intersubject variability and menstrual cycle changes." *J. Biomed. Opt.* 9(3) (2004): 541–552.

[13] Jakubowski, D. B., et al. "Monitoring neoadjuvant chemotherapy in breast cancer using quantitative diffuse optical spectroscopy: A case study." *J. Biomed. Opt.* 9(1) (2004): 230–238.

[14] Shah, N., J. E. Gibbs, D. Wolverton, A. Cerussi, N. Hylton, and B. Tromberg. "Combined diffuse optical spectroscopy and contrast-enhanced magnetic resonance imaging for monitoring breast cancer neoadjuvant chemotherapy: A case study." *J. Biomed. Opt.* 10(5) (2005): 051503.

[15] Hsiang, D., et al. "Coregistration of dynamic contrast enhanced MRI and broadband diffuse optical spectroscopy for characterizing breast cancer." *Technol. Canc. Res. Treat.* 4(5) (2005): 549–558.

[16] Pham, T. H., O. Coquoz, J. B. Fishkin, E. Anderson, and B. J. Tromberg. "Broad bandwidth frequency domain instrument for quantitative tissue optical spectroscopy." *Rev. Sci. Instr.* 71(6) (2000): 2500–2513.

[17] Bevilacqua, F., A. J. Berger, A. E. Cerussi, D. Jakubowski, and B. J. Tromberg. "Broadband absorption spectroscopy in turbid media by combined frequency-domain and steady-state methods." *Appl. Opt.* 39(34) (2000): 6498–6507.

[18] Browder, T., C. E. Butterfield, B. M. Kraling, B. Shi, B. Marshall, M. S. O'Reilly, and J. Folkman. "Antiangiogenic scheduling of chemotherapy improves efficacy against experimental drug-resistant cancer." *Canc. Res.* 60(7) (2000): 1878–1886.

[19] Lennernas, B., P. Albertsson, H. Lennernas, and K. Norrby. "Chemotherapy and antiangiogenesis—drug-specific, dose-related effects," *Acta Oncol.* 42(4) (2003): 294–303.

[20] Padhani, A. R. "Contrast agent dynamics in breast MRI." In R. Warren and A. Coulthard (eds.), *Breast MRI in practice*, 43–54. London: Martin Dunitz, 2002.

[21] Merritt, S., F. Bevilacqua, A. J. Durkin, D. J. Cuccia, R. Lanning, B. J. Tromberg, G. Gulsen, H. Yu, J. Wang, and O. Nalcioglu. "Coregistration of diffuse optical spectroscopy and magnetic resonance imaging in a rat tumor model." *Appl. Opt.* 42(16) (2003): 2951–2959.

[22] Martin, W. M., and N. J. McNally. "The cytotoxic action of adriamycin and cyclophosphamide on tumor cells in vitro and in vivo." *Int. J. Radiat. Oncol. Biol. Phys.* 5(8) (1979): 1309–1312.

[23] Cerussi, A., et al. "Predicting response to breast cancer neoadjuvant chemotherapy using diffuse optical spectroscopy." *Proc. Natl. Acad. Sci. USA* 104(10) (2007): 4014–4019.

[24] Arpino, G., et al. "Predictive value of apoptosis, proliferation, HER-2, and topoisomerase IIalpha for anthracycline chemotherapy in locally advanced breast cancer." *Breast Canc. Res. Treat.* 92 (2005): 69–75.

[25] Pogue, B. W., et al. "Quantitative hemoglobin tomography with diffuse near-infrared spectroscopy: Pilot results in the breast." *Radiology* 218 (2001): 261–266.

[26] Liu, H., B. Chance, A. H. Hielscher, S. L. Jacques, and F. K. Tittel. "Influence of blood vessels on the measurement of hemoglobin oxygenation as determined by time-resolved reflectance spectroscopy." *Med. Phys.* 22 (1995): 1209–1217.

[27] Fisher, E. R., et al. "Pathobiology of preoperative chemotherapy: Findings from the National Surgical Adjuvant Breast and Bowel Project (NSABP) protocol B-18." *Cancer* 95 (2002): 681–695.

CHAPTER 9
Optical Imaging and X-Ray Imaging

Qianqian Fang, Stefan Carp, Juliette Selb, and David Boas

9.1 Introduction

9.1.1 Current Clinical Approach to Breast Cancer Screening and Diagnosis

According to the American Cancer Society, 182,460 women will be diagnosed with invasive breast cancer in 2008, and 22% of them will die from the disease. During the same period, another 67,770 will be diagnosed with in situ breast cancer. In fact, approximately one in eight women will develop breast cancer during their lifetime [1].

While some tumors are still discovered by palpation, the majority of breast cancer diagnoses are made with X-ray mammography [2], which offers greater than 80% sensitivity [3, 4]. Still, over 20% of women with breast cancer have had a negative mammogram in the preceding year [5, 6], while nearly 25% of the women called back for additional imaging will prove to have had false-positive results [7]. Furthermore, mammography has significant difficulties in women with dense breasts [8] and in distinguishing malignant from benign tumors. Therefore, the need persists to detect cancers that might be missed by mammography and to improve specificity to reduce the number of unnecessary biopsies.

Other diagnostic methods offer means to address these concerns. Digital mammography has, in recent years, been shown to provide superior diagnostic information with respect to traditional film mammography and continues to gain acceptance [8, 9]. An even more sophisticated form of digital mammography, digital breast tomosynthesis (DBT), is currently in clinical trials; it is hoped that its three-dimensional imaging of the breast will improve the sensitivity and specificity of standard mammography [10–13]. Still, not all types of cancers reveal themselves to X-ray at an early stage [14].

Additional diagnostic techniques in use include color Doppler ultrasonography, which seeks to image blood flow associated with malignant tumors [15]; contrast-enhanced MRI, which is based on imaging before and after applying a gadolinium-based contrast agent [16–21]; and positron emission tomography, which is based on imaging of metabolic contrast [22–24]. These techniques generally offer high sensitivity but relatively low specificity.

Functional methods such as contrast-enhanced MRI and PET are gaining ground with respect to specificity. Schnall et al. [25] and Kuhl et al. [26] have reported that combining morphologic and kinetic data can improve the specificity of the former. Weisenberger et al. [27], Levine et al. [28], and Rosen et al. [29] have reported improved results with positron emission mammography (PEM): 86% sensitivity, 91% specificity for tumors smaller than 2.5 cm. Still, the cost and availability of these techniques inhibit their use for large-scale screening.

Diffuse optical tomography (DOT), an emerging technology for functional imaging [30], offers a relatively inexpensive alternative to more costly methods such as PET, MRI, and PEM. Pioneering work has been reported with respect to DOT-based breast optical imagers [31–40]. Nonetheless, while the technology provides unique opportunities for imaging breast cancer, it is clear that no single imaging modality will detect all cancers with high specificity.

9.1.2 The Importance of Fusing Function and Structural Information

Improved sensitivity and specificity in breast cancer imaging are likely to come from multimodal approaches combining structural and functional imaging technologies. The active development of such approaches has been one of the most notable signatures of medical imaging in the past decade [41]. Rapid advances in diffuse optical tomography [30], PET [42], MRI [43], electrical impedance imaging [44, 45], microwave tomography [46], and other techniques have opened a new frontier for detecting cancer by pinpointing unique functional biomarkers such as hemoglobin concentration [47], oxygenation [35], blood flow [48], and electrical [49] and mechanical [50] properties associated with the presence and growth of tumors. However, most of these functional imaging methods provide only low-resolution images. Combining low-resolution functional imaging with high-resolution structural imaging in a spatially/temporally coregistered manner creates a win-win strategy: for instance, utilizing the high-resolution structure images as a prior, the functional imaging modality could yield improved image quality and reduced artifacts [51, 52] to deliver more accurate representation of the functional status of tissue; at the same time, some existing limitations of the structural imaging modalities can be overcome or reduced by adding complementary physiological information from the functional imaging modality. Coregistration of the two modalities also facilitates interpretation of images and extrapolation of findings from one modality to the other, as well as acceptance by the radiology community of the new technologies.

PET/CT has established the paradigm of combining functional and structural imaging modalities and has fundamentally impacted the path of cancer-patient management [53, 54]. After more than 10 years of development, it is fast approaching maturity and has achieved massive deployment in clinical institutions worldwide. PET/CT has demonstrated significant advantages for accurate diagnosis and staging in certain cancers and offers detection rates substantially higher than MRI or PET or CT alone [55–57]. The success of PET/CT has established the importance of fusing functional and structural information for diagnosis and screening in the clinic.

Inspired by the success of PET/CT, researchers have begun to explore the possibility of combining DOT with structural imaging modalities for imaging breast cancer. Zhu et al. reported clinical application of an ultrasound transducer incorporated into an optical imaging system for imaging both healthy and cancer breasts [33, 58]. Brooksby et al. [59] used DOT/MRI to image healthy subjects and patients with tumors in their breasts, following the earlier work by Ntziachristos et al. [60]. Similar work was reported by Choe et al. [61] and Klifa et al. [62]. Combined DOT/MRI has also been used to monitor response to chemotherapy [34, 61, 63–66].

While combined DOT/MRI appears to be efficacious, incorporating functional imaging into X-ray mammography may provide a more practical alternative for large-scale application. X-ray is relatively inexpensive and, because it is the gold standard in mammographic screening and diagnosis, readily available in most clinics. The approach to integrated DOT and X-ray mammography has several advantages for widespread clinical implementation: (1) the two modalities complement each other very well with respect to image resolution and specificity; (2) the known advantages of X-ray mammography, including ease of access, established approaches to image interpretation, and the extensive knowledge base of the technique, combined with the low-cost and nonionizing radiation of DOT, produce a cost-efficient solution for implementing a multimodality system for breast cancer detection; and (3) the incremental fashion in which the additional diagnostic information from DOT is incorporated to the established X-ray technique may form a cultural bridge and lead to a lower barrier to acceptance by radiologists.

9.1.3 Recent Advances in DOT for Imaging Breast Cancer

The quickly evolving technique of diffuse optical tomography has become one of the most promising modalities for imaging breast cancer. Advanced imaging instruments with more flexible source/detector configurations [32, 36, 40, 67–69], improved portability [70], and faster data acquisition [40, 71, 72] have been reported. At the same time, increasingly sophisticated approaches to diffuse optical image reconstruction have been proposed, taking advantage of (1) prior information available from the use of multiple-wavelength data acquisition (i.e., "spectral priors") [73–75] and structural information available from alternate modalities such as MRI and CT (i.e., "structural priors") [51, 52]; (2) sophisticated online sensor calibration methods [76–78]; (3) 3D modeling [39, 61, 79–81]; and (4) improved algorithmic methods for stabilizing the reconstruction process against sensor noise and other uncertainty (known as the "regularization techniques") [59, 82–84], producing images with better accuracy and reduced artifacts. Following these advances in instrumentation and algorithms, clinical trials using DOT imaging systems have begun at multiple institutions on both healthy and lesion-bearing patients, exploring both the spectral signatures and spatial structures of breast tissues [33, 39, 61, 64, 65, 85, 86].

Recent trials have further demonstrated the sensitivity and specificity of DOT for the presence of breast cancer. The absorption spectra of hemoglobin and water have shown unique features that are specific to the presence of tumors [70]. Statistically significant discrimination of malignant and benign lesions was reported in a recent study involving 108 patients and a time-domain DOT system [35]. A recent study using a combined DOT/MR system demonstrated improvements in image contrast of tumor reconstruction using structural information [59, 85, 87], indicating that combining DOT with mammography will likely provide better sensitivity and specificity compared to either DOT or mammography alone. Ongoing development of optical molecular contrast agents will likely lead to further improvements in the sensitivity and specificity of the technique [88–90].

Other improvements have helped to boost the potential of the technique for breast cancer imaging. Importantly, recent technological advances have enabled the exploration of an additional dimension: time. Dynamic optical imaging, which measures the changes observed in biological tissue in a time-resolved fashion, allows access to a wealth of additional diagnostic information reflecting the tissue metabolic state as well as the response of tissue to external stimuli. Near-infrared optical systems have been developed to image both the intrinsic tissue dynamics [91, 92] and the response of tissue to external stimuli [93, 94]. In particular, we have recently shown that external compression of the breast allows the estimation of the tissue volumetric blood flow and oxygen consumption, which are known to correlate with malignancy [48, 95, 96]. Furthermore, the time evolution of tissue physiological parameters may hold the key to additional cancer markers—for example, the timescales for pressure relaxation after compression, as detected by surface measurement and its effect on hemodynamics, may offer an opportunity to assess tissue mechanical properties.

9.2 Instrumentation and Methods

9.2.1 Tomographic Optical Breast-Imaging System and Tomosynthesis

A combined X-ray/optical breast-imaging system was built at Massachusetts General Hospital (MGH) between 2001 and 2005. The original prototype of the system included only a radio frequency (RF)–modulated imaging unit [97]. After the first clinical trial of the system in 2004, significant modifications were applied. The current design of the tomographic optical breast-imaging (TOBI) system includes both RF-modulated and continuous-wave (CW) laser modules and can be operated in RF and CW modes simultaneously to acquire optical measurements. Figure 9.1(a) shows a photo of the system. The RF subsystem provides two laser wavelengths (685 and 830 nm) modulated at 70 MHz [36]. Optical switches (DiCon, California) multiplex the RF signals to 40 source locations on the probe; the transmitted light from the breast is collected by eight RF avalanche photodiode detectors (APD, Hamamatsu). The RF measurements were used to determine the bulk-optical properties and contribute to improved image resolution when used together with the CW data for image reconstruction.

The CW multiplexer unit (MUX) has six frequency-encoded lasers (685, 750, 808, 830, 906, and 980 nm). A fast Galvo scanner (Innovations in Optics, Inc., Massachusetts) is used to deliver the CW lasers to a maximum of 300 available locations on the optical probe with an average dwell time of 200 ms per location. An additional CW system (TechEn, Inc., Massachusetts) [98] provides 26 frequency-encoded lasers, split equally between 685 and 830 nm, which are used for continuous monitoring of tissue changes at 26 source locations. The CW units share 32 APD (Hamamatsu) detectors, and the CW signals are subsequently demodulated for each channel and wavelength. For all MUX CW signals, demultiplexing follows

9.2 Instrumentation and Methods

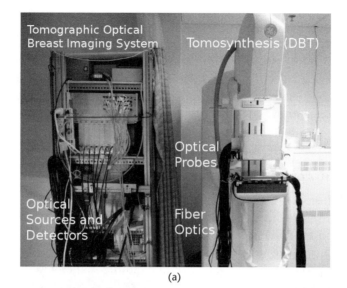

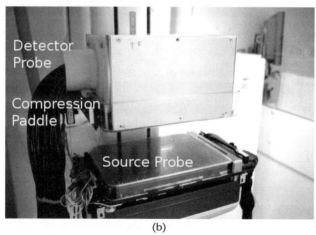

Figure 9.1 Photos of the TOBI/DBT system: (a) overview, and (b) probes.

to separate the signals for each multiplexed source location. In addition to the optical system, a high-resolution linear encoder (Unimeasure, Inc., Oregon) and four pressure transducers (Omigadyne, Inc., Ohio) are mounted on the optical probes to give accurate readings of source-detector separation and the applied pressure, respectively.

The TOBI optical probes [see Figure 9.1(b)] were meticulously designed to provide the capability of coregistration with 2D mammography or tomosynthesis. The anodized aluminum source probe covers a total area of 20 × 18 cm with fiber optics mounting locations over a 5 mm spacing grid. The metallic part of the probe can be securely attached to an optically transparent cassette modified from a standard mammography compression paddle. This cassette is fastened onto the mammography machine. Similarly, the metallic detector probe can be easily mounted onto and detached from the moving compression arm using a push-button lock. The source/detector probes are inserted into the cassettes before the optical measurement is taken and removed before X-ray scans are taken. In both cases, the compression paddles retain their positions to ensure no movement of the target breast.

The tomosynthesis unit used in our research was developed by GE Healthcare. It is capable of collecting 15 projections within a 90° swing angle. The 3D DBT images were reconstructed off-line by a maximum-likelihood-type algorithm [99, 100]. The spatial resolution for a typical DBT image is 0.1 mm in the transverse (x,y) plane with a z slice thickness of 1 mm.

9.2.2 3D Forward Modeling and Nonlinear Image Reconstruction

The diffusion equation was typically used as the mathematical model for the light propagation in human tissue. Various numerical models were implemented and evaluated for solving the diffusion model, including the finite-difference [83] and finite-element (FE) methods [39]. The finite-element approach was found to be particularly promising as it is superior in handling shapes with curved boundaries. This makes it suitable for this application where the geometry of the breast can be readily extracted from the coregistered 3D tomosynthesis scan and modeled as FE meshes. An efficient iterative multi-right-hand-side solver [101] was implemented to the evaluation of the FE solution, which provides 200% to 300% acceleration in solving speed compared to solving for each source and detector individually [102]. On a Pentium IV–class PC, the average computation time for obtaining one forward solution is about 1 second for a mesh with 20,000 nodes.

For accurate recovery of the absorption and scattering properties of breast tissue, a nonlinear parameter-estimation approach based on a Gauss-Newton method was implemented to fully account for the nonlinearity effect of the forward model [39]. With this method, the forward solutions from the initial guesses of optical properties were computed by the FE method, and the sensitivity matrix (i.e., the Jacobian) was calculated by a fast adjoint formulation [39]; using the differences between the measurement and model prediction, updates to the absorption and scattering coefficients were computed by solving a regularized pseudoinversion problem. This update scheme is repeated until a good match between the measurement and model prediction is found. This nonlinear approach was further extended to incorporate simultaneous calibration coefficient recovery and the spectral and structural prior in the reconstruction (see Sections 9.2.3 and 9.2.4).

The accuracy of our forward solver and the nonlinear reconstructor ensures a full exploitation of our measurement data. In the meantime, the flexibility and computational efficiency of the forward model and the adjoint approach for calculating the Jacobian also make 3D optical image reconstruction readily affordable under nondemanding computation conditions.

9.2.3 Simultaneous Image Reconstruction with Calibration Coefficient Estimation

Using a coupling liquid to submerge the breast and interface the optical fibers and the target is a common approach to reducing systematic error and is often found with stand-alone optical breast-imaging systems [35, 38, 61, 103]. However, this approach may add significant complication to the operating procedures for combining with X-ray in the clinic and is therefore not preferred for TOBI.

As described in Section 9.2.1, we designed a pair of removable probes that can be used to acquire optical measurements when attached to mammography compression paddles, and which allow an X-ray scan to be performed when detached from the paddles without altering the compression of the target breast. For most clinical experiments, we followed the subject measurement with a calibration phantom measurement. Due to variations in fiber contact, breast skin color, and probe alignment, the phantom measurement was often insufficient for removing all systematic errors; as a result, the reconstructed image often shows artifacts close to the locations of the sources or detectors [76]. Although similar artifacts also appear for some stand-alone DOT systems, they have a greater influence on image quality for compression configurations, like TOBI, where the regions of interests are close to the sources and detectors.

To improve image quality for measurement contaminated by large systematic error, Boas et al. proposed a simultaneous coupling-coefficient-estimation approach in conjunction with the image reconstruction [76]. In this method, one assumes a multiplicative model for the systematic error between the phantom and breast measurement. The optical measurement can be represented as

$$\Phi_{i,j} = s_i \times d_j \times \Phi_{i,j}^{model}(\mu_a, D) \tag{9.1}$$

where s_i and d_j are the unknown source and detector coupling coefficients (denoted as SD), respectively; $\Phi_{i,j}^{model}$ is the predicted measurement from the diffusion model; and $\Phi_{i,j}$ is the measurement. The image-reconstruction problem is now formulated as simultaneous estimation of optical absorption, scattering, and the SD coefficients.

Using this SD-estimation approach, the image artifacts near the sources and detectors were significantly reduced, resulting in dramatic improvement in image quality. Based on the initial work in [76], this model was further extended to a 3D nonlinear Bayesian framework by Oh et al. [77], to measurement systems with rotational symmetry by Tarvainen et al. [104], and to a log-amplitude/phase formulation by Schweiger et al. [78]. More recently, Fang et al. [39] added additional constraints in terms of regularization and postfiltering for SD estimation to reduce the cross talk between the SD distribution and the sample optical contrast. This approach has shown improvement in accurate recovery of target contrast, particularly for TOBI where the measurement sample space covers only a limited angle.

9.2.4 Utilizing Spectral Prior and Best Linear Unbiased Estimator

The absorption spectra of hemoglobin species, water, and lipid have been extensively studied and well documented by several researchers [47, 105, 106]. Incorporating the spectral information of the chromophores into the image reconstruction could: (1) reduce the number of estimated unknowns, and (2) synergistically use multispectral measurement at different wavelengths and subsequently improve the accuracy and robustness of the image reconstruction. Li et al. [107] implemented multispectral image-reconstruction algorithms to directly reconstruct hemoglobin, water, and lipid concentrations from multispectral data. This approach was recently extended to reconstructing scattering and SD coefficients [39].

Li et al. [108] further explained the theoretical implications and advantages of direct multispectral reconstruction by concluding that a best linear unbiased estimator (BLUE) can be achieved by incorporating the spectral prior directly into the reconstruction. Recently, we incorporated the direct SD-estimation approach into the direct chromophore/scattering reconstruction, which demonstrated robustness in processing clinical data measured from the TOBI/DBT system. In particular, reasonable hemoglobin images can be recovered using the 780 and 830 nm wavelength pair, which fails using the indirect approach.

9.2.5 Utilizing Spatial Prior from Tomosynthesis Image

The availability of coregistered high-resolution X-ray/tomosynthesis images brings the following advantages to the combined DOT/X-ray system: (1) the curved boundaries of the breast can be captured by tomosynthesis scans, allowing accurate geometric modeling; (2) the fine boundaries between the fibroglandular and adipose tissues, as well as those for lesions, can be traced by segmentation algorithms and used to explore the optical/physiological properties of different tissue types for constraining the image reconstruction to improve accuracy; and (3) the X-ray images can be used to guide the interpretation and fusion with functional images from optical data.

To exploit the a priori geometric information provided by DBT images, we have studied different mesh-generation methods [39, 102] and developed convenient meshing software to create 3D FE meshes from the coregistered tomosynthesis scans. It has been shown that using the correct breast geometry is important for accurate image reconstruction [102]. Improvements in image resolution and contrast-to-noise ratio using the spatial prior for synthetic data reconstructions have been demonstrated using the spatial prior from the segmented X-ray images as regularization [107]. For the clinical measurements from the TOBI/DBT system, binary and mixed segmentation approaches were developed, with the former representing the glandular and adipose tissue as distinct regions and the latter using a statistically derived weight where each pixel simultaneously includes both glandular and fatty content.

9.3 Clinical Trial of TOBI/DBT Imaging System

A pilot study of the combined X-ray/optical imaging system (22 patients) was conducted between 2001 and 2002 and guided hardware and software development for the TOBI/DBT system [36]. A new clinical trial started in August 2005, which has recruited 79 subjects for the combined TOBI/DBT study (for 53 of them, measurements were taken on both breasts). Of those subjects, 42 were recruited from the screening pool and 37 from patients recalled for biopsies. For the 65 processed patients, the diagnostic results indicated that 49 were healthy, 12 had tumors, and 4 had benign lesions. The averaged age of these patients was 59, and their average body mass index (BMI) was 29.1.

9.3.1 Image Reconstruction of Healthy Breasts

Using multiwavelength RF and CW measurements from TOBI and geometric priors from DBT images, we performed nonlinear bulk-tissue-property estimation and image reconstruction using the Gauss-Newton approach noted in Section 9.2.2. This work was recently extended to multispectral direct reconstruction and used for processing the clinical data [109]. The average reconstructed total hemoglobin concentration ([HbT]) from 80 healthy breast measurements was 16.9 μM, and the average oxygen saturation (SO_2) was 73.1%. The average [HbT] value is at the lower end of literature values (17 μM [86] to 40 μM [110]) for healthy breast tissue. The reduction in [HbT] is likely caused by the blood removal produced by the associated mammographic compression in our experiments. This result generally agreed with the estimate from our spectroscopic breast-compression study [94].

In Color Plate 20, we show representative reconstructed [HbT] images for breasts with different radiological densities, including fatty breasts, scattered density breasts, heterogeneously dense breasts, and extremely dense breasts [111]. By comparing the reconstructed optical hemoglobin images from optical measurements and the coregistered X-ray images, we can easily identify the chest-wall muscle, fibroglandular regions, and the surrounding adipose tissue, with muscle tissue normally presenting higher hemoglobin concentration and adipose tissue presenting lower concentrations. At the same time, we recognize that the optical images are influenced, to a certain extent, by mammographic compression: the optical images from a subset of patients (a, b, and j) show composite features from both tissue structure and pressure distribution. A 5% to 25% reduction in total hemoglobin in the central region of the breast is found for patients with very fatty or very dense breasts, likely a result of pressure-induced blood redistribution. We have conducted mechanical simulations that further confirm this hypothesis [39]. The correlation between the optical and X-ray images demonstrates reliable performance of the combined imaging system in a realistic environment. The findings on pressure-blood coupling provide new opportunities for tumor detection. Manipulating tissue pressure and investigating the dynamics of tissue optical properties represent promising new directions in obtaining improved contrast and specificity for combined mammography/optical breast imaging.

9.3.2 Imaging Breasts with Tumors or Benign Lesions

Applying a similar processing approach to our lesion-patient measurements, we found quite promising results. In Color Plate 21, we show the reconstructed image slices for a breast containing an invasive ductal carcinoma (IDC) (in this case, a large portion of the tumor is ductal carcinoma in situ, or DCIS). Color Plate 21(a) also provides the corresponding DBT image slice, the contours of the tumor (thick line), and the fibroglandular tissue (thin lines). Similarly, the reconstruction results of a breast with a smaller malignant tumor (1 cm in diameter) are shown in Color Plate 22.

The [HbT] image of the lesion-bearing breast in Color Plate 21(b) presents a positive contrast (about 2:1) with margins well fitted within the contours of the lesion. The scattering coefficient image shows a similar pattern. In Color Plate 21(c), the SO_2 values inside the tumor region demonstrate a lower value compared with the surrounding tissue. These findings agree with the published signatures of malignant lesions such as high vessel density and high metabolism. Similar findings can be observed in Color Plate 22, except that the SO_2 decrease inside the tumor is not significant due to tumor size. In this case, the chest-wall muscle tissue and fibroglandular tissue present higher [HbT]/scattering and lower SO_2, like those seen in the healthy subjects.

9.3.3 Region-of-Interest Analysis

Guided by the tissue segmentation from tomosynthesis scans of both healthy and lesion-bearing breasts, we created regions of interest (ROIs) for chest-wall muscle, fibroglandular, adipose, and tumor tissues. Using these ROI analyses, we derived the mean and standard deviations of [HbT], SO_2 and μ'_s for each tissue type. To reduce the intersubject variations, we normalized the optical properties of each tissue by those of the adipose tissue and performed statistical tests on the normalized optical properties [109].

Using the ROI data from 20 healthy breasts and 4 tumor breasts (only tumors larger than 1 cm were selected), we found that the tumor [HbT] is significantly greater than that of the fibroglandular tissue in the same breast (single-side, paired t-test, $p < 0.001$) or in the healthy population (single-side, two-sample t-test, $p = 0.009$). The mean [HbT] contrast between the tumor and adipose tissue is 1.7, which agrees with the values reported in [112]. Similarly, the μ'_s value (830 nm) of the tumor tissue is significantly greater (paired t-test, $p = 0.009$) than that of the fibroglandular tissue in the lesion-bearing breasts. The differences in SO_2 between the tumor and healthy muscle or fibroglandular tissue are not significant. This also agrees with published literature [35].

9.4 Dynamic Imaging of Breast Under Mechanical Compression

As mentioned in Section 9.3.1, the mammographic compression associated with the breast measurements seems to alter the static blood distribution as well as to add temporal dependence to the tissue physiological parameters from the optical measurements. Simulations in Boverman et al. [92] showed that, without correctly accounting for the dynamics in the tissue, the reconstructed contrast may become inaccurate under clinical circumstances. This motivates further investigation into these pressure-induced tissue transients and their impact on the performance of a combined X-ray/optical imaging system.

9.4.1 Experiment Setup

To begin to understand the compression-induced tissue dynamics, a pilot study was designed to measure the concentration of the hemoglobin species in the breast at various compression levels. For this purpose, we used a mammography-like compression system consisting of a set of plastic plates attached to a computer-controlled translation stage used to vary the interplate distance and, hence, the compression level. Optical fibers were integrated into the bottom plate in a

9.4 Dynamic Imaging of Breast Under Mechanical Compression

same-side reflective configuration and attached to an eight-wavelength frequency-domain spectrometer (ISS, Inc., Illinois). The entire system was mounted on a table such that the volunteer's breast rested on the bottom compression plate and was compressed craniocaudally. The upper plate was attached by means of two force transducers, providing online monitoring of the applied compression force. Carp et al. [94] have published a full description of the system and initial results.

9.4.2 Tissue Dynamic from Healthy Subjects

Figure 9.2 shows typical [HbT] and SO_2 recordings during the course of three 6 lb. compression cycles (the arrows between vertical bars indicate the periods during which the breast was under compression at constant interplate distance). An initial fast decrease in [HbT] was observed when compression was applied, followed by a slow recovery after the compression plates stopped moving (most likely as a result of pressure changes, described later). While SO_2 also showed a decrease as compression was applied, we also observed a continued slow decay with an approximately exponential profile. This could possibly result from tissue oxygen consumption *exceeding* oxygen delivery due to the compression-induced reduction in blood flow. Our modeling allows us to estimate volumetric blood flow and oxygen consumption from the measured temporal evolution of [HbT] and SO_2.

By considering a mass balance of [HbO] within the tissue volume (V_t) probed by the optical system, a partial breast occlusion model can be derived, predicting the temporal evolution of SO_2 as a function of two metabolic parameters: volumetric oxygen consumption (OC/V_t) and volumetric blood flow (BF/V_t). The [HbO] mass balance can be written as

$$\frac{d[HbO_2]}{dt} = -\frac{OC}{4V_t} + \frac{F_{in}[HbT]_b S_a O_2}{V_t} - \frac{F_{out}[HbT]_b S_v O_2}{V_t} \qquad (9.2)$$

where F_{in} and F_{out} are the blood inflow and outflow, respectively, into V_t, $[HbT]_b$ is the blood hemoglobin concentration, and S_aO_2 and S_vO_2 are the arterial and venous hemoglobin oxygen saturation, respectively. Taking advantage of real-time measurements of $[HbT]_t$, we note that F_{out} can be computed as follows:

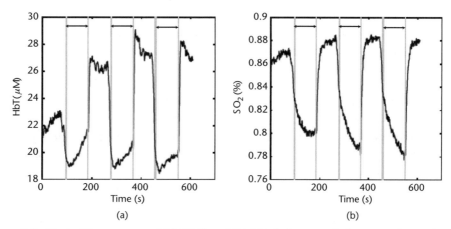

Figure 9.2 Typical time courses of (a) [HbT] and (b) SO_2 during repeated compression cycles.

$$F_{out} = F_{in} - \frac{d[HbT]_t}{dt}\frac{V_t}{[HbT]_b} \qquad (9.3)$$

Also, we assume $SO_2 = fS_aO_2 + (1 - f)S_vO_2$, with $f \approx 0.5$. Noting that $[HbO_2] = SO_2[HbT]_t$, substituting and rearranging, we can write the following equation for $SO_2(t)$:

$$\frac{dSO_2(t)}{dt} = a + bSO_2(t) \qquad (9.4)$$
$$SO_2(t=0) = SO_{2,init}$$

where

$$a = \frac{1}{[HbT]_t}\left(-\frac{OC}{4Vt} + \frac{F_{in}[HbT]_b S_aO_2}{V_t} - \left(\frac{F_{in}[HbT]_b}{V_t} - \frac{d[HbT]_t}{dt}\right)\frac{fS_aO_2}{1-f}\right)$$
$$b = -\frac{1}{[HbT]}\left(\left(\frac{F_{in}[HbT]_b}{V_t} - \frac{d[HbT]_t}{dt}\right)\frac{1}{1-f} + \frac{d[HbT]_t}{dt}\right) \qquad (9.5)$$

Equation (9.5) can be solved numerically to estimate OC/V_t and F_{in}/V_t at each voxel of the DOT image, or the numerical solution can provide a temporal basis function for SO_2 to be employed in a joint spatiotemporal reconstruction of the optical measurements. Equation (9.5) also depends on S_aO_2, $[HbT]_b$ and f. These can be set either from measurements (pulse oximeter for S_aO_2) or published values.

Fitting (9.5) to measurements in 10 normal volunteers, average values were 1.64 ±0.6 μmol/100 mL/min. for oxygen consumption and 1.97 ±0.6 mL/100 mL/min. for blood flow, in fairly good agreement with PET studies (see [94] for additional discussion).

As mentioned previously, mechanical tissue relaxation also appears to govern blood dynamics. Figure 9.3(a) shows a typical recording of the breast-tissue reaction force during three consecutive compression cycles. Several features can be distinguished. First, the force ramps up as the compression stage applies pressure to the tissue. Then, once the control system has determined that a force level of 6 lbs. has been reached, the compression plate stops, and the recorded force (hence, pressure) rapidly decreases over the first few seconds, followed by continued gradual reduction with an exponential-like profile during the rest of the compression plateau. For the specific example shown, the force decreased 39%, 24%, and 23%, respectively, during the slow phase, and the time constants of the corresponding exponential fits were 25, 39, and 49 seconds, respectively. The progressive increase in the time constant and the simultaneous decrease in the amount of pressure reduction is likely a conditioning effect on the breast-tissue-collagen matrix. The breast thickness at the beginning of the second and third compression cycles is lower than in the beginning of the previous corresponding cycle (data not shown)—also a conditioning effect [50, 113].

It is important to note that a plot of [HbT] versus pressure [shown in Figure 9.3(b)] reveals a small rate of change of [HbT] with respect to pressure at higher

9.4 Dynamic Imaging of Breast Under Mechanical Compression

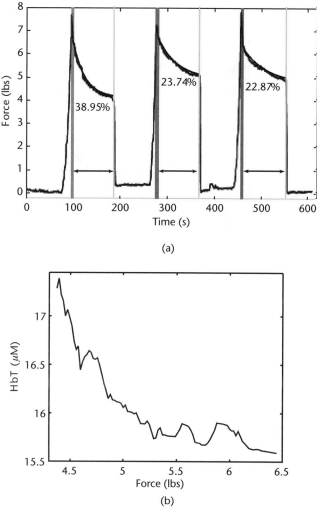

Figure 9.3 Typical (a) compression force recordings and (b) [HbT]-pressure relationship during repeated compressions.

pressures and a high rate of change with respect to pressure at the lower pressure. Since [HbT] is representative of the total blood volume (in the absence of significant hematocrit changes), the data in Figure 9.3(b) represents evidence that vascular compartments of varied compliance participate in the blood return process. At the initially high pressure, values compliance is low, likely representing volume changes in the arterial compartment, followed by increased compliance as the pressure relaxes, likely representing volume changes in the capillary and venous compartments.

9.4.3 Contact Pressure Map Under Compression

Figure 9.4 shows a normalized contact pressure map obtained from a volunteer breast using a Tekscan I-Scan pressure-distribution measurement system (Tekscan, Inc., Massachusetts) while the breast was immobilized by the tomosynthesis com-

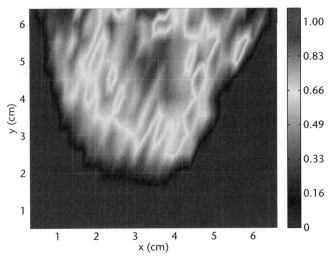

Figure 9.4 A measured pressure distribution (normalized) from a compressed breast.

pression plates in the same fashion as during an actual clinical measurement. The salient feature of this plot is the notably higher pressure in the center of the contact area, suggesting a larger pressure in the center of the breast compared to on the periphery, which is consistent with our observation of reduced [HbT] in the center of homogeneously fatty and homogeneously dense breasts as shown in Color Plate 20. In this particular case, the center pressure is almost 50% higher than the pressure near the tissue boundary. This difference is due to the higher stiffness of glandular tissue and will likely lead to a differentiation of the dynamic features of a postcompression measurement based on tissue type, which opens the door to additional biomarkers useful for tumor characterization, as the mechanical properties of tumor tissue are yet again different from both adipose and glandular parenchyma.

9.5 Conclusions

Initial clinical trials of a combined optical and tomosynthesis system have demonstrated great promise for providing functional-structural information fusion in breast cancer screening and diagnosis. Despite the low spatial resolution, the optically derived physiological parameters, such as [HbT], SO_2, and scattering coefficients, provide consistent indications of tissue vascular and metabolic status for both healthy and tumor-bearing breasts. The interpretation of these functional images becomes straightforward due to the coregistration nature of the functional and structural image components; thus, the findings from one of the images can easily be extrapolated to the other.

In future studies using this combined optical/tomosynthesis system, we will expand our effort to image lesion cases, not only for malignant but also for benign lesions, with the hope of identifying the sensitivity and specificity of this combined modality for various lesion types. We will further exploit the coregistered X-ray images in the form of structural priors to further enhance the accuracy of the parameter estimation. Furthermore, the dynamic signatures in the tissue under mechanical compression will be further explored to discover novel biomarkers that may bear higher specificity to the presence of certain lesions.

References

[1] American Cancer Society, *Cancer prevention and early detection facts and figures 2008*, http://www.cancer.org/downloads/STT/2008CAFFfinalsecured.pdf.

[2] Singletary, S. E., "Multidisciplinary frontiers in breast cancer management: A surgeon's perspective." *Cancer* 109(6) (2007): 1019–1029.

[3] Kerlikowske, K., et al., "Effect of age, breast density, and family history on the sensitivity of first screening mammography." *JAMA* 276(1) (1996): 33–38.

[4] Rosenberg, R. D., et al., "Effects of age, breast density, ethnicity, and estrogen replacement therapy on screening mammographic sensitivity and cancer stage at diagnosis: Review of 183,134 screening mammograms in Albuquerque, New Mexico." *Radiology* 209(2) (1998): 511–518.

[5] Elmore, G., et al., "Ten-year risk of false positive screening mammograms and clinical breast examinations." *NEJM* 338(16) (1998): 1089–1096.

[6] Fletcher, S. W., and J. G. Elmore, "Mammographic screening for breast cancer." *NEJM* 348(17) (2003): 1672–1680.

[7] Feig, S. A., et al., "American College of Radiology guidelines for breast cancer screening." *Am. J. Roentgenol.* 171(1) (1998): 29–33.

[8] Pisano, E. D., "Diagnostic performance of digital versus film mammography for breast-cancer screening." *NEJM* 353(17) (2005): 1773–1783.

[9] James, J. J., "The current status of digital mammography." *Clin. Radiol.* 59(1) (2004): 1–10.

[10] Dobbins, J. T., and D. J. Godfrey, "Digital X-ray tomosynthesis: Current state of the art and clinical potential." *Phys. Med. Biol.* 48(19) (2003): R65–R106.

[11] Reiser, I., et al., "Computerized detection of mass lesions in digital breast tomosynthesis images using two- and three-dimensional radial gradient index segmentation." *Technol. Canc. Res. Treat.* 3(5) (2004): 437–441.

[12] Rafferty, E. A., et al., "Tomosynthesis: A new tool for breast cancer detection." *Breast Canc. Res. Treat.* 94 (2005): S2.

[13] Chan, H. P., et al., "Computer-aided detection system for breast masses on digital tomosynthesis mammograms: Preliminary experience." *Radiology* 238(3) (2006): 1075–1080.

[14] Bird, R. E., T. W. Wallace, and B. C. Yankaskas, "Analysis of cancers missed at screening mammography." *Radiology* 184(3) (1992): 613–617.

[15] Lee, S. K., et al., "Evaluation of breast-tumors with color doppler imaging—a comparison with image-directed doppler ultrasound." *J. Clin. Ultrasound* 23(6) (1995): 367–373.

[16] Kuhl, C. K., et al., "Breast MR imaging screening in 192 women proved or suspected to be carriers of a breast cancer susceptibility gene: Preliminary results." *Radiology* 215(1) (2000): 267–279.

[17] Podo, F., et al., "The Italian multi-centre project on evaluation of MRI and other imaging modalities in early detection of breast cancer in subjects at high genetic risk." *J. Exp. Clin. Canc. Res.* 21(3) (2002): 115–124.

[18] Kriege, M., et al., "Efficacy of MRI and mammography for breast-cancer screening in women with a familial or genetic predisposition." *NEJM* 351(5) (2004): 427–437.

[19] Warner, E., et al., "Surveillance of BRCA1 and BRCA2 mutation carriers with magnetic resonance imaging, ultrasound, mammography, and clinical breast examination." *JAMA* 292(11) (2004): 1317–1325.

[20] Leach, M. O., et al., "Screening with magnetic resonance imaging and mammography of a UK population at high familial risk of breast cancer: A prospective multicentre cohort study (MARIBS)." *Lancet* 365(9473) (2005): 1769–1778.

[21] Lehman, C. D., et al., "Screening women at high risk for breast cancer with mammography and magnetic resonance imaging." *Cancer* 103(9) (2005): 1898–1905.

[22] Tse, N. Y., et al., "The application of positron emission tomographic imaging with fluorodeoxyglucose to the evaluation of breast disease." *Ann. Surg.* 216(1) (1992): 27–34.

[23] Adler, L. P., et al., "Evaluation of breast masses and axillary lymph-nodes with [F-18] 2-deoxy-2-fluoro-d-glucose PET." *Radiology* 187(3) (1993): 743–750.

[24] Gorres, G. W., H. C. Steinert, and G. K. von Schulthess, "PET and functional anatomic fusion imaging in lung and breast cancers." *Canc. J.* 10(4) (2004): 251–261.

[25] Schnall, M. D., and D. M. Ikeda, "Lesion Diagnosis Working Group report." *J. Mag. Res. Imag.* 10(6) (1999): 982–990.

[26] Kuhl, C. K., et al., "Dynamic breast MR imaging: Are signal intensity time course data useful for differential diagnosis of enhancing lesions?" *Radiology* 211(1) (1999): 101–110.

[27] Weisenberger, D. "Positron emission mammography." Jefferson Lab, 2006, www.jlab.org/div_dept/detector/pem.

[28] Levine, E. A., et al., "Positron emission mammography: Initial clinical results." *Ann. Surg. Oncol.* 10(1) (2003): 86–91.

[29] Rosen, E. L., et al., "Detection of primary breast carcinoma with a dedicated, large-field-of-view FDG PET mammography device: Initial experience." *Radiology* 234(2) (2005): 527–534.

[30] Gibson, A. P., J. C. Hebden, and S. R. Arridge, "Recent advances in diffuse optical imaging." *Phys. Med. Biol.* 50 (2005): R1–R43.

[31] Pogue, B. W., et al., "Quantitative hemoglobin tomography with diffuse near-infrared spectroscopy: Pilot results in the breast." *Radiology* 218(1) (2001): 261–266.

[32] Culver, J. P., et al., "Three-dimensional diffuse optical tomography in the parallel plane transmission geometry: Evaluation of a hybrid frequency domain/continuous wave clinical system for breast imaging." *Med. Phys.* 30(2) (2003): 235–247.

[33] Zhu, Q., N. G. Chen, and S. H. Kurtzman, "Imaging tumor angiogenesis using combined near infrared diffusive light and ultrasound." *Opt. Lett.* 28 (2003): 337–339.

[34] Jakubowski, D. B., et al., "Monitoring neoadjuvant chemotherapy in breast cancer using quantitative diffuse optical spectroscopy: A case study." *J. Biomed. Opt.* 9(1) (2004): 230–238.

[35] Intes, X., et al., "Time-domain optical mammography SoftScan: Initial results." *Acad. Radiol.* 12(8) (2005): 934–947.

[36] Zhang, Q., et al., "Coregistered tomographic X-ray and optical breast imaging: Initial results." *J. Biomed. Opt.* 10(2) (2005): 024033.

[37] Gulsen, G., et al., "Design and implementation of a multifrequency near-infrared diffuse optical tomography system." *J. Biomed. Opt.* 11(1) (2006): 014020.

[38] Nielsen, T., et al., "Image reconstruction and evaluation of system performance for optical fluorescence tomography." *Proc. SPIE* 6431 (2007): 64310801–64310810.

[39] Fang, Q., et al., "Combined optical imaging and mammography of the healthy breast: Optical contrast derived from breast structure and compression." *IEEE Trans. Med. Imag.*, 2007.

[40] Lee, K., S. D. Konecky, R. Choe, H. Y. Ban, A. Corlu, T. Durduran, and A. G. Yodh, "Transmission RF diffuse optical tomography instrument for human breast imaging." *Proc. SPIE* 6629 (2007): 66291R.

[41] Gould, P., "The rise and rise of medical imaging: The state of the art in medical imaging technology." *Phys. World*, http://www.physicsworld.com/ows/article/print/17968.

9.5 Conclusions

[42] Wahl, R. L., et al., "Primary and metastatic breast-carcinoma—initial clinical-evaluation with PET with the radiolabeled glucose analog 2-[F-18]-fluoro-2-deoxy-d-glucose." *Radiology* 179(3) (1991): 765–770.

[43] Morris, E. A., "Breast cancer imaging with MRI." *Radiolog. Clin. N. Am.* 40(3) (2002): 443–466.

[44] Wtorek, J., J. Stelter, and A. Nowakowski, "Impedance mammograph 3D phantom studies." In *Electrical Bioimpedance Methods: Applications to Medicine and Biotechnology*, 1999, 520–533.

[45] Kerner, T. E., et al., "Electrical impedance spectroscopy of the breast: Clinical imaging results in 26 subjects." *IEEE Trans. Med. Imag.* 21(6) (2002): 638–645.

[46] Meaney, P. M., et al., "A clinical prototype for active microwave imaging of the breast." *IEEE Trans. Microwave Theory Tech.* 48(11) (2000): 1841–1853.

[47] Quaresima, V., S. J. Matcher, and M. Ferrari, "Identification and quantification of intrinsic optical contrast for near-infrared mammography." *Photochem. Photobiol.* 67(1) (1998): 4–14.

[48] Durduran, T., et al., "Diffuse optical measurement of blood flow in breast tumors." *Opt. Lett.* 30(21) (2005): 2915–2917.

[49] Joines, W. T., Y. Zhang, C. Li, and R. L. Jirtle, "The measured electrical properties of normal and malignant human tissues from 50 to 900 MHz." *Med. Phys.* 21(4) (1994): 547–550.

[50] Wellman, P. S., and R. D. Howe, "The mechanical properties of breast tissues in compression." Harvard BioRobotics Laboratory Technical Report 99003 (1999).

[51] Li, A., et al., "Tomographic optical breast imaging guided by three-dimensional mammography." *Appl. Opt.* 42(25) (2003): 5181–5190.

[52] Dehghani, H., C. M. Carpenter, R. K. Yalavarthy, B. W. Pogue, and J. P. Culver, "Structural a priori information in near-infrared optical tomography." *Proc. SPIE* 6431(64310B) (2007): 6431001–6431005.

[53] Weir, L., D. Worsley, and V. Bernstein, "The value of FDG positron emission tomography in the management of patients with breast cancer." *Breast J.* 11(3) (2005): 204–209.

[54] Czernin, J., and H. R. Schelbert, "PET/CT in cancer patient management." *J. Nucl. Med.* 48 (2007): (JNM Supplement).

[55] Hany, T. F., et al., "PET diagnostic accuracy: Improvement with in-line PET-CT system: Initial results." *Radiology* 225(2) (2002): 575–581.

[56] Fakhry, N., et al., "Comparison between PET and PET/CT in recurrent head and neck cancer and clinical implications." *Eur. Arch. Oto-Rhino-Laryngology* 264(5) (2007): 531–538.

[57] Jeong, H. S., et al., "Use of integrated F-18-FDG PET/CT to improve the accuracy of initial cervical nodal evaluation in patients with head and neck squamous cell carcinoma." *Head Neck* 29(3) (2007): 203–210.

[58] Zhu, Q., et al., "Imager that combines near-infrared diffusive light and ultrasound." *Opt. Lett.* 24(15) (1999): 1050–1052.

[59] Brooksby, B., et al., "Combining near-infrared tomography resonance imaging to study in vivo and magnetic breast tissue: Implementation of a Laplacian-type regularization to incorporate magnetic resonance structure." *J. Biomed. Opt.* 10(5) (2005): 051504.

[60] Ntziachristos, V., et al., "MRI-guided diffuse optical spectroscopy of malignant and benign breast lesions." *Neoplasia* 4(2) (2002): 347–354.

[61] Choe, R., et al., "Diffuse optical tomography of breast cancer during neoadjuvant chemotherapy: A case study with comparison to MRI." *Med. Phys.* 32(4) (2005): 1128–1139.

[62] Klifa, C. S., et al., "Combination of magnetic resonance imaging and diffuse optical spectroscopy to predict radiation response in the breast: An exploratory pilot study." *Breast Canc. Res. Treat.* 100 (2006): S202.

[63] Wolmark, N., et al., "Preoperative chemotherapy in patients with operable breast cancer: Nine-year results from National Surgical Adjuvant Breast and Bowel Project B-18." *J. Natl. Canc. Inst. Monogr.* 2001(30) (2001): 96–102.

[64] Tromberg, B. J., et al., "Imaging in breast cancer—diffuse optics in breast cancer: Detecting tumors in pre-menopausal women and monitoring neoadjuvant chemotherapy." *Breast Canc. Res.* 7(6) (2005): 279–285.

[65] Cerussi, A. E., et al., "Can diffuse optical spectroscopy predict the final pathological response of neoadjuvant chemotherapy? A retrospective pilot study." *Breast Canc. Res. Treat.* 94 (2005): S50.

[66] Shah, N., et al., "Combined diffuse optical spectroscopy and contrast-enhanced magnetic resonance imaging for monitoring breast cancer neoadjuvant chemotherapy: A case study." *J. Biomed. Opt.* 10(5) (2005): 051503.

[67] McBride, T. O., et al., "A parallel-detection frequency-domain near-infrared tomography system for hemoglobin imaging of the breast in vivo." *Rev. Sci. Instr.* 72(3) (2001): 1817–1824.

[68] Piao, D. Q., et al., "Video-rate near-infrared optical tomography using spectrally encoded parallel light delivery." *Opt. Lett.* 30(19) (2005): 2593–2595.

[69] Nielsen, T., et al., "Image reconstruction and evaluation of system performance for optical fluorescence tomography." *Proc. SPIE* 6431 (2007): 643108-1–643108-10.

[70] Cerussi, A., et al., "In vivo absorption, scattering, and physiologic properties of 58 malignant breast tumors determined by broadband diffuse optical spectroscopy." *J. Biomed. Opt.* 11(4) (2006): 044005.

[71] Franceschini, M. A., et al., "Diffuse optical imaging of the whole head." *J. Biomed. Opt.* 11(5) (2006): 054007.

[72] Piao, D., et al., "Instrumentation for video-rate near-infrared diffuse optical tomography." *Rev. Sci. Instr.* 76(12) (2005): 124301–124301-13.

[73] Corlu, A., et al., "Uniqueness and wavelength optimization in continuous-wave multispectral diffuse optical tomography." *Opt. Lett.* 28(23) (2003): 2339–2341.

[74] Li, A., et al., "Reconstructing chromosphere concentration images directly by continuous-wave diffuse optical tomography." *Opt. Lett.* 29 (2004): 256–258.

[75] Srinivasan, S., et al., "Near-infrared characterization of breast tumors in vivo using spectrally constrained reconstruction." *Technol. Canc. Res. Treat.* 4(5) (2005): 513–526.

[76] Boas, D. A., T. Gaudette, and S. R. Arridge, "Simultaneous imaging and optode calibration with diffuse optical tomography." *Opt. Exp.* 8(5) (2001): 263–270.

[77] Oh, S., et al., "Source detector calibration in three-dimensional Bayesian optical diffusion tomography." *J. Opt. Soc. Am. A* 19 (2002): 1983–1993.

[78] Schweiger, M., et al., "Image reconstruction in optical tomography in the presence of coupling errors." *Appl. Opt.* 46 (2007): 2743–2756.

[79] Durduran, T., et al., "Algorithms for 3D localization and imaging using near-field diffraction tomography with diffuse light." *Opt. Exp.* 4(8) (1999): 247–262.

[80] Pogue, B. W., et al., "Three-dimensional simulation of near-infrared diffusion in tissue: Boundary condition and geometry analysis for finite-element image reconstruction." *Appl. Opt.* 40(4) (2001): 588–600.

[81] Dehghani, H., et al., "Multiwavelength three-dimensional near-infrared tomography of the breast: Initial simulation, phantom, and clinical results." *Appl. Opt.* 42(1) (2003): 135–145.

[82] Heilscher, A. H., and S. Bartel, "Use of penalty terms in gradient-based iterative reconstruction schemes for optical tomography." *J. Biomed. Opt.* 6 (2001): 183–192.

[83] Boverman, G., et al., "Quantitative spectroscopic diffuse optical tomography of the breast guided by imperfect a priori structural information." *Phys. Med. Biol.* 50(17) (2005): 3941–3956.

[84] Douiri, A., et al., "Anisotropic diffusion regularization methods for diffuse optical tomography using edge prior information." *Meas. Sci. Technol.* 18(1) (2007): 87–95.

[85] Brooksby, B., et al., "Imaging breast adipose and fibroglandular tissue molecular signatures by using hybrid MRI-guided near-infrared spectral tomography." *PNAS* 103(23) (2006): 8828–8833.

[86] Srinivasan, S., et al., "In vivo hemoglobin and water concentrations, oxygen saturation, and scattering estimates from near-infrared breast tomography using spectral reconstruction." *Acad. Radiol.* 13(2) (2006): 195–202.

[87] Brooksby, B., et al., "Magnetic resonance-guilded near infrared tomography of the breast," *Rev. Sci. Instrum.* 75 (2004): 5262–5270.

[88] Schwartz, G. K., et al., "Potentiation of apoptosis by flavopiridol in mitomycin-C-treated gastric and breast cancer cells." *Clin. Canc. Res.* 3(9) (1997): 1467–1472.

[89] Mahmood, U., et al., "Near-infrared optical imaging of protease activity for tumor detection." *Radiology* 213(3) (1999): 866–870.

[90] Licha, K., "Contrast agents for optical imaging." In *Contrast Agents II*, Berlin: Springer, 2002, 1–29.

[91] Barbour, R. L., et al., "Optical tomographic imaging of dynamic features of dense-scattering media." *J. Opt. Soc. Am. A—Opt. Image Sci. Vis.* 18(12) (2001): 3018–3036.

[92] Boverman, G., et al., "Spatio-temporal imaging of the hemoglobin in the compressed breast with diffuse optical tomography." *Phys. Med. Biol.* 52 (2007): 3619–3641.

[93] Jiang, S. D., et al., "In vivo near-infrared spectral detection of pressure-induced changes in breast tissue." *Opt. Lett.* 28(14) (2003): 1212–1214.

[94] Carp, S. A., et al., "Compression-induced changes in the physiological state of the breast as observed through frequency domain photon migration measurements." *J. Biomed. Opt.* 11(6) (2006).

[95] Beaney, R. P., et al., "Positron emission tomography for in vivo measurement of regional blood-flow, oxygen utilization, and blood-volume in patients with breast-carcinoma." *Lancet* 1(8369) (1984): 131–134.

[96] Wilson, C., et al., "Measurements of blood-flow and exchanging water space in breast-tumors using positron emission tomography—a rapid and noninvasive dynamic method." *Canc. Res.* 52(6) (1992): 1592–1597.

[97] Zhang, Q., et al., "Coregistered tomographic X-ray and optical breast imaging: Initial results." *J. Biomed. Opt.* 10(2) (2005): 024033.

[98] Joseph, D. K., et al., "Diffuse optical tomography system to image brain activation with improved spatial resolution and validation with functional magnetic resonance imaging." *Appl. Opt.* 45(31) (2006): 8142–8151.

[99] Wu, T., et al., "Tomographic mammography using a limited number of low-dose conebeam projection images." *Med. Phys.* 30 (2003): 365–380.

[100] Wu, T., et al., "Digital tomosynthesis mammography using a parallel maximum-likelihood reconstruction method." *Proc. SPIE* 5368 (2004): 1–11.

[101] Boyse, W. E., and A. A. Seidl, "A block QMR method for computing multiple simultaneous solutions to complex symmetric systems." *SIAM J. Sci. Comput.* 17 (1996): 263–274.

[102] Fang, Q., et al., "Nonlinear image reconstruction algorithm for diffuse optical tomography using iterative block solver and automatic mesh generation from tomosynthesis images." *Proc. SPIE* 6081 (2006): 608100.1–608100.10.

[103] Durduran, T., et al., "Bulk optical properties of healthy female breast tissue." *Phys. Med. Biol.* 47(16) (2002): 2847–2861.

[104] Tarvainen, T., et al., "Computational calibration method for optical tomography." *Appl. Opt.* 44 (2005): 1879–1888.

[105] Querry, G. M. H. a. M. R., "Optical constants of water in the 200-nm to 2000-μm wavelength region." *Appl. Opt.* 12 (1973): 555–563.

[106] Wray, S., et al., "Characterization of the near infrared absorption spectra of cytochrome aa3 and haemoglobin for the non-invasive monitoring of cerebral oxygenation." *Biochem. Biophys. Acta* 933(1) (1988): 184–192.

[107] Li, A., et al., "Reconstructing chromosphere concentration images directly by continuous-wave diffuse optical tomography." *Opt. Lett.* 29(3) (2004): 256–258.

[108] Li, A., et al., "Optimal linear inverse solution with multiple priors in diffuse optical tomography." *Appl. Opt.* 44(10) (2005): 1948–1956.

[109] Fang, Q., J. Selb, S. A. Carp, G. Boverman, E. L. Miller, D. H. Brooks, R. H. Moore, D. B. Kopans, and D. A. Boas, "Combined optical and X-ray tomosynthesis breast imaging." *Radiology*, 2008.

[110] Cerussi, A. E., et al., "Sources of absorption and scattering contrast for near-infrared optical mammography." *Acad. Radiol.* 8(3) (2001): 211–218.

[111] Liberman, L., and J. H. Menell, "Breast imaging reporting and data system (BI-RADS)." *Radiol. Clin. N. Am.* 40(3) (2002): 409–430.

[112] Poplack, S. P., et al., "Electromagnetic breast imaging: Results of a pilot study in women with abnormal mammograms." *Radiology* 243(2) (2007): 350–359.

[113] Kerdok, A. E., M. P. Ottensmeyerc, and R. D. Howe, "Effects of perfusion on the viscoelastic characteristics of liver." *J. Biomech.* 39(12) (2006): 2221–2231.

CHAPTER 10
Diffuse Optical Imaging and PET Imaging

Soren D. Konecky and Arjun G. Yodh

10.1 Introduction

In the preceding two chapters, diffuse optical imaging (DOI) was combined with magnetic resonance imaging (MRI) and X-ray imaging. The primary goal of that work was to combine higher-resolution imaging modalities with low-resolution diffuse optical imaging in order to use structural information from the former to improve upon the functional potential of DOI. In particular, the structural details acquired using MRI and X-ray imaging were used as a priori information to aid the optical reconstructions. The goal of the research described in this chapter is different. We will coregister DOI of human breast with positron emission tomography (PET). PET is a clinically useful imaging modality that employs the uptake of radiopharmaceuticals to measure physiological processes. In PET, the increased metabolic rate of most tumors compared to normal tissue provides a basis for their detectability via the radiopharmaceutical ^{18}F-fluorodeoxyglucose (^{18}F-FDG). Like PET, DOI also primarily measures the physiological characteristics of tissue. DOI is sensitive to changes in the absorption of near-infrared light due to variation of the concentrations of endogenous chromophores such as oxy- and deoxyhemoglobin, water, and lipid. Using exogenous fluorescence probes, DOI also has the potential to measure other physiological characteristics of tissue such as pH, intracellular calcium concentration, and tumor specific receptors. Thus, the combined use of DOI, fluorescence DOI (FDOI), and PET holds potential to expand the toolbox for researchers who study cancer in vivo. The goal of this chapter is to compare PET and DOI for breast tumor imaging, to demonstrate how these comparisons can be accomplished, and to suggest ways that the coregistration of these functional imaging techniques may be beneficial.

We begin by reviewing some research in both the PET and DOI literature. Clearly, the ability to detect physiological change is important for measuring and predicting tumor responses to cancer treatment. To date, clinicians primarily use tumor size to evaluate the response of tumors to therapy. Unfortunately, however, this approach requires clinicians to wait weeks to months for anatomical changes to occur, even though some physiological changes surely occur on shorter timescales. In addition, some of the newest therapies (e.g., hormone therapies for breast cancer) are potentially "cytostatic." These therapies may stop cancer growth without destroying the cancer and may be successful even when no significant reduction in tumor size occurs [1]. So while tumor size will always be important in evaluating treatment response, there is a need to predict and monitor cancer therapy on shorter timescales. PET scans taken after the first round of chemotherapy are demonstrably strong indicators of treatment efficacy in breast cancer patients [2–7]. Likewise, several case studies using optical methods to monitor neoadjuvant chemotherapy of locally advanced breast cancers have shown promise [8–10]. Unlike PET, continuous or repetitive treatment monitoring is feasible with optics due to its low cost and noninvasive nature. In all of these studies, the long-term clinical goal is to predict the outcome of treatment early on, while there remains enough time to modify treatment. This is especially important for breast cancer, where many treatment options can exist, even if the initial chemotherapy fails.

DOI and PET can identify resistance factors to cancer treatments. For example, hypoxic tumors [i.e., those having a low partial pressure of oxygen (pO_2)] are often more resistant to radiation and chemotherapy [11–14]. Several studies report that the determination of the oxygenation status of a tumor might afford improved disease management [15–18]. DOI detects tumor hypoxia by measuring decreases of tissue blood oxygenation (StO_2), and high/low values of StO_2 in a lesion with respect to the surrounding tissue imply high/low relative values of pO_2 in the lesion. Likewise, increased ^{18}F-FDG uptake measured with PET is associated with hypoxia. A lack of oxygen can lead to the anaerobic metabolism of glucose, which is inefficient and requires that cells increase glucose consumption. Thus, ^{18}F-FDG uptake could be correlated with tissue StO_2.

There are further potential benefits to be derived by combining DOI and PET. DOI data can facilitate more accurate determination of the tumor hypoxic state by PET. Some nonhypoxic tumors have high rates of glucose metabolism, and chronic hypoxia can lead to decreases in glucose metabolism. ^{18}F-FDG PET alone is therefore not always a reliable measure of tissue hypoxia. Indeed, this observation has lead to recent research using nitroimidazole PET tracers such as ^{18}F-fluoromisonidazole to measure tumor hypoxia in variety of cancers, including breast cancer [19, 20]. Diffuse optical methods measure tissue oxygenation using endogenous contrast. Thus, they are not subject to variations in tracer uptake due to physiological factors such as poor perfusion [21]; nor do they require the subject to return to the hospital on another day for injection and scan of a second tracer. In addition, simple models of the relative rate of oxygen metabolism in tumors can be employed by diffuse optical methods [22] and might in the future provide a means to study the relationship between FDG kinetics and oxygen metabolism. A high rate of glucose consumption that is not accompanied by a high rate of oxygen metabolism, for example, would imply that some glucose is being metabolized inefficiently, presumably due to an insufficient supply of oxygen.

Finally, PET techniques are well suited to validate DOI. This validation is important because, unlike PET, DOI is still in its initial research phase and has not as yet been fully translated to the clinic. It is reasonable to expect that increases in glucose metabolism require more blood for glucose and oxygen delivery and therefore should be accompanied by increases in total hemoglobin concentration. In fact, ^{18}F-FDG uptake has already been shown to correlate well with the uptake of a tumor blood-flow-specific tracer in breast cancer [23, 24]. If a strong correlation between hemoglobin concentration and glucose consumption exists, PET could be very well suited to validate DOI results.

The remainder of this chapter is organized as follows. We begin with an introduction to PET imaging for researchers in optical imaging. This is followed by sections on DOI and fluorescence DOI, with an emphasis on the methods used in recent work. Next, we show results from recent clinical research. Comparisons between DOI and PET imaging for breast cancer suggest correlations between ^{18}F-FDG uptake and optically measured parameters such as total hemoglobin concentration and scattering [25]. Fluorescence DOI (FDOI) of human breast using indocyanine green (ICG) suggests increased vascular permeability in breast cancers [26].

10.2 Positron Emission Tomography (PET)

10.2.1 PET Fundamentals

Positron emission tomography (PET) is a clinically accepted imaging modality that images the uptake of a pharmaceutical of physiological interest by tagging it with a positron emitting radioisotope. The tagged pharmaceutical, called a radiopharmaceutical, is injected or inhaled. It then distributes in the body in accordance with the biokinetics of the pharmaceutical, which are similar to those of its nonradioactively labeled analog. When a proton in the nucleus of the radioisotope decays into a neutron, it emits a positron and an antineutrino. The positron travels a short distance (~1 mm for ^{18}F) in the tissue losing energy through Coulomb interactions, and eventually annihilates with an electron. The annihilation produces a pair of 511-keV photons traveling in (nearly) opposite directions [Figure 10.1(a)]. Assuming neither photon is absorbed by tissue, the two photons will exit the body at almost the exact same time. PET tomographs are designed to detect these coincident photon pairs along all possible projection lines through the body [Figure 10.1(b)]. By measuring the number of photon pairs emitted along each projection line, one can reconstruct quantitative maps of the tracer distribution. The resulting image of tracer distribu-

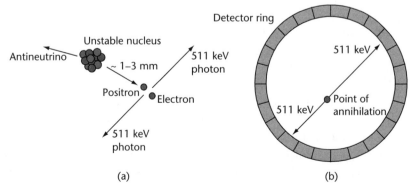

Figure 10.1 (a) Schematic of positron decay and annihilation. A proton in the unstable nucleus decays to neutron giving off a positron and antineutrino. The positron travels a few millimeters in tissue before annihilating with an electron to give off a pair of 511-keV photons traveling in opposite directions. (b) An annihilation event produces two 511-keV photons, which are detected by a ring of detectors.

tion thus serves as an indication of a physiologic process, which is interpreted by the physician.

The tracer used for most clinical studies is ^{18}F-fluorodeoxyglucose (^{18}F-FDG). As ^{18}F has a half-life of 109.8 minutes, a relatively large fraction of the ^{18}F decays may be detected during a typical 30-minute scan. In addition, the half-life is long enough so that the radioactive fluorine can be produced in a regional facility and flown to nearby hospitals. An analog of glucose, ^{18}F-FDG enters the cell and is phosphorylated in parallel to glucose to form ^{18}F-fluorodeoxyglucose-6-phosphate (^{18}F-FDG-6-P). However, once phosphorylated, it cannot be further broken down by the cell. Furthermore, the ^{18}F-FDG-6-P is not readily dephosphorylated and cannot cross the cell membrane. As a result, the ^{18}F-containing molecule is metabolically trapped in the cell. Over time, cells metabolizing larger amounts of glucose will accumulate more ^{18}F. An image of the ^{18}F distribution in the body taken about an hour after injection offers a quantitative mapping of ^{18}F-FDG uptake. It is therefore a good measure of glucose metabolism.

10.2.2 PET Image Reconstruction

Image-reconstruction methods in PET can be divided into two general categories: analytic and iterative (see [27, Chs. 21 and 22], for a more in-depth treatment). In the analytic approaches, the data for each pair of detectors (corrected for attenuation) is treated as the radon transform (line integral) of the tracer concentration across the line connecting the two detectors. The tracer concentration is determined by inverting the radon transform using filtered back-projection or a related algorithm. Analytic methods are computationally fast; however, they do not permit all effects of the measurement process to be modeled.

Iterative methods require a large amount of computation but permit more accurate modeling of the measurement process. These methods involve the inversion of a system matrix (similar to the weight matrix in DOI), which gives the sensitivity of each measurement to each voxel in the image. Unlike the weight matrix in DOI, however, the system matrix for PET is linear (i.e., the values of its elements do not depend on the tracer distribution for which we are solving). Also, in contrast to optical tomography, where the weight matrix is nearly singular, for most detector configurations, the PET system matrix is well posed and easily inverted. Each row corresponds to one detector pair and consists primarily of ones for voxels in a narrow volume connecting the pair of detectors and zeroes for other voxels, with adjustments that take into account the attenuation and scattering of the 511-keV photons, random coincidence events, and detector characteristics.

The principal difficulty in PET reconstructions is that only a small number of photons are collected. As a result, the data is noisy, and it is desirable to take into account photon statistics of the measurement. For this reason the system matrix is inverted using iterative algorithms that attempt to find the tracer distribution with the highest probability for producing the measured data. The maximum-likelihood expectation-maximization (ML-EM) algorithm, first used in emission tomography in the 1980s, is the best known [28, 29]. Several other algorithms have been developed to speed up the slow convergence of the ML-EM algorithm when reconstructing large 3D volumes. One of these, the three-dimensional row-action maximum likelihood algorithm (3D RAMLA), was used to generate the PET reconstructions for the work presented in this chapter [30].

10.2.3 PET Instrumentation

We will compare 3D DOI reconstructed breast images with PET images of the same breast acquired by two different PET scanners: a dedicated breast-only PET (BPET) scanner developed at the University of Pennsylvania and a commercially available whole-body PET scanner (Allegro, Philips Medical Systems). We briefly describe the scanners here. For a thorough discussion of PET system design, the reader is referred to the review by Lewellen and Karp [27, Ch. 10].

Commercially available whole-body PET tomographs achieve high sensitivity to 511-keV annihilation photon pairs using a cylindrical configuration of detectors surrounding the patient. The imaging instrument used for acquisition of whole-body PET images in this chapter was an Allegro scanner, with an axial field of view (FOV) of 18 cm, a transaxial FOV of 56 cm, and a ring diameter of 86.4 cm at the surface of the detectors. The scanner exhibits 5-mm spatial resolution (i.e., FWHM of a point source) and a sensitivity of 4.4 cps/kBq [31].

In our study, patients fasted for at least 4 hours prior to the scan. Each scan was initiated 60 minutes after intravenous administration of ^{18}F-FDG with a dose of 5.2 MBq/kg. Sequential overlapping scans were acquired to cover the body from neck to pelvis as the patient lay supine on the gantry. Transmission scans obtained with a ^{137}Cs point source were interleaved between the multiple emission scans to correct for nonuniform attenuation of the 511-keV photons by the patient's body and the gantry.

The ability to image breast cancer with ^{18}F-FDG PET has led to the development of a dedicated breast-imaging PET scanner, BPET [32, 33]. In a whole-body scanner, the 511-keV photons emitted from the breast are attenuated by the body, reducing the scanner's sensitivity to breast lesions. In contrast, a dedicated breast scanner permits the breast to be imaged with significant reduction in attenuation (i.e., about a factor of 10 reduction). The subject lies prone on a table with an opening to allow the breast to drop between two detectors whose separation distance can be adjusted to accommodate different-sized breasts [Color Plate 23(a)].

The scanner is composed of two curved-plate NaI(Tl) detectors of 1.9-cm thickness each with an active area of 28×21 cm^2. By positioning the detectors close to the breast, a large solid angle can be covered, thus optimizing the system's sensitivity for a split-ring configuration. However, this configuration leads to the loss of data from the 511-keV photons arriving at angles not covered by the detector plates. In fact, for a typical separation of 20 cm, the angular coverage of 180° corresponds to one-half of the complete angular acceptance. This geometry requires the use of a limited angle reconstruction, which we perform using a modified version of 3D RAMLA that compensates for the missing data.

The spatial resolution of the system varies from 3.8 mm (radially at center) to 4.5 mm (radially at $r = 5$ cm). The Allegro whole-body scanner has a uniform spatial resolution of 5 mm. Phantom measurements have demonstrated superior contrast recovery for BPET compared to the Allegro instrument as a result of the improved spatial resolution, even with the loss of data due to the limited angle geometry. A pilot study of 20 patients imaged with both Allegro and BPET demonstrated good correlation in lesion detectability, but better detail in the breast lesions was achieved in the BPET images [34].

10.3 Diffuse Optical Imaging (DOI)

10.3.1 DOI Instrumentation

There are two basic approaches for combining diffuse optical measurements with measurements from other medical imaging modalities. In one approach the DOI device is incorporated into the other device. This approach was described in Chapter 6 by Carpenter and Pogue (MRI) and in Chapter 9 by Fang, Carp, Selb, and Boas (X-ray tomosynthesis) [35–38]. The advantage of such a system is that measurements from the two modalities can be made concurrently in the same geometry, facilitating coregistration of the resulting images. However, integration of the DOI system into another instrument places restrictions on both instrumentation types. In the second approach, measurements are taken on separate stand-alone devices. Parameters are derived optimally from the respective images (taken separately) and compared. Then, as described by Azar in Chapter 7, software can be used to coregister the images for a more detailed comparison. This approach readily permits DOI measurements to be combined with more than one modality.

Our DOI imaging device is a hybrid system [Color Plate 23(b)]. The instrument takes both continuous-wave transmission and frequency-domain remission measurements at six near-infrared wavelengths in the parallel-plate soft-compression geometry. The patient lies in a prone position with her breasts inside a box with an antireflection coated glass window on the detector side. A compression plate holds the breast in place against the viewing window by mildly compressing the breast to a thickness of between 5.5 and 7.5 cm. The box is then filled with a matching fluid with optical properties similar to human breast. The matching fluid consists of water, India ink for absorption, and a fat emulsion for scattering.

Six diode lasers (650, 690, 750, 786, 830, and 905 nm), four of which (690, 750, 786, and 830 nm) are intensity-modulated at 70 MHz, are connected via optical fibers and series of optical switches (DiCon Fiber Optics, Richmond, California) to 45 source positions located on the compression plate. The source positions form a 9×5 grid with a separation of 1.6 cm between nearest neighbors. The breast is scanned by serially guiding the light from each laser to each source position.

For remission detection, nine homodyne frequency-domain detector units [39] are connected to the compression plate by a 3×3 grid of 3-mm detector fibers with a spacing of 1.6 cm. Each unit contains an avalanche photodiode and utilizes a homodyne technique to derive the amplitude and phase of the detected signal. For transmission detection, a CCD camera (Roper Scientific, Trenton, New Jersey, VersArray:1300F) is focused on the viewing window. It acquires an image for each source-position/laser combination with an exposure time of 500 ms. A 24×41 grid of 984 pixels is selected from the CCD chip. It measures the continuous wave light intensity at locations on the viewing window with a spacing of ~3 mm.

10.3.2 DOI Image Reconstruction

Our multispectral approach permits us to solve directly for oxy- and deoxyhemoglobin concentrations via decomposition of the absorption coefficient into contributions from individual chromophores, assuming a simple Mie-scattering approximation for the reduced scattering coefficient. We implemented this approach by modifying the Time-resolved Optical Absorption and Scattering Tomography (TOAST) software in order to utilize multispectral continuous wave data [40]. The method is described in detail in Corlu et al. [41].

The propagation of near-infrared light in biological media is modeled by a diffusion equation [42]. In the frequency domain, the equation has the form

$$-\nabla \cdot D(\mathbf{r},\lambda)\nabla\Phi(\mathbf{r},\lambda,\omega) + \left[\mu_a(\mathbf{r},\lambda) + \frac{i\omega n}{c}\right]\Phi(\mathbf{r},\lambda,\omega) = q_o(\mathbf{r},\lambda,\omega) \quad (10.1)$$

Here Φ is the photon fluence rate, λ is the wavelength of the light source, ω is the frequency at which the light source is intensity-modulated ($\omega = 0$ for continuous-wave measurements), q_o is the light source distribution, and c is the speed of light. The optical properties of the breast are described by the light diffusion coefficient $D \approx 1/3\mu'_s$ (μ'_s is the reduced scattering coefficient), the absorption coefficient μ_a, and the tissue index of refraction n.

We model the absorption coefficient as the sum of the absorption from the individual chromophores (Hb, HbO$_2$, water, and lipids) in the breast, that is,

$$\mu_a(\lambda) = \sum_i c_i \varepsilon_i(\lambda) \quad (10.2)$$

Here, each c_i is the concentration of the ith chromophore, and $\varepsilon_i(\lambda)$ is the corresponding wavelength-dependent extinction coefficient. We model the wavelength dependence of the reduced scattering coefficient using simplified Mie scattering theory [43, 44]. A scattering prefactor, A, depends primarily on the number and size of the scatterers, and a scattering exponent, b, depends on the size of the scatterers. They are combined as follows:

$$\mu'_s = A\lambda^{-b} \quad (10.3)$$

Our goal is to reconstruct spatial maps of A, b, and the chromophore concentrations by minimizing the difference between measured data and predictions of the photon diffusion model.

Two scans are made for each breast: a reference scan in which the tank is filled with matching fluid only and a scan with the breast immersed in matching fluid. We fit data from the frequency-domain measurements of the breast to an analytic solution of the diffusion equation for a homogeneous medium in the slab geometry in order to obtain estimates of the average chromophore concentrations, scattering prefactor A, and scattering power b inside the breast. The absorption due to volume concentrations of water (31%) and lipid (57%) in the breast is held fixed, based on values from the literature [45–47]. The optical properties of the matching fluid are determined independently by fitting to the frequency-domain measurements of the reference scan.

A photograph of the compressed breast is taken just before the scan. It allows us to segment the imaging volume into breast and matching fluid regions. Using average results for the breast as an initial guess, we then employ a nonlinear conjugate gradient algorithm to solve directly for 3D tomographic maps of the chromophore concentrations and scattering prefactor A inside the breast. The scattering amplitude b is held fixed at its bulk value, as are the optical properties of the matching-fluid region. At each iteration, a finite element solver predicts the detected continuous-wave light intensity based on the current maps of chromophore concentrations, and these maps are then updated in order to minimize χ^2, which represents the difference between measured and predicted values of light exiting the breast. Finally, the resulting maps are combined to form images of total hemoglobin concentration $[THC(\mathbf{r}) = C_{Hb}(\mathbf{r}) + C_{HbO_2}(\mathbf{r})]$, blood oxygen saturation $[StO_2(\mathbf{r}) = C_{HbO_2}(\mathbf{r})/THC(\mathbf{r})]$, reduced scattering coefficient $[\mu'_s(\mathbf{r}) = A(\mathbf{r})\lambda^{-b}]$, overall optical attenuation $[\mu_{eff}(\mathbf{r}) = \sqrt{\mu_a(\mathbf{r})/D(\mathbf{r})}]$, and an empirical optical index $[OI(\mathbf{r}) = rTHC(\mathbf{r}) \times r\mu'_s(\mathbf{r})/rStO_2(\mathbf{r})]$.

10.4 Fluorescence Diffuse Optical Imaging (FDOI)

The use of exogenous contrast agents holds potential to increase the number of physiological parameters that can be measured by diffuse optical methods. Fluorescent contrast agents have been used to measure tissue pH [48], intracellular calcium concentration [49], and a variety of tumor-specific receptors [50–56]. Many researchers have explored the use of fluorescence imaging in turbid media [57–61]. Because it is approved by the FDA, the most widely used contrast agent in the diffuse optics community has been indocyanine green (ICG). Several studies suggest that leaky vasculature in tumors delays the washout of ICG, raising the relative concentration between cancerous and normal tissue [35, 62, 63].

In our experiments, an additional ICG fluoresence scan is performed after the endogenous optical properties of the breast are measured using the methods described in Section 10.3. The fluorescence scan is performed with 786-nm excitation light. An 830-nm bandpass filter (OD = 4, CVI Laser Inc.) and a 785-nm notch filter (OD = 6, Semrock, Inc.) are placed in front of the CCD. The notch filter is put in front of the bandpass filter. In this way, the 786-nm excitation light is blocked before reaching the bandpass filter, preventing the detection of excitation-light-induced bandpass filter autofluorescence. The total extinction of 785-nm excitation light is 10 dB, and the transmission loss of 830-nm emission light is approximately 50% (mostly due to the bandpass filter).

The protocol for the fluorescence scan is as follows. A monitoring scan consisting of repeated measurements using a single source position begins 45 seconds before the administration of ICG. This scan is used later to derive the ICG pharmacokinetics. A bolus of sterile ICG is then given for 30 seconds, followed by a normal saline flush of 20 cc for 30 seconds. After 24 frames (i.e., 6 minutes) of the monitoring scan, a full tomographic scan using all 45 source positions (including the one used in the monitoring scan) is conducted.

For fluorescence image reconstruction, we attempt to determine the spatially varying concentration of fluorophore in the sample. The transport of the emitted light is governed by (10.1) at the emission wavelength. For a continuous-wave measurement ($\omega = 0$), the concentration of fluorophore is related to the source term on the right side of this equation by

$$q_0(\lambda_{fl}, \mathbf{r}) = C(\mathbf{r}) \times \varepsilon(\lambda_{ex}) \times \eta \times \Phi(\lambda_{ex}, \mathbf{r}) \tag{10.4}$$

That is, the amount of fluorescent light emitted $q_0(\lambda_{fl}, \mathbf{r})$ is proportional to the product of the fluorophore concentration $C(\mathbf{r})$ and the amount of excitation light $\Phi(\lambda_{ex}, \mathbf{r})$. The amount of excitation light inside the medium can be calculated by solving the diffusion equation with, for example, finite element methods using the reconstructed values of $\mu(\lambda_{ex}, \mathbf{r})$ and $\mu'_s(\lambda_{ex}, \mathbf{r})$ determined from the endogenous scan. (Here we are typically ignoring the small extra absorption due to the fluorescent probe.) The proportionality constants are the extinction coefficient $\varepsilon(\lambda_{ex})$ and the fluorescence quantum yield η of the fluorophore.

To solve for the fluorophore concentration, we convolve the source term (10.4) with the Green's function for the diffusion equation (10.1) given the optical properties of the medium. Since the excitation and emission wavelengths are close, it is a reasonably good approximation to use the optical properties determined at the excitation wavelength from the endogenous image reconstruction. Thus, the equation we must solve is

$$\Phi_m(\lambda_{fl}, \mathbf{r}_s, \mathbf{r}_d) = \int d^3r \Phi_c(\lambda_{ex}, \mathbf{r}_s, \mathbf{r}) G_c(\lambda_{ex}, \mathbf{r}, \mathbf{r}_d) \varepsilon(\lambda_{ex}) \eta C(\mathbf{r}) \tag{10.5}$$

It is common to account for systematic errors (e.g., varying detector efficiencies and light strengths between different source/detector pairs) by multiplying the measured emission data by the calculated excitation data divided by the measured excitation data [i.e., $\Phi_c(\lambda_{ex}, \mathbf{r}_s, \mathbf{r}_d)/\Phi_m(\lambda_{ex}, \mathbf{r}_s, \mathbf{r}_d)$] [64]. In addition, it is necessary to scale the emission data to account for the ICG washout that occurs during the (10-minute) fluorescence scan. Ideally, the scaled data should represent the signal that would be measured if the emission light for all the source positions could be measured at the same time. The scaling can be accomplished by monitoring the ICG kinetics using a single source position as described above, then fitting the measured fluorescent signal to a decaying exponential. For each CCD exposure, the measured value for all pixels is multiplied by $\exp[\beta(t_i - t_0)]$ where β is the decay rate of the monitored fluorescence signal, t_i is the time at which source i is measured, and t_0 is the time at which we are solving for the fluorophore concentration $C(\mathbf{r})$ [63].

Once the raw emission data has been adjusted, the simplest approach is to divide the sample into voxels with volume h^3, discretize (10.5), and solve the resulting matrix equation. For each measurement i and voxel j in the medium, we let

$$A_{i,j} = h^3 \Phi_c(\lambda_{fl}, \mathbf{r}_{si}, \mathbf{r}_j) G_c(\lambda_{fl}, \mathbf{r}_j, \mathbf{r}_{di}) \varepsilon(\lambda_{ex}) \eta \tag{10.6}$$

$$x_j = C(\mathbf{r}_j) \tag{10.7}$$

and

$$b_i = \frac{\Phi_c(\lambda_{ex}, \mathbf{r}_{si}, \mathbf{r}_{di})}{\Phi_m(\lambda_{ex}, \mathbf{r}_{si}, \mathbf{r}_{di})} \Phi_m(\lambda_{fl}, \mathbf{r}_{si}, \mathbf{r}_{di}) \quad (10.8)$$

We then solve the matrix equation

$$(\mathbf{A}^T \mathbf{A} + \alpha \mathbf{L})\mathbf{x} = \mathbf{A}^T \mathbf{b} \quad (10.9)$$

to get the fluorophore concentration for each voxel. The regularization term $\alpha \mathbf{L}$ can take many forms. In our reconstructions, α is constant, and $\mathbf{L}$ is a Laplacian matrix (for details, see [63, 65]).

In order for FDOI to be successful, the amount of detected emission light must be much greater than the amount of excitation light that is still detected. That is, we require that

$$\frac{\Phi(\lambda_{fl}, \mathbf{r}_s, \mathbf{r}_d)}{\Phi(\lambda_{ex}, \mathbf{r}_s, \mathbf{r}_d)} E \gg 1 \quad (10.10)$$

where E is the relative detection efficiency between the emission and excitation wavelengths ($E \sim 5 \times 10^9$ using the filters described earlier). The photon fluence rate at the emission wavelength can be calculated from (10.5). For simplicity, let us assume that the concentration of fluorophore is zero outside of a small region centered at $\mathbf{r}$ (e.g., outside a tumor at r), and that all spatially dependent variables in (10.5) are approximately constant in this region. The left-hand side of (10.10) then becomes approximately

$$\frac{\Phi(\lambda_{ex}, \mathbf{r}_s, \mathbf{r}) G(\lambda_{fl}, \mathbf{r}, \mathbf{r}_d) \varepsilon(\lambda_{ex}) \eta C(\mathbf{r}) V}{\Phi(\lambda_{ex}, \mathbf{r}_s, \mathbf{r}_d)} E \quad (10.11)$$

where V is the volume of this region. For ICG in water, $\varepsilon(\lambda_{ex}) = 0.254$ cm$^{-1}/\mu$M [66] and $\eta = 0.016$ [67]. For a source/detector pair located directly across from each other through a slab of thickness $L = 6$ cm, with $\mu_a = 0.05$ cm^{-1}, $\mu'_s = 8$ cm^{-1}, and a 1 cc fluorescent inclusion with an ICG concentration of 1 μM, (10.11) equals $\sim 10^7$ which is indeed > 1.

Unfortunately, this signal level also means that the amount of fluorescent emission light detected due to the fluorescent inclusion will be $\sim 10^{-3}$ less than the excitation photons detected during the endogenous scan. For this reason, the CCD exposure time must be increased from 500 ms to ~ 15 seconds for the fluorescent scan.

10.5 Clinical Observations

10.5.1 Whole-Body PET and DOI

The simplest way to compare images from two different modalities is to use stand-alone scanners, analyze the images from each modality separately, and then compare the results. Several studies have used this approach to compare the results of diffuse optical measurements of human breast with other modalities including, MRI [8, 35, 68], X-ray mammography [69–71], and ultrasound [70, 72].

In a recent study we compared DOI and whole-body PET images from 14 subjects with breast lesions [25]. Contrast was visible in both DOI and PET images for nine subjects, in neither DOI or PET for two subjects, and in PET only for three subjects. When contrast was seen in the DOI images it always appeared in THC, μ'_s, μ_{eff}, and optical index. Significant contrast was never observed in StO$_2$.

These results were compared with the pathology reports from biopsies taken after imaging. A summary of the results is found in Table 10.1. Of the nine subjects who showed both DOI and PET contrast, histopathology confirmed invasive ductal carcinoma (IDC) with ductal carcinoma in situ (DCIS) in seven subjects, DCIS only in one subject, and normal breast tissue in one subject. In one of the subjects with IDC, two distinct lesions were visible with PET, but only the larger one was visible with DOI. For the subject with normal breast tissue, the increase in FDG uptake was located at a previous surgical site and was due to a postexcisional inflammation. This inflammation was visible in the DOI images as well. Of the two subjects who showed neither DOI nor PET contrast, one had a possible lipoma (benign), and the other had a cyst. Of the three subjects who showed contrast in PET but not in DOI, one had IDC and DCIS, one had a cyst (superficial and probably infected), and one did not receive a biopsy after negative findings from both ultrasound and MRI. For this subject, the uptake of FDG was diffuse (i.e., no clear focus of FDG uptake was visible).

Table 10.1 Visibility of Lesions to DOI and Whole-Body PET Compared with Histopathology After Imaging

Subject	Age	Days Between DOI and PET Examination	Visible in PET	Visible in DOI	Histopathology (type, mBR grade, size)
1	48	4	Yes	Yes	IDC and DCIS, 3 + 3 + 3 = 9, 2 cm
2	45	0	Yes	Yes	IDC and DCIS, 3 + 3 + 3 = 9, 0.5 cm
3	39	0	Yes	Yes	IDC and DCIS, 2 + 2 + 2 = 6, 3.4 and 0.8 cm
4	44	0	Yes	Yes	IDC and DCIS, 3 + 3 + 1 = 7, 2.3 cm
5	44	0	Yes	Yes	IDC and DCIS, 3 + 2 + 2 = 7, 1.8 cm
6	51	0	Yes	No	None (superficial cyst)
7	64	0	Yes	Yes	DCIS, 0.9 cm
8	43	0	Yes	No	None (MRI and US negative results)
9	53	0	No	No	Cyst
10	59	0	Yes	Yes	Normal tissue (surgical inflammation)
11	44	0	Yes	Yes	IDC and DCIS, 3 + 3 + 3 = 9, 1.5 cm
12	50	13	No	No	Mature adipose tissue (possible lipoma)
13	61	0	Yes	No	IDC and DCIS, 1 + 2 + 1 = 4, 0.8 cm
14	37	0	Yes	Yes	IDC and DCIS, 3 + 3 + 3 = 9, 2.3 cm

IDC: invasive ductal carcinoma; DCIS: ductal carcinoma in situ. mBR grade: (modified) Bloom-Richardson grade.
Source: [25].

A quantitative comparison of tumor-to-background ratios between the DOI and whole-body PET images showed positive correlations (p value < 0.05) between FDG uptake and THC, μ'_s, μ_{eff} and optical index. However, correlation coefficients for these parameters were not particularly high ($R = 0.67$–0.76). These results are summarized in Figure 10.2. Using the mean and maximum standardized uptake values for the PET scans, as opposed to tumor-to-background ratios, had little effect on the correlations with DOI parameters. Comparison of tumor-to-background ratios for both PET and DOI did not show significant correlations with age, tumor grade, or tumor size.

10.5.2 Breast-Only PET and DOI

A more rigorous approach to comparing images from different modalities is to coregister the images. Coregistration of DOI and BPET images makes possible comparison of specific regions of the BPET images with their corresponding regions in DOI images. Coregistration also enables one to determine to what extent lesions appear in the same spatial locations for the two modalities. Reconstructed DOI images have been coregistered with MRI [36, 37, 73], ultrasound [74, 75], and X-ray mammography [38, 76].

In our study comparing DOI and PET [25], we had the opportunity to coregister DOI images of three subjects with breast abnormalities with PET images acquired on the dedicated breast-only PET scanner (BPET) described in Section 10.2. As described in Section 10.3, our DOI device is a stand-alone breast imager. Thus, PET and DOI images were not acquired concurrently. Instead, they were acquired at different times and in slightly different geometries. Fortunately, the similar geometries of the scanners made coregistration possible, though the problem was made more challenging because the breast hangs freely in the BPET scanner, while in the DOI scanner, the breast is mildly compressed (to a thickness of between 5.5 and 7.5 cm). Using the methods reported in [73] (and in Chapter 7), we were able to deform the DOI breast images and align them with the BPET breast images.

The coregistered images in Figure 10.3 show qualitatively that DOI parameters (with the exception of StO_2) are above average in the ROIs determined from BPET. To confirm this observation, we performed the following analysis. For each DOI image, we calculated the average value of particular image parameters for all voxels in the entire breast and for all voxels in the ROI. The tumor-to-background ratio (TBR) is defined as the ratio of these two parameters (i.e., TBR = <roi>/<breast>). The optical index parameter shows the greatest contrast (TBR = 1.5–1.7). THC, μ'_s, and μ_{eff} exhibit somewhat less contrast (TBR = 1.1–1.4), while very little variation in StO_2 is observed (TBR $\cong$ 1.0).

10.5.3 ICG Fluorescence

As mentioned previously, exogenous fluorophores expand the number of physiological parameters that can be measured with DOI and PET. One such parameter of recent interest is vascular permeability. Several studies have explored the use of ICG as a contrast agent to help the detection and imaging of breast tumors. Many rapidly growing tumors have increased vascularity and leaky blood vessels. Certain small

10.5 Clinical Observations

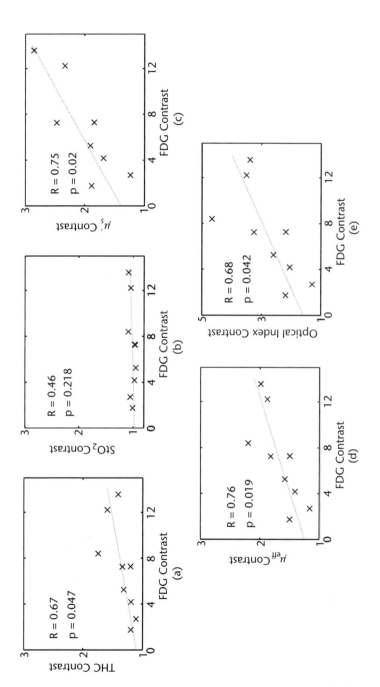

Figure 10.2 Correlations between contrast ratios in FDG uptake and DOI parameters for the nine patients with tumors visible to both DOI and PET. *R* and *p* denote the correlation coefficient and *p* value, respectively. (a) Total hemoglobin concentration (THC), (b) tissue blood oxygenation (StO$_2$), (c) scattering μ_s', (d) overall attenuation μ_{eff} and (e) optical index. (*From:* [25]. © 2008 American Institute of Physics. Reprinted with permission.)

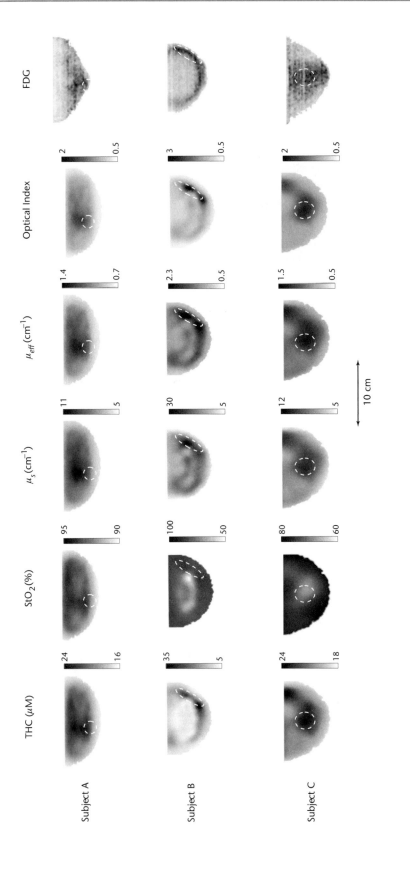

Figure 10.3 Images of the breasts from three females imaged with both DOI and BPET. Each image corresponds to a caudal-cranial slice taken from the 3D reconstruction of a breast after coregistration. Each row corresponds to a breast from one of the three patients. The columns correspond to total hemoglobin concentration (THC), tissue blood oxygenation (StO$_2$), reduced scattering coefficient μ_s' at 786 nm, overall attenuation (μ_{eff}), optical index, and FDG uptake measured with PET. The dashed ellipses enclose the regions of interest. (*From:* [25]. © 2008 American Institute of Physics. Reprinted with permission.)

molecules, such as the MRI contrast agent gadolinium chelate, can leak from these blood vessels and then accumulate in the intravascular space. Breast imaging with ICG is predicated on the hypothesis that ICG, a small molecule that binds to albumin in plasma, will accumulate in this space as well. Indeed, Ntziachristos et al. [35] imaged absorption contrast due to ICG in the breast of three subjects. Their measurements were made concurrently with gadolinium-enhanced MRI and exhibited agreement with respect to the localization and contrast of lesions. Intes et al. [62] were also able to localize breast tumors using ICG absorption. In addition, their research provided evidence that variation of the in vivo ICG pharmacokinetics between normal and diseased tissue may help to distinguish benign from malignant tumors.

Successful in vivo fluorescence DOI (FDOI) has been demonstrated in whole-body imaging in mice by several authors with a variety of fluorescent probes [51, 77–81]. Researchers have also explored fluorescence lymph imaging in mice [82], swine [83], and breast cancer patients [84]. Recently, Corlu et al. were able to translate FDOI into humans using ICG fluorescence to image breast tumors in three subjects [63]. Two of the three subjects were also measured using whole-body PET. The schematic in Color Plate 24(a) shows the location of an invasive ductal carcinoma in a 46-year-old premenopausal female. The tumor is clearly visible in the gadolinium-enhanced MR image [Color Plate 24(b)], which is also a measure of vascular permeability. To get a composite view of the raw data, the sum of the CCD exposures from all source positions during the fluorescent scan divided by the sum of all CCD exposures during the endogenous scan is shown in Color Plate 24(c). The right-hand side of the image corresponds to the lateral side of the right breast as viewed from the feet of the subject. Color Plate 24(d) shows an axial slice from the ^{18}F-FDG whole-body PET images of this subject. The right breast containing the tumor appears in the upper left corner. Color Plate 25(a) shows the reconstructed DOI images of this breast. The tumor is clearly visible in the total hemoglobin, reduced scattering, and ICG concentration images. However, as shown in Color Plate 25(b), the contrast in the ICG concentration image is significantly larger. ICG and ^{18}F-FDG uptake were visible in similar locations for the two subjects having both PET and FDOI scans. The maximum standardized uptake values of ^{18}F-FDG in the two subjects were 1.6 and 3.8, compared to ICG contrast ratios of 5.5 and 3.5, respectively. Further work is needed in order to determine what relationship, if any, exists between ICG contrast and the uptake of ^{18}F-FDG.

10.6 Summary

PET, DOI, and FDOI are functional imaging techniques that interrogate cancer physiology in deep tissue in vivo. Combined, they have the potential to measure a large number of functional parameters. Among these parameters, glucose metabolism, hypoxia, tissue hemoglobin concentration and saturation, tissue scattering, and vascular permeability were explored in this chapter. This work, the first to explore the potential of PET and DOI multimodal imaging, will likely stimulate further investigation along these lines for cancer-response characterization.

Acknowledgments

We wish to thank our PET collaborators R. Wiener, S. M. Srinivas, J. R. Saffer, R. Freifelder, and J. S. Karp. We also thank N. Hajjioui, A. Khamene, and F. Azar for developing the software used to coregister DOI and PET images. For patient recruitment, we thank M. D. Schnall, M. A. Rosen, B. J. Czerniecki, and J. C. Tchou. Finally, this work would not have been possible without the contributions of DOI researchers R. Choe, A. Corlu, T. Durduran, K. Lee, David Busch, M. Schweiger, S. R. Arridge, and M. Grosicka-Koptyra.

References

[1] Eubank, W. B., and D. A. Mankoff, "Evolving role of positron emission tomography in breast cancer imaging," *Sem. Nucl. Med.* 35 (2005): 84–99.

[2] Schwarz, J. D., et al., "Early prediction of response to chemotherapy in metastatic breast cancer using sequential ^{18}F-FDG PET," *J. Nucl. Med.* 46 (2005): 1144–1150.

[3] Smith, I. C., A. E. Welch, A. W. Hutcheon, I. D. Miller, S. Payne, F. Chilcott, S. Waikar, T. Whitaker, A. K. Ah-See, O. Eremin, S. D. Heys, F. J. Gilbert, and P. F. Sharp, "Positron emission tomography using [(18)F]-fluorodeoxy-d-glucose to predict the pathologic response of breast cancer to primary chemotherapy," *J. Clin. Onc.* 18 (2000): 1676–1688.

[4] Wahl, R. L., K. Zasadny, M. Helvie, G. D. Hutchins, B. Weber, and R. Cody, "Metabolic monitoring of breast cancer chemohormonotherapy using positron emission tomography: initial evaluation," *J. Clin. Onc.* 11 (1993): 2101–2111.

[5] Schelling, M., N. Avril, J. Nahrig, W. Kuhn, W. Romer, D. Sattler, M. Werner, J. Dose, F. Janicke, H. Graeff, and M. Schwaiger, "Positron emission tomography using [f-18]fluorodeoxyglucose for monitoring primary chemotherapy in breast cancer," *J. Clin. Oncol.* 18 (2000): 1689–1695.

[6] Mankoff, D. A., L. K. Dunnwald, J. R. Gralow, G. K. Ellis, E. K. Schubert, J. Tseng, T. J. Lawton, H. M. Linden, and R. B. Livingston, "Changes in blood flow and metabolism in locally advanced breast cancer treated with neoadjuvant chemotherapy," *J. Nucl. Med.* 44 (2003): 1806–1814.

[7] Gennari, A., S. Donati, and B. A. Salvadori, "Role of 2-[18F] fluorodeoxyglucose(FDG) positron emission tomography (PET) in the early assessment of response to chemotherapy in metastatic breast cancer patients," *Clinical Breast Cancer* 1 (2000): 156–161.

[8] Choe, R., A. Corlu, K. Lee, T. Durduran, S. D. Konecky, M. Grosicka-Koptyra, S. R. Arridge, B. J. Czerniecki, D. L. Fraker, A. DeMichele, B. Chance, M. A. Rosen, and A. G. Yodh, "Diffuse optical tomography of breast cancer during neoadjuvant chemotherapy: a case study with comparison to MRI," *Med. Phys.* 32(4) (2005): 1128–1139.

[9] Jakubowski, D. B., A. E. Cerussi, F. Bevilacqua, N. Shah, D. Hsiang, J. Butler, and B. J. Tromberg, "Monitoring neoadjuvant chemotherapy in breast cancer using quantitative diffuse optical spectroscopy: a case study," *J. Biomed. Opt.* 9 (2004): 230–238.

[10] Zhu, Q., S. H. Kurtzma, P. Hegde, S. Tannenbaum, M. Kane, M. Huang, N. G. Chen, B. Jagjivan, and K. Zarfos, "Utilizing optical tomography with ultrasound localization to image heterogeneous hemoglobin distribution in large breast cancers," *Neoplasia* 7(3) (2005): 263–270.

[11] Emmenegger, U., G. C. Morton, G. Francia, Y. Shaked, M. Franco, A. Weinerman, S. Man, and R. S. Kerbel, "Low-dose metronomic daily cyclophosphamide and weekly tirapazamine: a well-tolerated combination regimen with enhanced efficacy that exploits tumor hypoxia," *Cancer Research* 66 (2006): 1664–1674.

[12] Warenius, H. M., R. White, J. H. Peacock, J. Hanson, R. A. Britten, and D. Murray, "The influence of hypoxia on the relative sensitivity of human tumor cells to 62.5 MeV (p to Be) fast neutrons and MeV photons," *Radiation Research* 154 (2000): 54–63.

[13] Vaupel, P., and M. Hockel, "Blood supply, oxygenation status and metabolic micromilieu of breast cancers: characterization and therapeutic relevance (review)," *Int. J. Oncol.* 17 (2000): 869–879.

[14] Brown, J. M., "The hypoxic cell: a target for selective cancer therapy {eighteenth Bruce F. Cain memorial award lecture," *Cancer Research* 59 (1999): 5863–5870.

[15] Hockel, M., and P. Vaupel, "Tumor hypoxia: definitions and current clinical, biologic, and molecular aspects," *J. Natl. Cancer Inst.* 93 (2001): 266–276.

[16] Blagosklonny, M. V., "Hypoxia-inducible factor: Achilles heel of antiangiogenic cancer therapy," *Int. J. Oncol.* 19 (2001): 257–262.

[17] Moeller, B. J., Y. Cao, Z. Vujaskovic, C. Y. Li, Z. A. Haroon, and M. W. Dewhirst, "The relationship between hypoxia and angiogenesis," *Sem. Rad. Onc.* 14 (2004): 215–221.

[18] Denny, W. A., "Prospects for hypoxia-activated anticancer drugs," *Curr. Med. Chem. Anti-Canc. Agents* 4 (2004): 395–399.

[19] Rajendran, J. G., D. A. Mankoff, F. O'Sullivan, L. M. Peterson, D. L. Schwartz, E. U. Conrad, A. M. Spence, M. Muzi, D. G. Farwell, and K. A. Krohn, "Hypoxia and Glucose Metabolism in Malignant Tumors Evaluation by [18F] Fluoromisonidazole and [18F] Fluorodeoxyglucose Positron Emission Tomography Imaging," *Clin. Canc. Res.* 10 (2004): 2245–2252.

[20] Padhani, A. R., K. A. Krohn, J. S. Lewis, and M. Alber, "Imaging oxygenation of human tumours," *European Radiology* 17(4) (2007): 861–872.

[21] Thorwarth, D., S. M. Eschmann, F. Paulsen, and M. Alber, "A kinetic model for dynamic [18 F]-Fmiso PET data to analyse tumour hypoxia," *Phys. Med. Biol.* 50(10) (2005): 2209–2224.

[22] Zhou, C., R. Choe, N. Shah, T. Durduran, G. Q. Yu, A. Durkin, D. Hsiang, R. Mehta, J. Butler, A. Cerussi, B. J. Tromberg, and A. G. Yodh, "Diffuse optical monitoring of blood flow and oxygenation in human breast cancer during early stages of neoadjuvant chemotherapy," *J. Biomed. Opt.* 12 (2007): 051903.

[23] Zasadny, K. R., M. Tatsumi, and R. L. Wahl, "FDG metabolism and uptake versus blood flow in women with untreated primary breast cancers," *Eur. J. Nuc. Med. Mol. Imag.* 30 (2003): 274–280.

[24] Tseng, J., L. K. Dunnwald, E. K. Schubert, J. M. Link, S. Minoshima, M. Muzi, and D. A. Mankoff, "18F-FDG kinetics in locally advanced breast cancer: correlation with tumor blood flow and changes in response to neoadjuvant chemotherapy," *J. Nucl. Med.* 45 (2004): 1829–1837.

[25] Konecky, S. D., R. Choe, A. Corlu, K. Lee, R. Wiener, S. M. Srinivas, J. R. Saffer, R. Freifelder, J. S. Karp, N. Hajjioui, F. Azar, and A. G. Yodh, "Comparison of diffuse optical tomography of human breast with whole-body and breast-only positron emission tomography," *Med. Phys.* 35(2) (2008): 446–455.

[26] Corlu, A., R. Choe, T. Durduran, M. A. Rosen, M. Schweiger, S. R. Arridge, M. D. Schnall, and A. G. Yodh, "Three-dimensional in vivo fluorescence diffuse optical tomography of breast cancer in humans," *Opt. Exp.* 15(11) (2007): 6696–6716.

[27] Wernick, M. N., and J. N. Aarsvold, eds., *Emission Tomography: The Fundamentals of PET and SPECT*, New York: Elsevier Academic Press, 2004.

[28] Shepp, L. A., and Y. Vardi, "Maximum likelihood reconstruction for emission tomography," *IEEE Trans. Med. Imag.* 1 (1982): 113–122.

[29] Lange, K., and R. Carson, "EM reconstruction algorithms for emission and transmission tomography," *J. Comput. Assist. Tomogr.* 8 (1984): 306–316.

[30] Browne, J. A., and A. R. De Pierro, "A row-action alternative to the EM algorithm for maximizing likelihoods in emission tomography," *IEEE Trans. Med. Imag.* 15 (1996): 687–699.

[31] Surti, S., and J. S. Karp, "Imaging characteristics of a 3-D GSO whole-body PET camera," *J. Nucl. Med.* 45 (2004): 1040–1049.

[32] Freifelder, R., and J. S. Karp, "Dedicated PET scanners for breast imaging," *Phys. Med. Biol.* 42 (1997): 2453–2480.

[33] Freifelder, R., C. Cardi, I. Grigoras, J. R. Saffer, and J. S. Karp, "First results of a dedicated breast PET imager, BPET, using NaI(Tl) curve plate detectors," *IEEE Nuclear Science Symposium Conference Record* 3 (2001): 1241–1245.

[34] Srinivas, S. M., R. Freifelder, J. R. Saffer, C. A. Cardi, M. J. Geagan, M. E.Werner, A. R. Kent, A. Alavi, M. D. Schnall, and J. S. Karp, "A dedicated breast positron emission tomography (BPET) scanner: characterization and pilot patient study," *IEEE Nuclear Science Symposium and Medical Imaging Conference Record*, (San Diego, CA), (2006).

[35] Ntziachristos, V., A. G. Yodh, M. Schnall, and B. Chance, "Concurrent MRI and diffuse optical tomography of breast after indocyanine green enhancement," *Proc. Natl. Acad. Sci.* 97 (2000): 2767–2772.

[36] Hsiang, D., N. Shah, H. Yu, M. Su, A. Cerussi, J. Butler, C. Baick, R. Mehta, O. Nalcioglu, and B. Tromberg, "Coregistration of dynamic contrast enhanced MRI and broadband diffuse optical spectroscopy for characterizing breast cancer," *Technol. Cancer Res. Treat.* 4 (2005): 549–558.

[37] Brooksby, B., B. W. Pogue, S. Jiang, H. Dehghani, S. Srinivasan, C. Kogel, T. D. Tosteson, J.Weaver, S. P. Poplack, and K. D. Paulsen, "Imaging breast adipose and fibroglandular tissue molecular signatures using hybrid MRI-guided near-infrared spectral tomography," *Proc. Natl. Acad. Sci.* 103, pp. 8828–8833, (2006).

[38] Li, A., E. L. Miller, M. E. Kilmer, T. J. Brukilacchio, T. Chaves, J. Stott, Q. Zhang, T. Wu, M. Chorlton, R. H. Moore, D. B. Kopans, and D. A. Boas, "Tomographic optical breast imaging guided by three-dimensional mammography," *Appl. Opt.* 42 (2003): 5181–5190.

[39] Yang, Y. S., H. L. Liu, X. D. Li, and B. Chance, "Low-cost frequency-domain photon migration instrument for tissue spectroscopy, oximetry, and imaging," *Opt. Eng.* 36(5) (1997): 1562–1569.

[40] http://www.medphys.ucl.ac.uk/˜martins/toast/index.html, accessed January 2007.

[41] Corlu, A.,R. Choe, T. Durduran, M. Schweiger, E. M. C. Hillman, S. R. Arridge, and A. G. Yodh, "Diffuse optical tomography with spectral constraints and wavelength optimization," *Appl. Opt.* 44(11) (2005): 2082–2093.

[42] Yodh, A. G., and D. A. Boas, "Functional imaging with diffusing light," in *Biomedical Photonics Handbook*, T. Vo-Dinh, (ed.), Boca Raton, FL: CRC Press, 2003, pp. 21-1–21-45.

[43] Bevilacqua, F., A. J. Berger, A. E. Cerussi, D. Jakubowski, and B. J. Tromberg, "Broadband absorption spectroscopy in turbid media by combined frequency-domain and steady-state methods," *Appl. Opt.* 39 (2000): 6498–6507.

[44] J. R. Mourant, T. Fuselier, J. Boyer, T. M. Johnson, and I. J. Bigio, "Predictions and measurements of scattering and absorption over broad wavelength ranges in tissue phantoms," *Appl. Opt.* 36 (1997): 949–957.

[45] Woodard, H. Q., and D. R. White, "The composition of body tissues," *Br. J. Radiol.* 59 (1986): pp. 1209–1219.

[46] White, D. R., H. Q. Woodard, and S. M. Hammond, "Average soft-tissue and bone models for use in radiation dosimetry," *Br. J. Radiol.* 60 (1987): 907–913.

[47] Lee, N. A., H. Rusinek, J. C. Weinreb, R. Chandra, R. C. Singer, and G. M. Newstead, "Fatty and fibroglandular tissue volumes in the breasts of women 20-83 years old: comparison of x-ray mammography and computer-assisted MR imaging," *Am. J. Roentgenology* 168 (1997): 501–506.

[48] Kuwana, E., and E. M. Sevick-Muraca, "Fluorescence lifetime spectroscopy for ph sensing in scattering media," *Anal. Chem.* 75 (2003): 4325–4329.

[49] Lakowicz, J., H. Szmacinski, K. Nowaczyk, W. J. Lederer, M. S. Kirby, and M. L. Johnson, "Fluorescence lifetime imaging of intracellular calcium in cos cells using quin-2," *Cell Calcium* 15 (1994): 7–27.

[50] Tung, W. R. C., U. Mahmood, and A. Bogdanov, "In vivo imaging of tumors with proteaseactivated near-infrared fluorescent probes," *Nat. Biotechnol.* 17 (1999): 375–378.

[51] Ntziachristos, V., C. Tung, C. Bremer, and W. R. Weissleder, "Fluorescence molecular tomography resolves protease activity in vivo," *Nat. Med.* 8, pp. 757–760, (2002).

[52] Ke, S., X. Wen, M. Gurfinkel, C. Charnsangavej, S. Wallace, E. M. Sevick-Muraca, and C. Li, "Near-infrared optical imaging of epidermal growth factor receptor in breast cancer xenografts," *Cancer Res.* 63 (2003): 7870–7875.

[53] Foster, T. H., B. D. Pearson, S. Mitra, and C. E. Bigelow, "Fluorescence anisotropy imaging reveals localization of meso-tetrahydroxyphenyl chlorin in the nuclear envelope," *Photochem. Photobiol.* 81 (2005): 1544–1547.

[54] Ballou, B., G. W. Fisher, A. S. Waggoner, D. L. Farkas, J. M. Reiland, R. Jaffe, R. B. Mujumdar, S. R. Mujumdar, and T. R. Hakala, "Tumor labeling in vivo using cyanine-conjugated monoclonal antibodies," *Cancer Immunol. Immunother.* 41 (1995): 257–263.

[55] Achilefu, S., R. B. Dorshow, J. E. Bugaj, and R. R., "Novel receptor-targeted fluorescent contrast agents for in vivo tumor imaging," *Invest. Radiol.* 35 (2000): 479–485.

[56] Kwon, S., S. Ke, J. P. Houston, W. Wang, Q. Wu, C. Li, and E. M. Sevick-Muraca, "Imaging dose-dependent pharmacokinetics of an rgd-fluorescent dye conjugate targeted to alpha v beta 3 receptor expressed in Kaposi's sarcoma," *Mol. Imaging.* 4 (2005): 75–87.

[57] O'Leary, M. A., D. A. Boas, B. Chance, and A. G. Yodh, "Reradiation and imaging of diffuse photon density waves using fluorescent inhomogeneities," *J. Lumin.* 60 (1994): 281–286.

[58] O'Leary, M. A., D. A. Boas, X. D. Li, B. Chance, and A. G. Yodh, "Fluorescent lifetime imaging in turbid media," *Opt. Lett.* 21 (1996): 158–160.

[59] Wu, J., L. Perelman, R. R. Dasari, and M. S. Feld, "Fluorescence tomographic imaging in turbid media using early-arriving photons and Laplace transforms," *Proc. Natl. Acad. Sci.* 94 (1997): 8783–8788.

[60] Das, B. B., F. Liu, and R. R. Alfano, "Time-resolved fluorescence and photon migration studies in biomedical and model random media," *Rep. Prog. Phys.* 60 (1997) 227–292.

[61] Hull, E. L., M. G. Nichols, and T. H. Foster, "Localization of luminescent inhomogeneities in turbid media with spatially resolved measurements of CW diffuse luminescence emittance," *Appl. Opt.* 37 (1998): 2755–2765.

[62] Intes, X., J. Ripoll, Y. Chen, S. Nioka, A. G. Yodh, and B. Chance, "In vivo continuous-wave optical breast imaging enhanced with indocyanine green," *Med. Phys.* 30 (2003): 1039–1047.

[63] Corlu, A., R. Choe, T. Durduran, M. A. Rosen, M. Schweiger, S. R. Arridge, M. D. Schnall, and A. G. Yodh, "Three-dimensional in vivo fluorescence diffuse optical tomography of breast cancer in humans," *Opt. Exp.* 15(11) (2007): 6696–6716.

[64] Ntziachristos, V., and W. R. Weissleder, "Experimental three-dimensional fluorescence reconstruction of diffuse media by use of a normalized born approximation," *Opt. Lett.* 26 (2001): 893–895.

[65] Schweiger, M., S. R. Arridge, and I. Nissila, "Gauss-Newton method for image reconstruction in diffuse optical tomography," *Phys. Med. Biol.* 50 (2005): 2365–2386.

[66] Prahl, S., "Optical properties spectra," http://omlc.ogi.edu/spectra/index.html, 2001, accessed February 2008.

[67] Sevick-Muraca, E., G. Lopez, J. Reynolds, T. Troy, and C. Hutchinson, "Fluorescence and absorption contrast mechanisms for biomedical optical imaging using frequency-domain techniques," *Photochem. Photobiol.* 66 (1997): 55–64.

[68] Shah, N., J. Gibbs, D. Wolverton, A. Gerussi, N. Hylton, and B. J. Tromberg, "Combining diffuse optical spectroscopy and contrast-enhanced magnetic resonance imaging for monitoring breast cancer neoadjuvant chemotherapy: a case study," *J. Biomed. Opt.* 10 (2005): 051503.

[69] Pogue, B. W., S. P. Poplack, T. O. McBride, W. A.Wells, K. S. Osterman, U. L. Osterberg, and K. D. Paulsen, "Quantitative hemoglobin tomography with diffuse near-infrared spectroscopy: Pilot results in the breast," *Radiology* 218 (2001): 261–266.

[70] Gu, X. J., Q. Z. Zhang, M. Bartlett, L. Schutz, L. L. Fajardo, and H. B. Jiang, "Differentiation of cysts from solid tumors in the breast with diffuse optical tomography," *Acad. Radiol.* 11 (2004): 53–60.

[71] Pifferi, A., P. Taroni, A. Torricelli, F. Messina, R. Cubeddu, and G. Danesini, "Four-wavelength time-resolved optical mammography in the 680-980-nm range," *Opt. Lett.* 28 (2003): 1138–1140.

[72] Zhu, Q., E. Conant, and B. Chance, "Optical imaging as an adjunct to sonograph in differentiating benign from malignant breast lesions," *J. Biomed. Opt.* 5(2) (2000): 229–236.

[73] Azar, F. S., K. Lee, A. Khamene, R. Choe, A. Corlu, S. D. Konecky, F. Sauer, and A. G. Yodh, "Standardized platform for coregistration of nonconcurrent diffuse optical and magnetic resonance breast images obtained in different geometries," *J. Biomed. Opt.* 12 (2007).

[74] Holboke, M. J., B. J. Tromberg, X. Li, N. Shah, J. Fishkin, D. Kidney, J. Butler, B. Chance, and A. G. Yodh, "Three-dimensional diffuse optical mammography with ultrasound localization in a human subject," *J. Biomed. Opt.* 5 (2000): 237–247.

[75] Zhu, Q. I., M. M. Huang, N. G. Chen, K. Zarfos, B. Jagjivan, M. Kane, P. Hedge, and S. H. Kurtzman, "Ultrasound-guided optical tomographic imaging of malignant and benign breast lesions: Initial clinical results of 19 cases," *Neoplasia* 5 (2003): 379–388.

[76] Zhang, Q., T. J. Brukilacchio, A. Li, J. J. Stott, T. Chaves, E. Hillman, T. Wu, A. Chorlton, E. Rafferty, R. H. Moore, D. B. Kopans, and D. A. Boas, "Coregistered tomographic x-ray and optical breast imaging: initial results," *J. Biomed. Opt.* 10(2) (2005): 024033.

[77] Graves, E. E., J. Ripoll, R. Weissleder, and V. Ntziachristos, "A submillimeter resolution fluorescence molecular imaging system for small animal imaging," *Med. Phys.* 30 (2003): 901.

[78] Pogue, B. W., S. L. Gibbs, B. Chen, and M. Savellano, "Fluorescence imaging in vivo: raster scanned point-source imaging provides more accurate quantification than broad beam geometries," *Technol. Cancer Res. Treat.* 3 (2004): 15–21.

[79] Patwardhan, S. V., S. R. Bloch, S. Achilefu, and J. P. Culver, "Time-dependent whole-body fluorescence tomography of probe bio-distributions in mice," *Opt. Express* 13 (2005): 2564–2577.

[80] Hwang, K., J. P. Houston, J. C. Rasmussen, A. Joshi, S. Ke, C. Li, and E. M. Sevick-Muraca, "Improved excitation light rejection enhances small-animal fluorescent optical imaging," *Mol. Imaging* 4 (2005): 194–204.

[81] Bloch, S., F. Lesage, L. McIntosh, A. Gandjbakhche, K. Liang, and S. Achilefu, "Whole-body fluorescence lifetime imaging of a tumor-targeted near-infrared molecular probe in mice," *J. Biomed. Opt.* 10 (2005): 54003.

[82] Kwon, S., and E. M. Sevick-Muraca, "Non-invasive imaging of lymph propulsion in mice," *Lymphatic Research and Biology* 5 (2007): 219–231.

[83] Sharma, R., W. Wang, J. C. Rasmussen, A. Joshi, J. P. Houston, K. E. Adams, A. Cameron, S. Ke, M. E. Mawad, and E. M. Sevick-Muraca, "Quantitative lymph imaging," *Am. J. Physiol. Heart Circ. Physiol.* 292 (2007): 3109–3118.

[84] Sevick-Muraca, E. M., R. Sharma, J. C. Rasmussen, M. V. Marshall, J. A. Wendt, H. Q. Pham, E. Bonefas, J. P. Houston, L. Sampath, K. E. Adams, D. K. Blanchard, R. E. Fisher, S. B. Chiang, R. Elledge, and M. E. Mawad, "Imaging of lymph flow in breast cancer patients after microdose administration of a near-infrared fluorophore: feasibility study," *Radiology* 246 (2008): 734–741.

CHAPTER 11
Photodynamic Therapy

Margarete K. Akens and Lothar Lilge

11.1 Introduction

Photodynamic therapy (PDT) describes the use of light-activated drugs, called photosensitizers, to produce oxygen radicals, which result in cell death and tissue necrosis. Hence, the reader may ask why there is a chapter on a therapeutic technology in a book of translational optical multimodal imaging. Photodynamic therapy is often referenced throughout this book as an application to which the presented imaging techniques may be applied to evaluate the treatment outcome. This is not surprising given that Photodynamic therapy is, at its heart, an optical technique. Thus, optical access to the treatment site is provided a priori, be it via the dermis, endoscopes for body cavities, or small optical fibers placed interstitially.

Optical and other imaging modalities are often employed to enable or improve PDT. All photosensitizers, the drug component in PDT, have an optical signature. The compounds possess characteristic absorption spectra, and most are also fluorescent. Thus, photosensitizers may also act as contrast agents and can be exploited for the localization and delineation of malignancies. Furthermore, photobleaching of the photosensitizer can be used as a measure for tumor response in a high-photon-density field [1]. Optical techniques also provide tools to determine the tissue optical properties required for photodynamic therapy delivery planning and monitoring of therapy progress as well as the immediate and delayed tissue response. Optical imaging techniques, possibly in combination with other imaging techniques, are used to guide placement of light sources, such as optical fibers and cavity illuminators. Conversely, PDT provides a model therapy in which novel multimodal imaging techniques can be demonstrated and evaluated because of considerable a priori knowledge of the immediate and short-term tissue responses following PDT, such as inflammation, vascular shutdown, apoptosis, autophagy, and necrosis [2, 3]. The close association between PDT and optical imaging follows from the simultaneous development of the therapeutic and diagnostic techniques, which often occurs within the same laboratories. The approaches exploit similar concepts within the framework that is now referred to as "biophotonics."

Examples of current indications for PDT include diseases of the skin, eye (age-related macular degeneration), organ linings, and solid tissue, mirroring the increased complexity of PDT delivery. This division of treatment targets points also to the ability to use only optical technologies or the need for nonoptical imaging technologies for increasing PDT delivery accuracy. For example, for imaging of the skin, fluorescence, confocal microscopy, optical coherence tomography (OCT) [4], and polarization-based optical imaging technologies have been demonstrated in vivo. For solid tissue, only diffuse optical tomography (fluorescent or scattering and absorption based) is appropriate; however, X-ray, CT, MRI, and PET often present preferable nonoptical imaging tools [5, 6]. For cavities that are endoscopically accessible, a range of optical technologies can be employed, particular for carcinoma in situ, in addition to other nonoptical imaging tools, given that the tumor volume is not too small.

Approved oncological PDT applications in the United States, Canada, and Europe can be divided into two groups. The first encompasses precancerous conditions, such as Barrett's esophagus, actinic keratosis, and early-stage bladder, lung, and other head and neck cancers [2, 7]. In Japan PDT is approved for all early-stage cancers. The second group comprises palliative therapies for obstructive tumors, particularly in the esophagus, lung, and bladder. The first group of indications represents thin layered disease. For these applications, surface-sensitive imaging technologies are preferable, as they will typically provide better contrast within the first millimeters. Often these imaging techniques do not require extensive image-reconstruction algorithms and are thus inexpensive and robust. Solid tumors and palliative therapy require volume-sensitive imaging techniques with great tissue penetration depth, for which optical techniques are not well suited.

Current PDT research is focusing on indications and therapies that will require a combination of surface- and volumetric-sensitive imaging techniques, as in the case of PDT adjuvant to surgical resection of brain tumors or fluorescence-guided resection [8–10]. In these cases, intraoperative MRI guidance will improve bulk-tissue removal, which will be followed by fluorescence-guided resection for remaining surface coverage by tumor cells, followed by PDT of surface proximal destruction of tumor cells.

Some optical imaging techniques employed in PDT research transcend the division between early- and late-stage malignancies, particularly when exploiting genetically modified organisms producing high-contrast optical imaging agents such as bioluminescence imaging (BLI) and green fluorescent protein (GFP)–based contrast and their variants employed preclinically for either surface lesions or solid tumors. However, these techniques are not necessarily suitable for clinical multimodal imaging as their clinical use is at present highly uncertain.

This chapter provides a very brief historical overview of PDT, and its principal promise as a highly targeted oncological intervention technique. We will highlight the photophysical, photochemical, and photobiological sequence of energy transfer at the heart of PDT and show how it may be readily adapted as to provide imaging contrast. This is followed by a presentation of the PDT basis, then by examples where imaging techniques have impacted on PDT, concentrating in particular on the delivery of light and monitoring the treatment outcome. We will also look at the reverse, where PDT has provided a model system for the development of imaging technologies.

In 1900, J. Prime, a French neurologist, used orally administered eosin for the treatment of epilepsy. He discovered, however, that this induced dermatitis in sun-exposed areas of skin. In 1905, Oscar Raab [11], a medical student working with Professor Herman von Tappeiner showed that the combination of acridine red and light had a lethal effect on Infusoria, a species of paramecium. Von Tappeiner and A. Jodlbauer went on to demonstrate the requirement of oxygen in this photosensitization reaction [12], and in 1907 they introduced the term *photodynamic action* to describe this phenomenon [13]. The first report of human photosensitization was in 1913 by the German Friedrich Meyer-Betz [14]. In order to determine whether humans were subject to the same effects seen in mice, he injected himself with 200 mg of hematoporphyrin and subsequently noticed prolonged pain and swelling in light-exposed areas. No further therapeutic applications of photodynamic action were investigated for close to 60 years, so the tumor-localizing abilities of a range of porphyrins, including hematoporphyrin, coproporphyrin, protoporphyrin, and zinc hematoporphyrin, were demonstrated by F. H. J. Figge in 1948 [15]. In 1955, S. K. Schwartz treated crude hematoporphyrin with acetic and sulfuric acids and derived a substance with twice the phototoxicity of hematoporphyrin, which became known as hematoporphyrin derivative (HpD). HpD was tested in clinical trails initially only for the photodetection of malignancies. In 1975, T. J. Dougherty et al. [16] reported the first successful complete tumor cure following administration of HpD and activation with red light from a xenon arc lamp for three 1 hour periods over 5 days in the treatment of experimental animal tumors, finally reinvigorating PDT research [17].

11.2 Basics of PDT

Today, the clinical attraction of PDT is given by the dual localization of the therapy, based on photosensitizer selectivity and light fluence confinement, providing the potential for a truly minimally invasive, surgery-equivalent therapy. Additionally, through the selection of the photosensitizer and the time delay between injection of the photosensitizer and light exposure, the surgeon or physician has the ability to evoke either a vascular or cellular tissue response, and the latter can come in the form of necrosis, apoptosis, or autophagy, further reducing the burden on the host if required. The localization by the exposure of the target to optical photons required for PDT also limits PDT to nonsystemic disease indications because in oncology or infectious-disease control, all affected tissue volumes need to be exposed to light.

The first photosensitizer to obtain regulatory approval was Porfimer Sodium, more commonly known under its trade name Photofrin, in 1993 for the treatment of bladder cancer in Canada. Four additional photosensitizers have been approved for clinical use in various jurisdictions: 5-aminolevulinic acid (ALA, 5-ALA); Levulan, the methyl ester of 5-aminolevulinic acid (Metvix); meso-tetra-hydroxyphenyl-chlorin (mTHPC, temoporfin, Foscan); and benzoporphyrin-derivative monoacid ring A (BPD-MA, verteporfin, Visudyne). Several other photosensitizers have been or are undergoing clinical trials. Among these are tin ethyl etiopurpurin (SnET2), mono-L-aspartyl chlorin e6 (Npe6) and other chlorins, lutetium texaphyrin (Lu-Tex), and the palladium bacteriopherophoribide photosensitizer TooKad, which are often chosen for their absorption bands at longer wavelengths (660, 664, 732, and 762 nm, respectively) (see Figure 11.1). A milder and shorter skin photosensitivity is the most common side effect of the newer

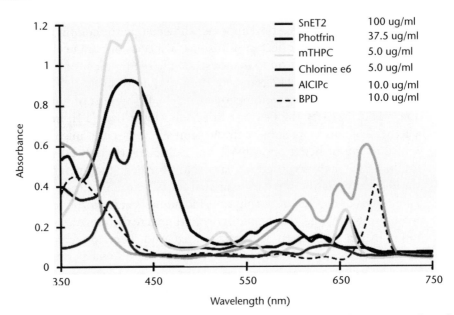

Figure 11.1 Absorption spectra of various approved photosensitizers and some currently under development.

generation of photosensitizers, as compared to Photofrin, which caused skin photosensitivity lasting several weeks. Levulan and Metvix do not represent the photoactive drug, but they are the chemical precursors synthesized by the target cells into protoporphyrin IX (PpIX), the actual photosensitizer, via the heme biosynthesis pathway [18].

The photosensitizer is commonly administered systemically by intravenous (IV) injection, except when used on skin or for 5-ALA, which is currently administered orally. For all IV-injected photosensitizers, the administered dose is over an order of magnitude below the toxicity level in the absence of photon exposure (dark toxicity). A favorable specific uptake ratio (SUR) is achieved for most photosensitizers by a higher metabolic uptake of the drug and a longer retention of the photosensitizers by malignant cells. 5-ALA can present very high SURs as the heme synthesis is increased in malignant cells, which often have down-regulated ferrochelatase, which adds iron (II) to protoporphyrin IX, converting it to heme. Hence, normal cells have a higher capacity in effectively chemically depleting the photosensitizer from the cells. The synthesis of PpIX occurs in the mitochondria, and most tumor cells have a higher concentration of mitochondria.

All currently approved photosensitizers are exerting their cytotoxic effects via a type II or oxygen-mediated mechanism (see Figure 11.2). The photon's quantum energy absorbed by the photosensitizer in the singlet ground state (^{1}PS) excites it into the singlet excited state (^{1}PS). Deexcitation is via internal conversion or fluorescence back to ^{1}PS or via intersystem crossing to its triplet state (^{3}PS), which is required for the photodynamic effect. Hence, high-quality photosensitizers have a high intersystem-crossing quantum yield. The excited molecule can react directly with biomolecules, such as protein and lipids, via proton or electron transfer, forming radicals or radical ions, which in turn interact with oxygen to produce oxygenated products. These reactions are typically referred to as type I photodynamic reactions. Alternatively, the energy of the excited photosensitizer can be directly transferred to

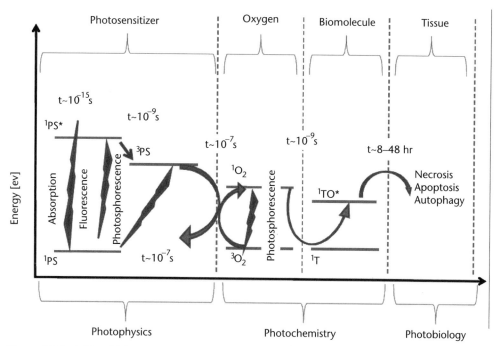

Figure 11.2 Jablonski diagram indicating the energy transitions from the photophysical effects via photochemical effects to photobiological effects.

molecular oxygen ($^3O_2$), which is in its triple state, exchanging energy and molecular spin, generating singlet oxygen ($^1O_2$), in the so-called type II reaction. Singlet oxygen is the most damaging species generated during PDT; it presents an extremely short lifetime (on the order of nanoseconds) and very short diffusion length in cells (<1 μm) [19]. Type I photosensitization generally invokes a reaction of the ^3PS directly with the substrate and will rapidly photochemically deplete the photosensitizer. In type II photoreactions, the sensitizer acts as a catalyst, potentially producing 1,000 $^1O_2$ molecules. Current estimates are that 10^7 $^1O_2$ molecules are required for cell destruction, or about 10^4 photosensitizing molecules per cell.

The efficacy of PDT depends on the type of photosensitizer used, including its particular vascular or subcellular localization, depending on the time delay between administration and light activation, drug concentration and SUR between the target and the surrounding normal tissue, light dose (fluence) and dose rate (fluence rate), and oxygen availability. PDT is delivered clinically in a single dose fraction lasting from a few minutes to 1 hour or slightly longer; hence, it is best described as a surgical intervention. Recent research has also demonstrated that PDT induced modifications to the immune system, and the immunological response can be exploited for therapy. To fully understand and optimize the efficacy for any given indication and photosensitizer concentration, the physical pharmacokinetics of the drug and its biological interplay need to be understood. That PDT requires orders of magnitude more radiation energy per volume tissue treated (Jcm^{-3}) than ionizing radiation demonstrates that nuclear damage is rarely observed, and PDT-induced mutagenic effects have not been demonstrated clinically. While ionizing radiation also requires knowledge of the physics and biology involved, the advantage of using high-energy photons (>1 keV), as compared to optical photons in the 1 to 3 eV range, is that the former undergo little scattering in biological tissues, and the variance in the tissue's stopping power for high-energy photons is very small for all soft tissues. Conversely, use of optical photons makes their transmission through tissue subject to light scattering and absorption, which not only vary significantly between various soft tissues but, for a given tissue, also between patients and within patients. Hence, treatment planning for particular large, solid tumors, for curative or palliative applications, is far more challenging. Thus, it is not surprising that current approved indications for curative PDT relate only to the treatment of thin lesions, as in early cancers, age-related macular degeneration in the eye, and precancerous conditions.

Following the photodiagnostic work in the 1940s to 1970s, it was well established that through the use of selective accumulation of the HpD and other porphyrins in malignant tissue, their fluorescent properties could be exploited for the detection and delineation of malignancies in the skin and other organs, such as the bladder, using direct illumination with a UVA-blue-emitting light source, as most of these photosensitizers have their Soret-Band absorption at about 400 nm. Good clinical surface delineation of the lesions is attainable independently of their thickness by the very limited penetration depth (μ_{eff}^{-1} ~1–3 mm) of these wavelengths into the tissue and through the high SUR between normal tissue and the malignancies. Color Plate 26 shows an example of a 5-ALA-enhanced Barrett's esophagus illuminated with broadband blue light. Using the q-band excitation, in the red-to-NIR portion of the spectrum, the photons interrogate a larger tissue volume, resulting in increased background fluorescence from the normal surrounding tissue, even when the photosensitizer presented a favorable SUR, reducing the contrast of the fluorescent imaging technique.

Various tissue-response models for PDT have been developed, taking one or possibly two of the major efficacy-determining parameters—light fluence, oxygen, and photosensitizer—into consideration. Within these PDT response models, one can differentiate between those using consumption (or change) of any of these three efficacy-determining parameters as an "implicit" dose metric or absolutely quantifying their presence as an "explicit" dose metric. The explicit dose metric thus assumes spatial and temporal colocalization of the three efficacy-determining parameters and can provide a forward calculation of the tissue response, whereas the implicit dose metric assumes that the observed change in consumption following onset of therapy is only due to the PDT effect and provides an integrated dose delivered up to that point in the treatment. The most commonly used implicit PDT models are based on photobleaching of the photosensitizer [20, 21] or oxygen consumption [22, 23]. Singlet oxygen luminescence must also be considered in this group, as it is also a measure of the oxygen consumption [24]. Models based on explicit physical parameters include the critical fluence [25], the effective dose [26], or the photodynamic threshold model [27].

11.3 Superficial Applications

Superficial targets, such as early cancer, are those in which the target thickness is short compared to the penetration depth of the PDT activation wavelength. Application can be found in the skin, bladder, esophagus, lungs, oral cavity, and eyes. In the latter, the target is the choroidal neovascularization in age-related macular degeneration. It is still considered a superficial application due to the transparent nature of the optical imaging system of the eye. Viral inactivation is also considered a superficial application as local infections are usually limited to the first few millimeters in depth [28]. For quantification of the tissue response in superficial tumors, the total effective fluence, proposed by Moseley [26], can be used. Another approach to describing tissue response can be based on the concentration of oxidizing radicals $[O_r]$ generated by PDT, given as

$$[O_r] = \Phi(r) k_{ref} t \frac{\lambda}{hc} \varepsilon C f \qquad (11.1)$$

where $\Phi(r)$ is the fluence rate at the surface, k_{ref} is the backscattered light from lower tissue layers, ε is the photosensitizer's molar extinction coefficient, C is the local concentration, and f is a conversion factor accounting for the quantum yield of oxygen-radical generation. Note that no tissue depth dependence or oxygen information is included as the tissue thickness is very small compared to the light's penetration depth, and oxygen is considered ubiquitously available.

In the skin, PDT mediated by topical application of 5-ALA or its ester Metrix is a very good alternative to surgery. PDT has demonstrated superb cosmetic tissue healing [29, 30], while permitting considerable safety margins [31]. 5-ALA is applied locally about 4 hours prior to illumination of the tumor. The local application provides for an increased SUR as the intact stratum corneum inhibits the penetration of 5-ALA into the skin, whereas most carcinomas have a broken stratum corneum. For basal cell carcinoma, the most common skin malignancy, complete response rates in the high 80% to 100% have been reported. Recurrences are often due to limited 5-ALA penetration into the tumor, which can be overcome by using weak solutions of dimethylsulfoxide or desferrioxamine applied before 5-ALA [32] to reduce the skin absorption of ALA. Another application for 5-ALA-induced, PpIX-mediated PDT is Bowen's disease. While most PDT applications on the skin are local, systemic photosensitizers (porfimer sodium or mTHPC) are required for treatment of multiple lesions.

One recent report noted cure rates of 91% and 94% for early laryngeal and oral cancers, respectively, in a rather large patient cohort [33], making a compelling argument for its use in oral cancers. Conversely, the use of PDT as an antimicrobial modality for oral infections is not that compelling, despite the fact that several photosensitizers are effective against microbiological organisms without inducing damage to the host tissues. However, the oral cavity requires a fine balance of native microflora, equally affected by PDT, which when lost could potentially lead to the overgrowth of opportunistic organisms [34].

11.4 PDT in Body Cavities

PDT in body cavities is an extension of the surface treatment from a physics point of view. Early-stage tumors represent only a thin target, and the source emission can be structured in such a fashion that a large portion or the entire surface of the organ is illuminated, resulting in a one-dimensional attenuation of the fluence rate Φ with depth d.

Historically, the first approved indication for PDT was early-stage bladder cancer. Focal exposure of small papillary carcinoma in situ in the bladder via a cystoscope through the urethra resulted in reasonable response rates, but recurrence was common, possibly due to residual tumor outside of the treatment field. Whole-bladder PDT resulted in very high incidence of side effects (urinary frequency, persistent reduction in bladder capacity, and pain), preventing PDT from becoming an established clinical treatment for bladder cancer. Nseyo et al. [35] showed that using a lower drug and light dose or using 514 nm illumination, which is stronger when absorbed by tissue, and limits PDT's effect to smaller depths, resulted in good tumor response rates without bladder injury or treatment-related morbidity [36]. Due to the very shallow nature of these tumors, whole-bladder PDT using short-wavelength green light for confinement of the PDT effect is an attractive treatment option. Currently, the focus is shifting slightly to combination therapies. More recently, 5-ALA and Hypericin, a photochemical thought to have antimicrobial and antiviral properties, have been proposed in combination with mitomycin C or Avastin [37] for recurrent superficial bladder cancer with close to 50% response rates for up to 24 months.

Muller and Wilson proposed the use of balloon irradiators for adjuvant intracranial PDT following surgical removal of the bulk tissue [38]. An inflatable balloon is filled with a 0.1% Intralipid solution and a cut-end, 600 mm diameter optical fiber is placed into the center of the balloon. The Intralipid solution randomizes the photo directions, and the balloon surface acts as a Lambertian emitter of the PDT activation light. The low structural support found in the brain allows the resection cavity to collapse equally around the balloon if it is inflated sufficiently. Similar approaches have been used, for example, in the cervix for endometrium ablation [39] and the bladder [40]. While in these indications the balloon serves both to conform the target tissue to the desired shape and to provide light scattering, the aspect ratio (diameter over length) of the esophagus would not provide a sufficient homogenization of the fluence rate at the balloon surface from a single cut-end light source. Hence, balloons used for esophageal PDT mainly serve to distend the normally collapsed esophagus into a cylindrical shape, which is then irradiated by a cylindrical, linear, light-diffusing fiber, in effect, a continuous line of point sources, placed centrally into the balloon. In PDT for carcinoma in the lung and early nonsmall-cell lung carcinomas, the physical size constraints will not permit the use of balloons for fiber-diffuser centering. However, given the small diameter of the bronchial tree and the permanent open lumen, a balloon is not required for source centering from a light dosimetry point. Additionally, most lesions are located at the branching points of the bronchial tree and often can be illuminated by a single fiber equipped with a distal microlense, achieving a fairly homogenous illumination of the lesion surface.

Patients with Barrett's esophagus who are also presenting with high-grade dysplasia can certainly benefit from PDT. Previously, these patients were routinely referred for resection surgery based upon the assumption of inevitable progression to cancer. Today, Photofrin-mediated PDT provides an excellent alternative without loss in quality of life. For Barrett's esophagus patients with low-grade dysplasia, the benefit is not as clear as their progression to cancer is not as certain [41].

11.5 PDT for Solid Tumors

PDT is initially an adjuvant therapy to surgical bulk-tissue removal, as described above, which it will certainly remain for various indications where edema and inflammation post PDT are major concerns, such as the brain. For some solid tumors, particularly for interstitial prostate therapy, PDT is gaining ground. One of PDT's main limitations, as compared to surface or cavity applications, is the thickness and volume of the target tissue. In PDT for solid tumors, the target can no longer be considered thin compared to the light penetration depth; hence, the tissue optical properties, comprised of absorption, μ_a, and light scattering, μ_s, tend to determine the treatable volume. Unless the volume is small and has a spherical or cylindrical shape that can be matched by the emitting profile from a single point or cylindrical source, multiple sources are required for successful treatment. A single, flat-cut, optical fiber can treat only 0.05 to 0.72 cm^3 at 630 nm, depending on the tissue optical properties, whereas a 3 cm long cylindrical diffuser can treat 6.25 to 22 cm^3. The former requires an interfiber spacing of 12 mm in two dimensions, whereas the latter permits an interfiber separation of 25 mm in only one dimension. Consequently, isotropic sources find limited use today in clinical interstitial PDT.

The fluence rate Φ inside the tissue as a function of distance r from the point source emitting with power S_0 follows:

$$\Phi(r) = \frac{3S_0 \mu_{eff}^2}{4\pi r \mu_a} e^{-\mu_{eff} r} \tag{11.2}$$

where the effective tissue attenuation, μ_{eff}, determines the fluence-rate gradient at larger distances from the source. For multiple sources, (11.2) has to be executed over all sources and summed. Through the high light scattering and absorption in tissue, the effect on the fluence-rate distribution within the tissue is comparable to a low pass filter, complicating the conformation of the fluence rate to the treatment target's boundary. Additionally, large intra- and interpatient variability in the other two efficacy-determining parameters has been observed. Photosensitizer (PS) concentration is homogenous [42] in neither human nor canine prostate [43]. Using Photofrin labeled with Indium-111 to image photosensitizer drug uptake directly by SPECT with MRI and contrast-enhanced CT structural imaging in a study involving 20 patients showed that the most effective photodynamic therapy for brain tumors may need to be tailored for each patient by correlating SPECT images with anatomical data produced by CT or MRI [5]. The magnitude of the tissue optical-property variations reported depends on the method use for their determination. At one extreme, using 762 nm and employing 3- to 5-cm-long cylindrical diffusers as source-detector optode pairs showed very homogenous tissue optical properties [44], whereas using cut-end fiber optode pairs and considering only the closest neighbors of any source showed demonstrable variations within the photosensitizer concentration at 730 nm [45]. Spatial-temporal monitoring of oxygen and photosensitizer concentration is difficult in solid tissues. Blood-oxygenation-level-dependent magnetic resonance imaging (MRI-BOLD) [46, 47] was demonstrated only in preclinical models, and the verdict as to its clinical utility is still out. Due to the variability in photosensitizer concentration in the target tissue—particularly for vascular-acting photosensitizers such as TOOKAD (WST09) and benzoporphyrin derivative (Verteporfin)–mediated PDT, which provide no selectivity in tissue uptake, aside from differences in vascularities—detailed planning and control of the fluence-rate field throughout the solid tumor appears the preferred approach to improve efficacy. Various treatment-planning platforms have been proposed for up to 12 source fibers to be inserted, for example, into the prostate. Most groups developing treatment-planning software prefer the prostate as it presents a relatively simple cylindrical geometry, apart from the apex, and the clinical standard of care aims at ablating the entire glandular tissue, which becomes a well-circumscribed and easily imaged clinical target volume.

The optimization process relies either on the Cimmino algorithm and a cost function given by the desired fluence-rate dose in the target volume and organs at risk, defined, for example, by the PDT threshold model mentioned above, as introduced by Altschuler et al. [48], or on a weighted gradient descent algorithm introduced by Rendon et al. [49]. The parameter space over which the optimization can be executed comprises the number of light sources, their position within the target volume, and the power per length for diffusers or the total power for flat-cut fibers, and possibly also on the emission profile of the cylindrical diffusers [50]. Figure 11.3 shows the result of a treatment-planning exercise for which the effective treatment volume was matched to CT images of a prostate. One would anticipate that the advances obtained in PDT treatment planning for the prostate could be applied in the near future also to other solid tumors, such as head and neck or brain tumors, so the planning software will need to consider organs at risk to a far greater extent than currently required for the prostate. Imaging of the 3D volume by standard clinical techniques is required at a resolution comparable to the effective attenuation distance in the target tissue and its surrounding organ at risk. Additionally, verification of the placement of the light source fibers within the 3D treatment volume is

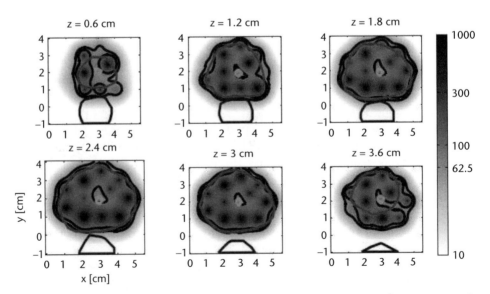

Figure 11.3 Isodose lines for the use of 11 tailored diffusers with $\mu_{eff} = 2.5$ cm^{-1}. The 100% and 62.5% isodose contours are shown in black.

paramount. Rendon et al. [49] showed that a 3 mm displacement can have significant impact on dose-volume histograms.

11.6 Delivery and Monitoring of PDT

Superficial and cavity-based placement of the source relative to the treatment target is commonly accomplished under direct visual guidance and does not benefit from additional imaging technologies. In the case of interstitial PDT, there is tremendous need and opportunity for imaging to impact the realization and accuracy of the a priori optimized treatment plan. Standard clinical imaging is required for establishing the clinical treatment volume. Additionally, optical fibers provide contrast in ultrasound- and X-ray-based imaging [51] and are compatible also with MRI. Hence, placement of optical fibers should be executed under image guidance, or at least verified, as displacement can significantly reduce the treatment's efficacy.

Biological tissue-response monitoring during or immediately at completion of PDT light activation would be the preferred method to validate completeness of the therapy. However, since PDT is commonly delivered as an acute treatment within a short period, biological effects are limited to vascular responses and early signs of edema. The former can be imaged using a host of techniques, such as contrast-enhanced MRI [46], optoacoustic imaging [52], or optical coherence tomography [53, 54]. Color Plate 27 shows the time evolution of the vascular tree following BPD-mediated PDT in a rat window chamber model using a speckle variance OCT approach, and Color Plate 28 shows similar measurements with an interstitial OCT probe for solid tumors [55]. Conversely, the well-known and well-controlled vascular shutdown is also used to demonstrate the performance of these imaging techniques. The relationship between the magnitude of PDT-induced vascular damage and the response rates observed is well documented. Failure to achieve complete vascular shutdown for at least 24 hours will not result in long-term cure [56, 57]. Inhibition of inflammatory responses and vasoconstriction decrease tumor response to PDT [58]; conversely, inhibition of angiogenesis through adjuvant chemotherapy enhances the PDT response [59, 60]. All of these studies demonstrate the importance of vascular-mediated damage in obtaining tumoricidal effect after in vivo PDT and the need to image the changes in the vascular dynamics throughout and post PDT. If the tumor vasculature is the primary target for PDT, the therapeutic benefit results from differences in vascular integrity in the tumors versus the surrounding normal tissues as opposed to from specific drug uptake in the tumor cells. The intrinsically high sensitivity of endothelial cells appears not to be promoting vascular stasis by itself.

Some of the other known early morphological changes following PDT are too subtle to detect with optical or other means in vivo. These include, for example, swelling of the astrocyte foot ends attached to the blood-brain barrier [61].

Other real-time monitoring of tumor response to PDT was demonstrated by dynamic ^{18}F-FDG PET imaging to correlate with the known mechanisms of action of photosensitizing drugs in vivo [62, 63]. For follow-up of TOOKAD-mediated PDT a few days posttreatment of canine prostate, it was shown that gadolinium-DPTA contrast-enhanced MRI is superior to DWI and T2 imaging in assessing the boundary of necrosis [64]. While these imaging methods cannot be used to modify the first PDT treatment, they can certainly be used to validate its performance early on to determine if the tissue response was sufficient to achieve tumor eradication.

11.7 The Future of PDT and Imaging

PDT will certainly continue to make inroads into interstitial therapies for indications such as the pancreas, the breast, or percutaneous, interperitoneal ovarian cancer. So, the assistance required by imaging techniques will increase. The prostate is a rather well-located and fixed organ, particularly when using transrectal ultrasound for fiber source placement. Thus, the clinical treatment volume is equivalent to the treatment planning volume, when using ionizing radiation terminology, as organ shift between imaging for treatment planning and fiber placement is minimal. However, this is not the case for the pancreas, bile duct, and peritoneal cavity, and imaging and image-analysis techniques that can track organ motion and deformation in real time will become paramount for keeping the clinical treatment volume equivalent to the treatment planning volume, which is one of the major advantages of using PDT in an ablative surgical manner.

Conversely, if PDT will be used in a gentler, nonablative manner, stretched over several days, to overcome imminent strong immune responses, such as edema, which are detrimental in immune-privileged sites like the brain, imaging of the volumes by optical tomography [65, 66], optical analogs, or nonoptical techniques will become paramount to validate the efficacy of the treatment, particularly as PDT is such a localized treatment. These long-term PDT treatments, termed *metronomic PDT* (mPDT), are currently under development [67, 68]. Thus, we believe that without strong support from optical and nonoptical imaging techniques for source placement and treatment monitoring, significant further inroads in interstitial PDT will not materialize. However, if therapeutic and treatment monitoring and validation of imaging techniques can be combined, the benefits of PDT as a minimally invasive therapy with extremely low mortality and negative effects on the quality of life can be exploited to their maximum.

Acknowledgments

We wish to thank Ms. Barbara Nelson and Dr. Hazel Collins for their assistance in preparing this chapter.

References

[1] Ma, L. W., et al. "A new method for photodynamic therapy of melanotic melanoma—effects of depigmentation with violet light photodynamic therapy," *J. Environ. Pathol. Toxicol. Oncol.* 26 (2007): 165–172.

[2] Hasan, T., et al. "Photodynamic therapy of cancer," in D. Kufe, R. Pollock, R. Weichselbaum, R. Bast, T. Gansler, J. Holland, and E. Frei, (eds.), *Holland-Frei cancer medicine 6*, 6th ed., 605–622, Hamilton, ON: BC Decker, 2003.

[3] Buytaert, E., et al. "Molecular effectors of multiple cell death pathways initiated by photodynamic therapy," *Biochem. Biophys. Acta* 1776 (2007): 86–107.

[4] Aalders, M. C., et al. "Doppler optical coherence tomography to monitor the effect of photodynamic therapy on tissue morphology and perfusion," *J. Biomed. Opt.* 11 (2006): 044011.

[5] Origitano, T. C., et al. "Photodynamic therapy for intracranial neoplasms: Investigations of photosensitizer uptake and distribution using indium-111 Photofrin-II single photon emission computed tomography scans in humans with intracranial neoplasms," *Neurosurgery* 32 (1993): 357–363; see discussion 363–364.

[6] Schaffer, M., et al. "Application of Photofrin II as a specific radiosensitising agent in patients with bladder cancer—a report of two cases," *Photochem. Photobiol. Sci.* 1 (2002): 686–689.

[7] Plaetzer, K., et al. "Photophysics and photochemistry of photodynamic therapy: Fundamental aspects," *Lasers Med. Sci.* (2008).

[8] Muller, P. J., and B. C. Wilson. "Photodynamic therapy of malignant primary brain tumours: Clinical effects, post-operative ICP, and light penetration of the brain," *Photochem. Photobiol.* 46 (1987): 929–935.

[9] Wagnieres, G. A., et al. "In vivo fluorescence spectroscopy and imaging for oncological applications," *Photochem. Photobiol.* 68 (1998): 603–632.

[10] Eljamel, M. S., et al. "ALA and Photofrin fluorescence-guided resection and repetitive PDT in glioblastoma multiforme: A single centre Phase III randomised controlled trial," *Lasers Med. Sci.* (2007).

[11] Raab, O. "Ueber die Wirkung fluoreszierender Stoffe auf Infusorien," *Z. Biol.* 39 (1900): 524–546.

[12] von Trappeiner, H., and A. Jodlbauer, "Ueber Wirkung der photodynamischen (fluoreszierenden) Stoffe auf Protozoan und Enzyme," *Dtsch. Arch. Klin. Med.* 80 (1904): 427–487.

[13] von Trappeiner, H., and A. Jodlbauer, *Die sensibilisierende Wirkung fluoreszierender Substanzen. Gesamte Untersuchungen ueber photodynamische Erscheinung*, Leipzig: F.C.W. Vogel, 1907.

[14] Meyer-Betz, F. "Untersuchungen ueber die biologische (photodynamische) Wirkung des Haematoporphyrins und andere Derivate des Blut- und Gallenfarbstoffs," *Dtsch. Arch. Klin. Med.* 112 (1913): 476–503.

[15] Figge, F. H. J., et al. "Studies on cancer detection and therapy—the affinity of neoplastic, embryonic, and traumatized tissue for porphyrins, metalloporphyrins, and radioactive zinc hematoporphyrin," *Anatom. Rec.* 101 (1948): 657–657.

[16] Dougherty, T. J., et al. "Photoradiation therapy. II. Cure of animal tumors with hematoporphyrin and light," *J. Natl. Cancer Inst.* 55 (1975): 115–121.

[17] Ackroyd, R., et al. "The history of photodetection and photodynamic therapy," *Photochem. Photobiol.* 74 (2001): 656–669.

[18] Peng, Q., et al. "5-aminolevulinic acid-based photodynamic therapy: Clinical research and future challenges," *Cancer* 79 (1997): 2282–2308.

[19] Niedre, M., et al. "Direct near-infrared luminescence detection of singlet oxygen generated by photodynamic therapy in cells in vitro and tissues in vivo," *Photochem. Photobiol.* 75 (2002): 382–391.

[20] Georgakoudi, I., et al. "The mechanism of Photofrin photobleaching and its consequences for photodynamic dosimetry," *Photochem. Photobiol.* 65 (1997): 135–144.

[21] Kunz, L., and A. J. MacRobert, "Intracellular photobleaching of 5,10,15,20-tetrakis(m-hydroxyphenyl) chlorin (Foscan) exhibits a complex dependence on oxygen level and fluence rate," *Photochem. Photobiol.* 75 (2002): 28–35.

[22] Foster, T. H., et al. "Oxygen consumption and diffusion effects in photodynamic therapy," *Radiat. Res.* 126 (1991): 296–303.

[23] Nichols, M. G., and T. H. Foster, "Oxygen diffusion and reaction kinetics in the photodynamic therapy of multicell tumour spheroids," *Phys. Med. Biol.* 39 (1994): 2161–2181.

[24] Jarvi, M. T., et al. "Singlet oxygen luminescence dosimetry (SOLD) for photodynamic therapy: Current status, challenges and future prospects," *Photochem. Photobiol.* 82 (2006): 1198–1210.

[25] Jankun, J., et al. "Optical characteristics of the canine prostate at 665 nm sensitized with tin etiopurpurin dichloride: Need for real-time monitoring of photodynamic therapy," *J. Urol.* 172 (2004): 739–743.

[26] Moseley, H. "Total effective fluence: A useful concept in photodynamic therapy," *Lasers Med. Sci.* 11 (1996): 139–143.

[27] Farrell, T. J., et al. "Comparison of the in vivo photodynamic threshold dose for photofrin, mono- and tetrasulfonated aluminum phthalocyanine using a rat liver model," *Photochem. Photobiol.* 68 (1998): 394–399.

[28] Wainwright, M. "Local treatment of viral disease using photodynamic therapy," *Int. J. Antimicrob. Agents* 21 (2003): 510–520.

[29] Hur, C., et al. "Cost-effectiveness of photodynamic therapy for treatment of Barrett's esophagus with high grade dysplasia," *Dig. Dis. Sci.* 48 (2003): 1273–1283.

[30] Ris, H. B., et al. "Photodynamic therapy with chlorins for diffuse malignant mesothelioma: Initial clinical results," *Br. J. Cancer* 64 (1991): 1116–1120.

[31] Grant, W. E., et al. "Photodynamic therapy: An effective, but non-selective treatment for superficial cancers of the oral cavity," *Int. J. Cancer* 71 (1997): 937–942.

[32] Fijan, S., et al. "Photodynamic therapy of epithelial skin tumours using delta-aminolaevulinic acid and desferrioxamine," *Br. J. Dermatol.* 133 (1995): 282–288.

[33] Biel, M. A. "Photodynamic therapy treatment of early oral and laryngeal cancers," *Photochem. Photobiol.* 83 (2007): 1063–1068.

[34] Komerik, N., and A. J. MacRobert, "Photodynamic therapy as an alternative antimicrobial modality for oral infections," *J. Environ. Pathol. Toxicol. Oncol.* 25 (2006): 487–504.

[35] Nseyo, U. O., et al. "Photodynamic therapy (PDT) in the treatment of patients with resistant superficial bladder cancer: A long-term experience," *J. Clin. Laser Med. Surg.* 16 (1998): 61–68.

[36] Nseyo, U. O., et al. "Green light photodynamic therapy in the human bladder," *Clin. Laser Mon.* 11 (1993): 247–250.

[37] Bhuvaneswari, R., et al. "Hypericin-mediated photodynamic therapy in combination with Avastin (bevacizumab) improves tumor response by downregulating angiogenic proteins," *Photochem. Photobiol. Sci.* 6 (2007): 1275–1283.

[38] Muller, P. J., et al. "Intracavitary photo-dynamic therapy (Pdt) of malignant primary brain-tumors using a laser-coupled inflatable balloon," *J. Neuro-Oncol.* 4 (1986): 113–113.

[39] Tadir, Y., et al. "Intrauterine light probe for photodynamic ablation therapy," *Obstet. Gynecol.* 93 (1999): 299–303.

[40] van Staveren, H. J., et al. "Integrating sphere effect in whole-bladder wall photodynamic therapy: III. Fluence multiplication, optical penetration and light distribution with an eccentric source for human bladder optical properties," *Phys. Med. Biol.* 41 (1996): 579–590.

[41] Wolfsen, H. C. "Present status of photodynamic therapy for high-grade dysplasia in Barrett's esophagus," *J. Clin. Gastroent.* 39 (2005): 189–202.

[42] Yu, G. Q., et al. "Real-time in situ monitoring of human prostate photodynamic therapy with diffuse light," *Photochem. Photobiol.* 82 (2006): 1279–1284.

[43] Jankun, J., et al. "Diverse optical characteristic of the prostate and light delivery system: Implications for computer modelling of prostatic photodynamic therapy," *BJU Int.* 95 (2005): 1237–1244.

[44] Weersink, R. A., et al. "Techniques for delivery and monitoring of TOOKAD (WST09)—mediated photodynamic therapy of the prostate: Clinical experience and

practicalities," in *Optical Methods for Tumor Treatment and Detection: Mechanisms and Techniques in Photodynamic Therapy XIV*, 5689 (2005): 112–122.

[45] Johansson, A., et al. "Real-time light dosimetry software tools for interstitial photodynamic therapy of the human prostate," *Med. Phys.* 34 (2007): 4309–4321.

[46] Gross, S., et al. "Monitoring photodynamic therapy of solid tumors online by BOLD-contrast MRI," *Nat. Med.* 9 (2003): 1327–1331.

[47] Woodhams, J. H., et al. "The role of oxygen monitoring during photodynamic therapy and its potential for treatment dosimetry," *Photochem. Photobiol. Sci.* 6 (2007): 1246–1256.

[48] Altschuler, M. D., et al. "Optimized interstitial PDT prostate treatment planning with the Cimmino feasibility algorithm," *Med. Phys.* 32 (2005): 3524–3536.

[49] Rendon, A., et al. "Treatment planning using tailored and standard cylindrical light diffusers for photodynamic therapy of the prostate," *Phys. Med. Biol.* 53 (2008): 1131–1149.

[50] Rendon, A., et al. "Towards conformal light delivery using tailored cylindrical diffusers: Attainable light dose distributions," *Phys. Med. Biol.* 51 (2006): 5967–5975.

[51] Lilge, L., et al. "Light dosimetry for intraperitoneal photodynamic therapy in a murine xenograft model of human epithelial ovarian carcinoma," *Photochem. Photobiol.* 68 (1998): 281–288.

[52] Xiang, L., et al. "Real-time optoacoustic monitoring of vascular damage during photodynamic therapy treatment of tumor," *J. Biomed. Opt.* 12 (2007): 014001.

[53] Rogers, A. H., et al. "Optical coherence tomography findings following photodynamic therapy of choroidal neovascularization," *Am. J. Ophthalmol.* 134 (2002): 566–576.

[54] Batioglu, F., et al. "Optical coherence tomography findings following photodynamic therapy of idiopathic subfoveal choroidal neovascularization," *Ann. Ophthalmol.* (Skokie) 39 (2007): 232–236.

[55] Standish, B. A., et al. "Interstitial Doppler optical coherence tomography monitors microvascular changes during photodynamic therapy in a Dunning prostate model under varying treatment conditions," *J. Biomed. Opt.* 12 (2007): 034022.

[56] Triesscheijn, M., et al. "Outcome of mTHPC mediated photodynamic therapy is primarily determined by the vascular response," *Photochem. Photobiol.* 81 (2005): 1161–1167.

[57] Chen, B., et al. "Blood flow dynamics after photodynamic therapy with verteporfin in the RIF-1 tumor," *Radiat. Res.* 160 (2003): 452–459.

[58] Chen, B., and P. A. de Witte, "Photodynamic therapy efficacy and tissue distribution of hypericin in a mouse P388 lymphoma tumor model," *Canc. Lett.* 150 (2000): 111–117.

[59] Fingar, V. H., et al. "The effects of thromboxane inhibitors on the microvascular and tumor response to photodynamic therapy," *Photochem. Photobiol.* 58 (1993): 393–399.

[60] Korbelik, M., and I. Cecic. "Contribution of myeloid and lymphoid host cells to the curative outcome of mouse sarcoma treatment by photodynamic therapy," *Canc. Lett.* 137 (1999): 91–98.

[61] Dereski, M. O., et al. "Normal brain tissue response to photodynamic therapy: Histology, vascular permeability and specific gravity," *Photochem. Photobiol.* 50 (1989): 653–657.

[62] Berard, V., et al. "Dynamic imaging of transient metabolic processes by small-animal PET for the evaluation of photosensitizers in photodynamic therapy of cancer," *J. Nucl. Med.* 47 (2006): 1119–1126.

[63] Lapointe, D., et al. "High-resolution PET imaging for in vivo monitoring of tumor response after photodynamic therapy in mice," *J. Nucl. Med.* 40 (1999): 876–882.

[64] Huang, Z., et al. "Magnetic resonance imaging correlated with the histopathological effect of Pd-bacteriopheophorbide (Tookad) photodynamic therapy on the normal canine prostate gland," *Lasers Surg. Med.* 38 (2006): 672–681.

[65] Pogue, B. W., and K. D. Paulsen, "High-resolution near-infrared tomographic imaging simulations of the rat cranium by use of a priori magnetic resonance imaging structural information," *Opt. Lett.* 23 (1998): 1716–1718.

[66] Tromberg, B. J. "Optical scanning and breast cancer," *Acad. Radiol.* 12 (2005): 923–924.

[67] Bisland, S. K., et al. "Metronomic photodynamic therapy as a new paradigm for photodynamic therapy: Rationale and preclinical evaluation of technical feasibility for treating malignant brain tumors," *Photochem. Photobiol.* 80 (2004): 22–30.

[68] Bogaards, A., et al. "Fluorescence image-guided brain tumour resection with adjuvant metronomic photodynamic therapy: Pre-clinical model and technology development," *Photochem. Photobiol. Sci.* 4 (2005): 438–442.

CHAPTER 12
Optical Phantoms for Multimodality Imaging

Shudong Jiang and Brian W. Pogue

12.1 Introduction

Testing new and developing optical imaging and multimodality imaging systems requires the simultaneous development of objects that physically simulate the properties of human or animal tissues pertinent to system performance. In the first stage of system development, these tissue phantoms are used for initially testing system designs and optimizing the signal-to-noise ratio. Then, in existing systems, phantoms can be used to perform frequent quality control or to compare performance between systems [1–3]. When systems are established and in routine clinical use with regulatory approval, there are generally requirements or recommendations for quality-control phantoms that need to be imaged for validation of system performance and use or are recommended by the manufacturer of the system. The benefits of these procedures are that system performance can then be made more uniform between institutions and over time and that the performance of systems can be objectively compared [4]. The added complexity of optical imaging often requires a spectral signature similar to that of tissue as well, indicating that the molecular composition should be as predominantly similar to tissue as is feasible. This added complexity is not always a primary constraint, but as the use of multimodality imaging grows, the value of optical measurements will become increasingly focused on molecular spectroscopy capabilities. Thus, this chapter outlines the basics of tissue phantoms and then discusses the specific features required for multimodality systems, such as optical spectroscopy.

Tissue-simulating phantom development for optical imaging began with the initial interest in breast transillumination for cancer imaging [5–8]. In the early 1990s, the introduction of spatially resolved, time-resolved, and frequency-domain light signals spurred a large number of researchers to investigate spectroscopy and imaging of tissue, leading to the generation of many different types of tissue phantoms with increasingly better properties [9–17]. There has been a significant increase of interest in newer types of medical optical imaging systems, such as tomography (NIR) [18–23], luminescence imaging [24–26], fluorescence molecular imaging [27–29], and optical coherence tomography (OCT) [30], and this keeps the area of tissue-phantom design advancing. Experimental progress toward molecular imaging applications requires tissue phantoms that have some of the specific molecular features of human tissue. At the same time, the multimodality imaging systems, such as NIR-MRI [31–34], NIR-tomosynthesis [35], and NIR-ultrasound [36–38], are requiring that tissue phantoms be able to mimic multiple properties of each modality for system comparison, evaluation, and quality control.

Over the past several decades, the phantoms for optical imaging and multimodal imaging have been developed with considerably superior designs; yet, routine, widespread clinical use of optical imaging has not been established for many systems. In addition, the spectral range and geometrical configuration of optics applications is so diverse that development of systems and tissue phantoms has not been a straightforward, linear progression. This chapter gives an overview of the various types of tissue-simulating phantoms and their applications, with a particular focus on the developing phantoms for MR and optical combinations.

12.2 Absorption and Scatter Phantom Composition

For each imaging modality, phantoms need to match the key physical and biochemical characteristics of the target tissue being imaged. The key optical properties of tissue are absorption and scattering. For small-scale (<1 mm) optical imaging, it is more important to match the absorption coefficient, $\mu_a(\lambda)$, the scattering coefficient, $\mu_s'(\lambda)$, and the anisotropy coefficient, $g(\lambda)$, which is defined as the average cosine of the scattering angle. Over larger distances (more than three to five scattering lengths [15], a scattering length being defined as the reciprocal of the scattering coefficient, $1/\mu_s$), matching the reduced scattering coefficient, μ_s' (also called the transport scattering coefficient and defined as $\mu_s' = (1 - g)\mu_s$) is all that is required. Over long distances, diffusive processes appear to be attenuated exponentially with this single coefficient [39], and only when boundaries or temporal signals are introduced is there a discernable separation of the effects of μ_a and μ_s'. An excellent compendium of tissue optical properties was compiled in the late 1980s by Cheong et al. [40] and updated in 1995 [41]. Figure 12.1 shows the spectrum of the main absorbers and

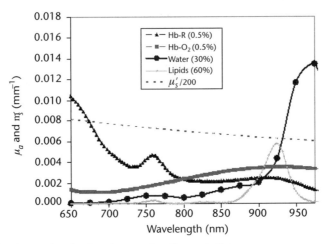

Figure 12.1 Spectrum of main absorbers and scatterers in tissue.

scatterers in tissue with representative concentrations that mimic average normal breast tissue.

In addition to matching the known coefficients of absorption, μ_a, and reduced scattering, μ'_s, of tissue at a certain wavelength or over broader wavelength ranges, phantoms are often required to mimic biologically important molecules, such as hemoglobin and melanin, endogenous fluorophores, such as NADH and FAD [42], or exogenous fluorophores, such as porphyrins or cyanine dyes [43]. Generations of hybrid phantoms with specific characteristics for multimodality imaging, such as elastic properties [44], biochemical properties, water/lipid concentrations [45], electrical properties [46], magnetic resonance properties, and thermal properties, together with optical properties, are becoming increasingly useful [47]. Table 12.1 shows some of the main absorbers and fluorophores used for optical tissue phantoms. The most common material used to match the tissue's μ_a, which has little wavelength dependence, is India ink [48]. Since μ_a is increased proportionally to the ink concentration, any of the value can be obtained by adjusting the concentration of the ink, although the problem with India ink is that its absorption comes from larger-sized particles of carbon, which scatter nearly as much as they absorb. Hence, the absorption coefficient of India ink cannot be exactly know without measuring it as mixed up within a highly scattering phantom. Besides India ink, molecular dyes are another common absorber to mimic the absorption, but they have the particular issue of typically having a peak wavelength dependence to their absorption, so they must be chosen for a specific wavelength range [49–51]. Multiple dyes can be used to broaden the wavelength coverage [52], and their absorption can be known exactly because they are typically single molecules. So, their extinction spectra are entirely due to absorption and can be measured in a standard spectrophotometer, and the concentration used in a phantom can be used to estimate exactly what the phantom absorption is. For short-term-usage phantoms,

Table 12.1 Absorbers and Fluorophores of Optical Tissue Phantoms [4]

Absorber or Fluorophore	Function	Limitations	Stability	References
Whole blood	Provide realistic tissue spectra and oxygenation function	—	Hours to days	[55–58]
Ink	Provide nearly flat absorption spectra	Ink is not stable or repeatable unless taken from a calibrated sample.	Days (if remixed)	[48, 59–61]
Molecular dyes	Provide spectra with wavelength peaks	—	Days to weeks	[61, 62]
Fluorophores	Provide compatibility with aqueous dissolving compounds	It may be necessary to avoid aggregation effects with addition of other agents.	Days to weeks	[63]
Heterogeneities (scattering/absorption/fluorescent)	Test tomography and imaging capabilities Fill inclusions in solid phantoms	Clear enclosures need to be avoided due to light channeling. Index-of-refraction changes may be significant for solid inclusions.	Days	[64]

where the spectrum of tissue is desired, the blood obtained from an animal may be the best absorber, and this can either be used in small pores within a larger scattering medium [53] or embedded throughout an aqueous gelatin-based phantom [54]. Figure 12.2 shows an example of the attenuation spectra of the major type of phantoms at NIR-wavelength range.

Many commonly used fluorophores can be readily dissolved in aqueous solution; however, some are hydrophilic molecules and require predissolving with organic solvents or in combination with monomerizing compounds. Although aggregation of certain hydrophobic dyes, such as protoporphyrin IX, is possible, addition of 5% Tween-29 (Fisher Scientific, United States) as an emulsifying agent has been found to correct this and result in a monomerized form of the fluorophore. The absorption and fluorescence spectra are similar to those observed when the dye is dissolved in a dilute organic solvent; however, care must be taken to appreciate that the absorption and emission spectra of all organic dyes tend to shift in each solvent. As such, directly measuring the dye absorption or emission in the matrix material, ideally without scatterer, is the best way to know the true basis spectra to expect.

There have been three main choices for the scattering agents used to mimic the multiple microscopic scattering from cellular organelles and extracellular constituents. The materials used have typically matched the physical process of scattering without exactly matching the nature of cellular scattering at the submicroscopic level. The key choices have been lipid microparticles, polymer microparticles, or white metal-oxide powders. The interesting feature of lipid microparticles is that they are biologically similar to the lipid membranes in subcellular organelles, which are thought to cause much of the scattering in tissue. However, lipid microparticles can only be used in short-term-usage phantoms because they decompose after periods of time, depending upon the sanitary and refrigeration conditions used. The polymer microspheres are an excellent choice from a scientific perspective due to their controllable size distribution and index of refraction. However, their cost is typically much higher than those of the other scattering agents, which limits the number of places in which they are actually used. The third choice, titanium-dioxide or aluminum-oxide powder, is commonly used, although perhaps the least controllable in terms of creating exact scattering values [49, 65]. These oxides are often the

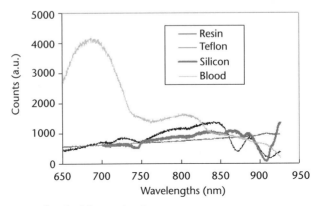

Figure 12.2 Spectrum of optical tissue phantoms.

main pigment in white paint and white plastics due to their high scattering coefficients, and they can be obtained in well-controlled spherical formulations, although their use is less established. Finally, in recent years scattering gold nanoparticles have been developed, and their use in tissue diagnostics and therapy has potential promise, due to their high scattering cross section and potential biocompatibility [66, 67]. While their use in phantoms is not well established, their significant Mie-like scatter cross section makes them a good potential scattering agent. Table 12.2 provides a summary of each of these agents.

12.3 Typical Tissue Phantoms for Multimodal and Optical Imaging

Table 12.3 summarizes the major types of tissue phantoms based on: (1) hydrogel, (2) polyester resin and RTV silicon, and (3) aqueous suspension. The choice of the phantom base is mostly dependent upon what the purpose of the phantom is. In the following sections, detailed procedures, multimodality images, and the main applications of these four types of phantoms are discussed.

12.3.1 Hydrogel-Based Phantoms

The hydrogel-based phantom is the most useful type of phantom for multimodal imaging. Since the water is encapsulated as its main component, and the water mobility has been limited by the stiff hydrogel matrix, in addition to optical imaging, this type of phantom can be imaged by MR [76], CT, ultrasound [77], PET, and other new modalities under development. The most common examples, gelatin (Type A, ~175 Bloom, Sigma Chemical Co., St. Louis, Missouri) and agarose, are two easily handled materials. By adding different contrast agents, agar and gelatin phantoms can be easily used for multimodal imaging. In addition, agar and gelatin allow inclusion of organic molecules and cellular-based constituents, while providing a semisolid object that can have a variety of shapes. For example, a cylindrical gelatin phantom with an inclusion on the edge was made for discussing the combining information of four model-based imaging systems under development that are being used to study breast cancer (magnetic resonance elastography, electrical impedance spectroscopy, microwave imaging spectroscopy, and NIR spectroscopic imaging) [46]. Another example is gelatin phantoms, which are used for validating the MRI-NIR breast cancer–detection system by adding the contrast agents both for optical and MR imaging. A photograph of the phantom, alongside another spherical inclusion, is shown in Color Plate 29(a). Color Plate 29(b) shows a T1-weighted MRI (25 ms TR, 450 flip angle) cross section of this phantom in the plane of the optical fibers. Different concentrations of gadolinium are used for the contrast of MR imaging. For optical contrast of the different tissue layers, India ink is used as the absorber, and titanium oxide is used as the scatterer. As in real tissue, the gelatin phantom's 60% to 90% water concentration provides great MR contrast. The NRI images reconstructed by using the layered structure information from the MRI are shown in Color Plate 29(c). The agreement between the images from two modalities verified this combined system, and the improvement of NIR images by using MRI information indicates the necessity of combining NIR and MRI.

Table 12.2 Scattering Agents Used in Phantoms [4]

Scatterer Material	Permanent	Biologically Compatible	Organic-Chemical Compatible	Particle Size	Index of Refraction	Particle Distribution Function	Recommended Use	References
Lipids	No	Yes	Yes	10 to 500 nm	1.45	Exponentially weighted to smaller sizes; impossible to get a single-size distribution	Intralipid, milk mixture Theory/experimental tests and multiple-phantom contrast studies	[8, 39, 45, 68–71]
Polymer microspheres	Yes	Yes	Yes	50 nm to 100 μm	1.59	Single-size function as ordered with possible 1% to 2% variance	Most accurate theoretical prediction of properties Use with all aqueous, resin, and RTV phantoms	Bangs Laboratories, Fishers, Indiana; Polysciences, Inc., Warrington, Pennsylvaria, and Eppelheim, Germany; Duke Scientific, Inc, Palo Alto, California [42, 49, 72, 73]
TiO_2 and Al_2O_3 powders	Yes	Yes	Yes	20 to 70 nm	2.4 to 2.9	Exponentially weighted or single size can be ordered	Use with gelatin, RTV, and resin phantoms	Sigma-Aldrich, Inc., commonly cited Many possible manufacturers and distributors Many different forms
Quartz-glass microspheres	Yes	Yes	Yes	250 nm	N/A	Single-size function with 10% variance	Use with resin phantoms	[60]

12.3 Typical Tissue Phantoms for Multimodal and Optical Imaging

Table 12.3 Main Classes of Tissue Phantoms [4]

Phantom Matrix Material	Permanent	Solid/ Liquid/ Flexible	Biologically Compatible	Organic-Chemical Compatible	Inclusions Possible?	Adjustable Absorption	Adjustable Scattering	Index of Refraction	Recommended Use	References
Aqueous suspensions	Yes/No	L	Yes	Yes	Yes	Yes	Yes	1.34	Initial use and multiple-phantom contrast studies	[8]
Gelatin/agar matrix base	No	F	Yes	Yes	Yes	Yes	Yes	1.35	Detailed heterogeneity phantom studies bioabsorbers and fluorophores	[42]
Polyester or epoxy resin base	Yes	S	No	No	Yes	Yes	Yes	1.54	Calibration and routine validation Intersystem comparisons	[49, 60, 65, 74]
RTV silicone base	Yes	F	No	No	Yes	Yes	Yes	1.4	Complex geometries with permanent flexible phantoms	[75]

Table 12.4 shows the recipe and mixture procedure to make the type of gelatin phantoms shown in Color Plate 29(a). An inclusion was made in these phantoms by creating inner regions with a small mold and then embedded in other mixtures prior to hardening. After hardening an adipose tissue–like material in a cylindrical mold, the center may be removed and filled with glandular tissue–like gelatin, which is then allowed to harden. The complex part of working with gelatin is making sure new gelatin mixtures are cooled sufficiently before using them with gelled layers; otherwise, the gelled layers will melt and cause a blurring of the intended layers. In addition, instead of using ink or blood to mimic the absorption of the tissue, add the dissolved fluorophores to the gelatin before it hardens but after it has cooled sufficiently to below 45°C. The phantoms to mimic tissue fluorescence are readily made with this procedure, with multiple fluorophores.

The main disadvantage of gelatin is its relatively short shelf life, which can be prolonged by refrigerating in airtight containers and/or by submersing in vegetable

Table 12.4 A Recipe and Mixing Procedure for Making a Gelatin Phantom

Gelatin Phantom Recipe

Mixtures make approximately 500 mL (fill an 82 mm beaker to a height of 80 mm)

Ingredients	Adipose Tissue	Glandular Tissue	Tumor Tissue
Gelatin (g)	50	75	100
Water (mL)	450	425	400
TiO_2 (g)	0.6	1.1	2
India ink (mL)	0.2	0.7	1.25
EDTA (g)	1	1	1
Gadolinium (mL)	0	1	0
Absorption coefficient (1/mm)	0.006	0.01	0.015
Reduced scattering coefficient (1/mm)	0.6	1	1.3

Alternative recipe (developed for MRE stiffness properties)

Ingredients	Adipose Tissue	Glandular Tissue	Tumor Tissue
Gelatin (g)	50	50	100
Vegetable oil (mL)	225	90	0
Water (mL)	225	360	400
Triton x-100	1	1	0

Mixing Procedure

1. Stir gelatin into water in large beaker with magnetic stir bar.
2. Microwave to approximately 40°C.
3. Let stand for 5 minutes, then spoon off bubbles from top.
4. Mix on stir plate until slight thickening is observed.
5. Pour off 50 mL into small beaker containing TiO_2, mix vigorously, and replace (repeat as necessary until all TiO_2 is transferred).
6. Add ink, EDTA, and gadolinium.
7. Apply thin coat of Vaseline to mold (so phantom can be easily removed).
8. When mixture reaches 30°C, pour into mold and refrigerate until semisolid.

oil. One important way to increase the melting point of the gelatin is to add 0.2% formalin, which increases the cross-linking of the gelatin. For multilayered phantoms, however, where one gelatin object is embedded in a background with a different composition, diffusion will decrease object-to-background contrast on the timescale of days. Adding oil to individual layers could limit this diffusion.

12.3.2 Polyester Resin and RTV Silicone Phantoms

Polyester resin phantoms were introduced by Firbank et al. using both TiO_2 [17] and polystyrene particle scatterers [49]; RTV silicone-based soft phantoms were introduced by Bays et al. [78] and Beck et al. [79]. The most common material for the resin phantoms is epoxy resin combined with a hardener, ink, and titanium oxide (Sigma Chemical Co., St. Louis, Missouri: titanium(IV) oxide, TiO_2, T-8141). The RTV-based compounds can be obtained from a number of manufacturers (RTV Elastosil 604, Wacker, Munich, Germany [75, 79]; Rhodorsil RTV 141, Rhone-Poulenc, France [78]; RTV-141, Medford Silicone, Medford, New Jersey [44]). Besides using inks such as 900NP [65, 80, 81] as absorbers, many types of nonorganic dyes have been successfully added to the resin and silicone phantoms; they provide wavelength-dependent absorption across the near-infrared and have no significant scattering coefficient as they are smaller molecules.

Figure 12.3 is a CT image of a group of homogenous and heterogeneous resin and silicone phantoms. Although the purpose of these phantoms is to validate the optical imaging system, the contrast of the inclusion to the background is shown clearly in this CT image, and the TiO_2 is thought to provide good imaging contrast, so the homogeneity of the phantom can be assessed with this approach.

A recipe and mixing procedure for making resin phantoms is listed in Table 12.5. The recipe for the RTV phantom is similar to that for the resin phantom, although the weights of the RTV (RTV-141, Medford Silicone, Medford, New Jersey) and hardener are changed to 500g and 17g, respectively. In addition, instead of the 24 hour curing time of the resin-based phantom, RTV silicone phantoms can need to be cured for 5 to 6 days. Furthermore, once cured, this material is not easily machined but can be cut with razor blades. Since mixing the resin or RTV with its

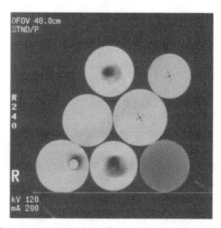

Figure 12.3 CT images of a group of homogenous and heterogeneous resin and silicone phantoms.

Table 12.5 Resin Phantom Recipe and Procedure [82]

Ingredients	330g resin (GY502 Araldite resin, D. H. Litter, Elmsford, New York)
	99g hardener (HY832 Araldite hardener, D. H. Litter)
	1.4g titanium dioxide powder
	0.5 mL 2% ink (predissolved as a 2% stock solution from the 100% ink)
Procedure	Mix resin, ink, and TiO2 well in container (10 minutes).
	Degas mixture in bell jar/break vacuum; repeat three to four times.
	Add 50% of hardener and mix well, especially the bottom (10 minutes).
	Add remaining hardener; mix well (10 minutes).
	Degas again in bell jar as before; repeat three to four times.
	Remove from bell jar before it gets hot or starts to react.
	Let cure 24 hours in fume hood (not under vacuum or it will foam up).
	When hardened, smooth the exterior by machining with a lathe into a finished cylinder.
	Interior holes for objects can be created by drilling into the cylinder.

hardener initiates a chemical process that solidifies the compound, careful preparation in a vacuum is required to prevent bubbles and allow proper curing.

Unlike gelatin phantoms, resin and silicone phantoms may for last many years and are excellent for repeatability studies. Figure 12.4 shows the optical properties of an RTV phantom measured by an NIR tomography system over 5 years. μ_a and μ'_s at six wavelengths of 661, 761, 785, 808, 826, and 849 nm are shown by different shapes of the data points. It can be seen that the fluctuation (st. dev./average) of

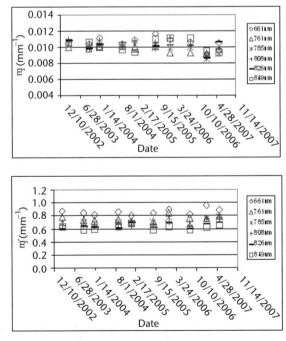

Figure 12.4 The optical properties of an RTV phantom measured by an NIR tomography system over 5 years. μ_a and μ'_s at six wavelengths are shown with different shapes of data points for each wavelength.

μ_a and μ'_s over 5 years is less than 6% of μ_a and 7% of μ'_s. Both are within the range of the imaging accuracy of the tomography imaging system.

Compared to the resin-based phantom, the merit and flexibility for the multimodality of the silicone phantom are its adjustable stiffness due to the amount of hardener. From a series of the mechanical test, it has been observed that the stiffness is in the same range as normal breast tissue when the hardener concentration is lowered below 6% [44, 59]. Balancing the desired stiffness with the practical need to limit the hardening time, a hardener concentration of about 3.4% was optimum for the phantom to mimic normal breast tissue. Like gelatin phantoms, a multilayer RTV phantom can be made with careful attention to procedure.

12.3.3 Aqueous Suspension Phantoms

Examining the needs of multimodality imaging of NIR with MRI, water-based phantoms are perhaps the ideal choice because they can employ any of the main absorbers, scatterers, and fluorophores mentioned in Section 12.2. In addition to the absorption of the absorbers added into the phantom, water is also a main source to affect the entire absorption spectrum throughout most of the visible and near-infrared wavelengths. The water absorption spectrum can be reliably assumed to match the measurements of Hale and Querry [83], and an excellent overview of the water spectra available and their conversion is available on the Web site of the Oregon Medical Laser Center [43].

Figure 12.5(a) shows the estimated total hemoglobin values of a homogenous phantom, as measured through an NIR tomography system. The phantom was a circular plastic container with a diameter of 70 mm and a height of 200 mm. It was filled with an Intralipid saline solution of human blood. The Intralipid concentration was fixed at 1% to maintain $\mu'_s = 0.9$ mm^{-1} at 785 nm. The blood was obtained heparinized as a liquid additive [heparin volume: 0.07 mL of 15% solution (buffered); weight: 10.5 mg EDTA (k3)]. The data indicates that tomographic measurement can be used to estimate total hemoglobin values accurately, as compared to the hematocrit values that were measured spectrophotometrically with a clinical cooximeter system. Phantoms with increasing blood added show increases proportional to the actual blood concentration.

In addition to mimicking the static properties of the tissue, the aqueous suspension phantoms have the unique advantage of mimicking the dynamic process of the tissue property change. Figure 12.5(b) is a plot of the measured results of oxygen saturation (S_tO_2) of a blood deoxygenation process. By adding a small amount of yeast into the container (1% Intralipid and 1% blood) and taking measurements over a period of time, S_tO_2 values for the complete range of partial oxygen pressure (pO_2) values from 150 to 0 mm Hg are measured by the same tomographic system. The pO_2 was measured using a chemical microelectrode (Diamond General, Inc., Ann Arbor, Michigan) after calibration of the electrode overnight in saline solution. The solid curve is the oxygen dissociation curve calculated from the pO_2 values. The agreement between measured S_tO_2 and the calculated values from a theoretical Hill curve prediction helps to validate the spectral response of the tomography system and reconstruction algorithm.

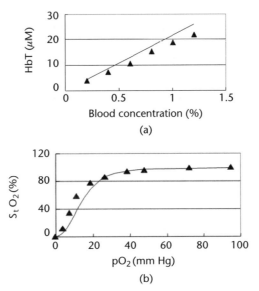

Figure 12.5 Estimated total hemoglobin and blood oxygen saturation of the homogenous blood phantoms measured by an NIR tomographic imaging system. (a) The estimated total hemoglobin values versus the blood concentrations. The Intralipid concentration of this phantom was fixed at 1% to maintain $\mu'_s = 0.9$ mm^{-1} at 785 nm. (b) A plot of the measured results of oxygen saturation (S_tO_2) of a blood deoxygenation process. Intralipid concentration is the same as above, and the blood concentration is 1%. The pO_2 was measured using a chemical microelectrode, and the solid curve is the theoretical oxygen dissociation curve for hemoglobin calculated from pO_2 values.

As an example of the phantom for molecular imaging, a heterogeneous aqueous suspension phantom with imperfect inclusion-to-background uptake has been imaged by a fluorescence tomography imaging system [84]. The phantom was composed of DPBS, 1% Intralipid, and India ink, resulting in background optical properties of $\mu_a = 0.005$ mm^{-1} and $\mu'_s = 1.4$ mm^{-1}. The nontargeted fluorophore indocyanine green (ICG) dissolved in DI water was added to the phantom volume to obtain a 300 nM ICG solution. A thin-walled plastic cylinder was positioned between the edge and center of the phantom to simulate a 2 cm diameter tumor region. The inclusion consisted of the same solution found in the phantom background, though the ICG concentration was elevated to 1 μM, providing a total contrast of just over 3:1. The excitation and fluorescence emission spectrums have been acquired at 240 source-detection positions. The integrated intensities acquired at these positions were calibrated to the model, and images were reconstructed using the soft-spatial-priors implementation. Figure 12.6 is the reconstructed image of this phantom. The estimated contract of inclusion-to-background contrast is approximately 2:1. The estimated contrast is lower than the true contrast, which may be due to the mismatch between the reconstruction model and the measured data.

An important complication in the use of aqueous-suspension, solution-based phantoms is the choice of container and the possibility of light channeling through the container walls, rather than through the solution. This is especially problematic over longer distances and in cases when inclusions or heterogeneities are to be incorporated into phantoms. Glass containers or containers with transparent,

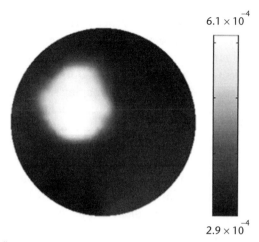

Figure 12.6 Image of fluorescence yield for a 70 mm diameter liquid phantom containing the nontargeted flourophore indocyanine green (ICG) heterogeneity. Inclusion-to-background concentration of ICG was 3:1. Images reconstructed using soft-spatial-prior implementation.

nonscattering walls need to be avoided for this use. Translucent nalgene containers (e.g., polypropylene, Lab Safety Supply, Janesville, Wisconsin) are good for liquid phantoms as these are relatively thin walled (1 mm) and cloudy in appearance, allowing minimal light "channeling" laterally around the walls of the bottle. Also, the addition of an inclusion to a liquid phantom requires an additional container, which is more problematic due to the smaller inclusion size and the reflection index mismatch. Furthermore, light channeling along the top surface of Intralipid over long distances has also been noted. Shielding the surfaces of the phantom with black can reduce this type of light channeling by forcing the light to enter and exit the phantom only at desired locations.

12.4 Conclusions

The choices for tissue optical phantoms are complex and developing steadily at present. There are few options for commercially available phantoms, largely because there are few commercially available systems for optical imaging of tissue. However, as optical spectroscopy and imaging become integrated into specific clinical systems, the need for established, repeatable calibration and reliability standards will grow. At present, there are largely three classes of phantoms in common usage: resin based, silicone based, and aqueous or gelatin based. The need for molecular spectroscopy of hemoglobin leads to the usage of the latter composition because the inclusion of hemoglobin is only possible with these. However, some phantoms, such as one available from Xenogen, Inc. (anthropomorphic mouse phantom for their IVIS imaging system), are available and have similar spectra to that of hemoglobin. While this is not exactly the same spectrum, the match can be sufficiently close within a narrow wavelength band that the phantom is a realistic simulation for imaging. However, the target of multimodality imaging requires the ability to match tissue properties from both imaging systems, and gelatin- or aqueous-based phantoms will always have a preference in this approach because they allow the easy incorporation of organic molecules that are present in tissue. In research and development, it is likely that gelatin-based phantoms will be the primary method for multimodality imaging between MR and optical as they allow easy contrast changes in both. In the area of CT and optical imaging, it may be that resin- or silicone-based phantoms are sufficient as the CT contrast is readily changed with nonorganic materials and the rigidity allows for stable, reproducible use in sequential studies.

In summary, there is no clear consensus on the usage of tissue phantoms, but as the systems that use them are developed, it is essential that the appropriate tissue phantoms be established at the same time. Examples in this chapter illustrate successful usage of multimodality phantoms for MR and optical imaging and point to the need for continued development in this area.

Acknowledgments

This study was supported through grants PO1CA84203, PO1CA80139, and K25CA106863.

References

[1] Cohen, G., "Contrast-detail-dose analysis of six different computed tomographic scanners," *J. Comput. Assist. Tomog.* 3(2) (1979): 197–203.

[2] Seltzer, S. E., R. G. Swensson, P. F. Judy, and R. D. Nawfel, "Size discrimination in computed tomographic images. Effects of feature contrast and display window," *Investig. Radiol.* 23(6) (1988): 455–462.

[3] Olsen, J. B., and E. M. Sager, "Subjective evaluation of image quality based on images obtained with a breast tissue phantom: Comparison with a conventional image quality phantom," *Br. J. Radiol.* 68(806) (1995): 160–164.

[4] Pogue, B. W., and M. S. Patterson, "Review of tissue simulating phantoms for optical spectroscopy, imaging and dosimetry," *J. Biomed. Opt.* 11(4) (2006): 041102.

[5] Watmough, D. J., "Diaphanography: Mechanism responsible for the images," *Acta Radiolog. Oncol.* 21(1) (1982): 11–15.

[6] Watmough, D. J., "Transillumination of breast tissues: Factors governing optimal imaging of lesions," *Radiology* 147(1) (1983): 89–92.

[7] Drexler, B., J. L. Davis, and G. Schofield, "Diaphanography in the diagnosis of breast cancer," *Radiology* 157 (1985): 41–44.

[8] Linford, J., S. Shalev, J. Bews, R. Brown, and H. Schipper, "Development of a tissue-equivalent phantom for diaphanography," *Med. Phys.* 13(6) (1986): 869–875.

[9] Delpy, D. T., M. Cope, P. Van der Zee, S. R. Arridge, S. Wray, and J. S. Wyatt, "Estimation of optical pathlength though tissue from direct time of flight measurement," *Phys. Med. Biol.* 33 (1988): 1433–1442.

[10] Patterson, M. S., B. Chonce, "Time resolved reflectance and transmittance for the non-invasive measurement of tissue optical properties," *Appl. Opt.* 28 (1989): 2331–2336.

[11] Jacques, S. L., "Time-resolved reflectance spectroscopy in turbid tissues," *IEEE Trans. Biomed. Eng.* 36(12) (1989): 1155–1161.

[12] Jacques, S. L., "Time-resolved propagation of ultrashort laser-pulses within turbid tissues," *Appl. Opt.* 28(12) (1989): 2223–2229.

[13] Wilson, B. C., and S. L. Jacques, "Optical reflectance and transmittance of tissues—principles and applications," *IEEE J. Quant. Electron.* 26(12) (1990): 2186–2199.

[14] Wilson, B. C., T. J. Farrell, and M. S. Patterson, "An optical fiber-based diffuse reflectance spectrometer for non-invasive investigation of photodynamic sensitizers in vivo," in *Future Directions and Applications in PDT*. SPIE Inst. Series. (1990): 219–232.

[15] Farrell, T. J., M. S. Patterson, and B. C. Wilson, "A diffusion theory model of spatially resolved, steady-state diffuse reflectance for the noninvasive determination of tissue optical properties," *Med. Phys.* 19(4) (1992): 879–888.

[16] Madsen, S. J., B. C. Wilson, M. S. Patterson, Y. D. Park, S. L. Jacques, and Y. Hefetz, "Experimental tests of a simple diffusion-model for the estimation of scattering and absorption-coefficients of turbid media from time-resolved diffuse reflectance measurements," *Appl. Opt.* 31(18) (1992): 3509–3517.

[17] Firbank, M., and D. T. Delpy, "A design for a stable and reproducible phantom for use in near-infrared imaging and spectroscopy," *Phys. Med. Biol.* 38 (1993): 847–853.

[18] Gratton, E., S. Fantini, M. A. Franceschini, G. Gratton, and M. Fabiani, "Measurements of scattering and absorption changes in muscle and brain," *Philosoph. Trans. Royal Soc. London—Series B: Biolog. Sci.* 352(1354) (1997): 727–735.

[19] Cooper, C. E., and R. Springett, "Measurement of cytochrome oxidase and mitochondrial energetics by near-infrared spectroscopy," *Philosoph. Trans. Royal Soc. London—Series B: Biolog. Sci.* 352(1354) (1997): 669–676.

[20] Hebden, J. C., "Advances in optical imaging of the newborn infant brain," *Psychophysiology* 40(4) (2003): 501–510.

[21] Hawrysz, D. J., and E. M. Sevick-Muraca, "Developments toward diagnostic breast cancer imaging using near-infrared optical measurements and fluorescent contrast agents," *Neoplasia* 2(5) (2000): 388–417.

[22] Pogue, B. W., J. D. Pitts, M. A. Mycek, R. D. Sloboda, C. M. Wilmot, J. F. Brandsema, and J. A. O'Hara, "In vivo NADH fluorescence monitoring as an assay for cellular damage in photodynamic therapy," *Photochem. Photobiol.* 74(6) (2001): 817–824.

[23] Chance, B., S. Nioka, J. Zhang, E. F. Conant, E. Hwang, S. Briest, S. G. Orel, M. Schnall, and B. J. Czerniecki, "Breast cancer detection based on incremental biochemical and physiological properties of breast cancers: A six-year, two-site study," *Acad. Radiol.* 12(8) (2005): 925–933.

[24] Walenta, S., T. Schroeder, and W. Mueller-Klieser, "Metabolic mapping with bioluminescence: Basic and clinical relevance," *Biomolec. Eng.* 18(6) (2002): 249–262.

[25] Contag, C. H., and M. H. Bachmann, "Advances in in vivo bioluminescence imaging of gene expression," *Ann. Rev. Biomed. Eng.* 4 (2002): 235–260.

[26] Contag, C. H., and B. D. Ross, "It's not just about anatomy: In vivo bioluminescence imaging as an eyepiece into biology," *J. Mag. Res. Imag.* 16 (2002): 378–387.

[27] Sevick-Muraca, E. M., J. P. Houston, and M. Gurfinkel, "Fluorescence-enhanced, near infrared diagnostic imaging with contrast agents," *Curr. Opin. Chem. Biol.* 6(5) (2002): 642–650.

[28] Ntziachristos, V., C. H. Tung, C. Bremer, and R. Weissleder, "Fluorescence molecular tomography resolves protease activity in vivo," *Nat. Med.* 8(7) (2002): 757–760.

[29] Ntziachristos, V., C. Bremer, E. E. Graves, J. Ripoll, and R. Weissleder, "In vivo tomographic imaging of near-infrared fluorescent probes," *Mol. Imag.* 1(2) (2002): 82–88.

[30] Fujimoto, J. G., C. Pitris, S. A. Boppart, and M. E. Brezinski, "Optical coherence tomography: An emerging technology for biomedical imaging and optical biopsy," *Neoplasia* 2(1–2) (2000): 9–25.

[31] Ntziachristos, V., A. G. Yodh, M. Schnall, and B. Chance, "Concurrent MRI and diffuse optical tomography of breast after indocyanine green enhancement," *Proc. Natl. Acad. Sci. USA* 97(6) (2000): 2767–2772.

[32] Ntziachristos, V., A. G. Yodh, M. D. Schnall, and B. Chance, "MRI-guided diffuse optical spectroscopy of malignant and benign breast lesions," *Neoplasia* 4(4) (2002): 347–354.

[33] Brooksby, B., B. W. Pogue, S. Jiang, H. Dehghani, S. Srinivasan, C. Kogel, T. Tosteson, J. B. Weaver, S. P. Poplack, and K. D. Paulsen, "Imaging breast adipose and fibroglandular tissue molecular signatures using hybrid MRI-guided near-infrared spectral tomography," *Proc. Natl. Acad. Sci. USA* 103(23) (2006): 8828–8833.

[34] Brooksby, B., S. Jiang, H. Dehghani, B. W. Pogue, K. D. Paulsen, C. Kogel, M. Doyley, J. B. Weaver, and S. P. Poplack, "Magnetic resonance-guided near-infrared tomography of the breast," *Rev. Sci. Instr.* 75(12) (2004): 5262–5270.

[35] Boverman, G., Q. Fang, S. A. Carp, E. L. Miller, D. H. Brooks, J. Selb, R. H. Moore, D. B. Kopans, and D. A. Boas, "Spatio-temporal imaging of the hemoglobin in the compressed breast with diffuse optical tomography," *Phys. Med. Biol.* 52(12) (2007): 3619–3641.

[36] Zhu, Q., E. Conant, and B. Chance, "Optical imaging as an adjunct to sonograph in differentiating benign from malignant breast lesions," *J. Biomed. Opt.* 5(2) (2000): 229–236.

[37] Zhu, Q., N. G. Chen, D. Piao, P. Guo, and X. Ding, "Design of near-infrared imaging probe with the assistance of ultrasound localization," *Appl. Opt.* 40(19) (2001): 3288–3303.

[38] Zhu, Q., S. H. Kurtzma, P. Hegde, S. Tannenbaum, M. Kane, M. Huang, N. G. Chen, B. Jagjivan, and K. Zarfos, "Utilizing optical tomography with ultrasound localization to image heterogeneous hemoglobin distribution in large breast cancers," *Neoplasia* 7(3) (2005): 263–270.

[39] Moes, C. J. M., M. J. van Gemert, W. M. Star, J. P. A. Marijnissen, and S. A. Prahl, "Measurements and calculations of the energy fluence rate in a scattering and absorbing phantom at 633 nm," *Appl. Opt.* 28(12) (1989): 2292–2296.

[40] Cheong, W. F., S. A. Prahl, and A. J. Welch, "A review of the optical properties of biological tissues," *IEEE J. Quant. Electr.* 26(12) (1990): 2166–2185.

[41] Cheong, W. F., "Summary of optical properties," in A. J. Welch (ed.), *Optical-thermal response of laser-irradiated tissue*. New York: Plenum Press, 1995, appendix to ch. 8.

[42] Durkin, A. J., S. Jaikumar, and R. Richardskortum, "Optically dilute, absorbing, and turbid phantoms for fluorescence spectroscopy of homogeneous and inhomogeneous samples," *Appl. Spectrosc.* 47(12) (1993): 2114–2121.

[43] Prahl, S. A., Oregon Medical Laser Center Web site, http://omlc.ogi.edu.

[44] Jiang, S., B. W. Pogue, T. O. McBride, M. M. Doyley, S. P. Poplack, and K. D. Paulsen, "Near-infrared breast tomography calibration with optoelastic tissue simulating phantoms," *J. Elec. Imag.* 12(4) (2003): 613–620.

[45] Merritt, S., G. Gulsen, G. Chiou, Y. Chu, C. Deng, A. E. Cerussi, A. J. Durkin, B. J. Tromberg, and O. Nalcioglu, "Comparison of water and lipid content measurements using diffuse optical spectroscopy and MRI in emulsion phantoms," *Technol. Canc. Res. Treat.* 2(6) (2003): 563–569.

[46] Li, D., P. M. Meaney, T. D. Tosteson, S. Jiang, T. E. Kerner, T. O. McBride, B. W. Pogue, A. Hartov, and K. D. Paulsen, "Comparisons of three alternative breast modalities in a common phantom imaging experiment," *Med. Phys.* 30(8) (2003): 2194–2205.

[47] D'Souza, W. D., E. L. Madsen, O. Unal, K. K. Vigen, G. R. Frank, and B. R. Thomadsen, "Tissue mimicking materials for a multi-imaging modality prostate phantom," *Med. Phys.* 28(4) (2001): 688–700.

[48] Madsen, S. J., M. S. Patterson, and B. C. Wilson, "The use of India ink as an optical absorber in tissue-simulating phantoms," *Phys. Med. Biol.* 37 (1992): 985–993.

[49] Firbank, M., M. Oda, and D. T. Delpy, "An improved design for a stable and reproducible phantom material for use in near-infrared spectroscopy and imaging," *Phys. Med. Biol.* 40(5) (1995): 955–961.

[50] Vernon, M. L., J. Frechette, Y. Painchaud, S. Caron, and P. Beaudry, "Fabrication and characterization of a solid polyurethane phantom for optical imaging through scattering media," *Appl. Opt.* 38(19) (1999): 4247–4251.

[51] Iizuka, M. N., M. D. Sherar, and I. A. Vitkin, "Optical phantom materials for near infrared laser photocoagulation studies," *Lasers Surg. Med.* 25(2) (1999): 159–169.

[52] Wagnieres, G., S. G. Cheng, M. Zellweger, N. Utke, D. Braichotte, J. P. Ballini, and H. vandenBergh, "An optical phantom with tissue-like properties in the visible for use in PDT and fluorescence spectroscopy," *Phys. Med. Biol.* 42(7) (1997): 1415–1426.

[53] Kurth, C. D., H. Liu, W. S. Thayer, and B. Chance, "A dynamic phantom brain model for near-infrared spectroscopy," *Phys. Med. Biol.* 40(12) (1995): 2079–2092.

[54] Brooksby, B., S. Jiang, H. Dehghani, B. W. Pogue, K. D. Paulsen, J. Weaver, C. Kogel, and S. P. Poplack, "Combining near-infrared tomography and magnetic resonance imaging to study in vivo breast tissue: Implementation of a Laplacian-type regularization to incorporate magnetic resonance structure," *J. Biomed. Opt.* 10(5) (2005): 051504.

[55] Kienle, A., M. S. Patterson, L. Ott, and R. Steiner, "Determination of the scattering coefficient and the anisotropy factor from laser Doppler spectra of liquids including blood," *Appl. Opt.* 35(19) (1996): 3404–3412.

[56] Hull, E. L., M. G. Nichols, and T. H. Foster, "Quantitative broadband near-infrared spectroscopy of tissue-simulating phantoms containing erythrocytes," *Phys. Med. Biol.* 43(11) (1998): 3381–3404.

[57] Srinivasan, S., B. W. Pogue, S. Jiang, H. Dehghani, and K. D. Paulsen, "Spectrally constrained chromophore and scattering NIR tomography improves quantification and robustness of reconstruction," *Appl. Opt.* 44(10) (2004): 1858–1869.

[58] Bednov, A., S. Ulyanov, C. Cheung, and A. G. Yodh, "Correlation properties of multiple scattered light: Implication to coherent diagnostics of burned skin," *J. Biomed. Opt.* 9(2) (2004): 347–352.

[59] Jiang, S., B. W. Pogue, T. O. McBride, and K. D. Paulsen, "Quantitative analysis of near-infrared tomography: Sensitivity to the tissue-simulating precalibration phantom," *J. Biomed. Opt.* 8(2) (2003): 308–315.

[60] Sukowski, U., F. Schubert, D. Grosenick, and H. Rinneberg, "Preparation of solid phantoms with defined scattering and absorption properties for optical tomography," *Phys. Med. Biol.* 41 (1996): 1823–1844.

[61] Cubeddu, R., A. Pifferi, P. Taroni, A. Torricelli, and G. Valentini, "A solid tissue phantom for photon migration studies," *Phys. Med. Biol.* 42(10) (1997): 1971–1979.

[62] Ebert, B., U. Sukowski, D. Grosenick, H. Wabnitz, K. T. Moesta, K. Licha, A. Becker, W. Semmler, P. M. Schlag, and H. Rinneberg, "Near-infrared fluorescent dyes for enhanced contrast in optical mammography: Phantom experiments," *J. Biomed. Opt.* 6(2) (2001): 134–140.

[63] Patterson, M. S., and B. W. Pogue, "Mathimatical model for time-resolved and frequency-domain fluorescence spectroscopy in biological tissues," *Appl. Opt.* 33(10) (1994): 1963–1974.

[64] Dehghani, H., B. W. Pogue, J. Shudong, B. Brooksby, and K. D. Paulsen, "Three-dimensional optical tomography: Resolution in small-object imaging," *Appl. Opt.* 42(16) (2003): 3117–3128.

[65] Hebden, J. C., D. J. Hall, M. Firbank, and D. T. Delpy, "Time-resolved optical imaging of a solid tissue-equivalent phantom," *Appl. Opt.* 34(34) (1995): 8038–8047.

[66] Sokolov, K., J. Aaron, V. Mack, T. Collier, L. Coghlan, A. Gillenwater, M. Follen, and R. Richards-Kortum, "Vital molecular imaging of carcinogenesis with gold bioconjugates," *Med. Phys.* 30(6) (2003): 1539–1539.

[67] Tkaczyk, T. S., M. Rahman, V. Mack, K. Sokolov, J. D. Rogers, R. Richards-Kortum, and M. R. Descour, "High resolution, molecular-specific, reflectance imaging in optically dense tissue phantoms with structured illumination," *Opt. Exp.* 12(16) (2004): 3745–3758.

[68] Wilson, B. C., P. J. Muller, and J. C. Yanch, "Instrumentation and light dosimetry for intra-operative photodynamic therapy (PDT) of malignant brain tumours," *Phys. Med. Biol.* 31(2) (1986): 125–133.

[69] van Staveren, H. J., C. J. M. Moes, J. van Marle, S. A. Prahl, and M. J. C. van Gemert, "Light scattering in Intralipid-10% in the wavelength range of 400–1100 nm," *Appl. Opt.* 30(31) (1991): 4507–4514.

[70] Flock, S. T., S. L. Jacques, B. C. Wilson, W. M. Star, and M. J. C. Vangemert, "Optical-properties of Intralipid—a phantom medium for light-propagation studies," *Lasers Surg. Med.* 12(5) (1992): 510–519.

[71] Waterworth, M. D., B. J. Tarte, A. J. Joblin, T. van Doorn, and H. E. Niesler, "Optical transmission properties of homogenised milk used as a phantom material in visible wavelength imaging," *Australasian Phys. Eng. Sci. Med.* 18(1) (1995): 39–44.

[72] Bays, R., G. Wagnieres, D. Robert, J. F. Theumann, A. Vitkin, J. F. Savary, P. Monnier, and H. vandenBergh, "Three-dimensional optical phantom and its application in photodynamic therapy," *Lasers Surg. Med.* 21(3) (1997): 227–234.

[73] Ramella-Roman, J. C., P. R. Bargo, S. A. Prahl, and S. L. Jacques, "Evaluation of spherical particle sizes with an asymmetric illumination microscope," *IEEE J. Sel. Top. Quant. Electron.* 9(2) (2003): 301–306.

[74] Firbank, M., and D. T. Delpy, "A phantom for the testing and calibration of near-infrared spectrometers," *Phys. Med. Biol.* 39(9) (1994): 1509–1513.

[75] Lualdi, M., A. Colombo, B. Farina, S. Tomatis, and R. Marchesini, "A phantom with tissue-like optical properties in the visible and near infrared for use in photomedicine," *Lasers Surg. Med.* 28(3) (2001): 237–243.

[76] Brooksby, B., S. Srinivasan, S. Jiang, H. Dehghani, B. W. Pogue, K. D. Paulsen, J. Weaver, C. Kogel, and S. P. Poplack, "Spectral-prior information improves near-infrared diffuse tomography more than spatial-prior," *Opt. Lett.* 30(15) (2005): 1968–1970.

[77] Doyley, M. M., J. B. Weaver, E. E. Van Houten, F. E. Kennedy, and K. D. Paulsen, "Thresholds for detecting and characterizing focal lesions using steady-state MR elastography," *Med. Phys.* 30(4) (2003): 495–504.

[78] Bays, R., G. Wagnieres, D. Robert, J. F. Theumann, I. A. Vitkin, J. F. Savary, P. Monnier, and H. van den Bergh, "Three-dimensional optical phantom and its application in photodynamic therapy," *Lasers Surg. Med.* 21 (1997): 227–234.

[79] Beck, G. C., N. Akgun, A. Ruck, and R. Steiner, "Design and characterisation of a tissue phantom system for optical diagnostics," *Lasers Med. Sci.* 13(3) (1998): 160–171.

[80] Schmidt, F. E. W., J. C. Hebden, E. M. C. Hillman, M. E. Fry, M. Schweiger, H. Dehghani, D. T. Delpy, and S. R. Arridge, "Multiple-slice imaging of a tissue-equivalent phantom by use of time-resolved optical tomography," *Appl. Opt.* 39(19) (2000): 3380–3387.

[81] Gibson, A., R. M. Yusof, H. Dehghani, J. Riley, N. Everdell, R. Richards, J. C. Hebden, M. Schweiger, S. R. Arridge, and D. T. Delpy, "Optical tomography of a realistic neonatal head phantom," *Appl. Opt.* 42(16) (2003): 3109–3116.

[82] McBride, T. O., *Spectroscopic reconstructed near infrared tomographic imaging for breast cancer diagnosis*, Hanover NH: Dartmouth College, 2001.

[83] Hale, G. M., and M. R. Querry, "Optical constants of water in the 200-nm to 200-um wavelength region," *Appl. Opt.* 12(3) (1973): 555–563.

[84] Davis, S. C., B. W. Pogue, R. Springett, C. Leussler, P. Mazurkewitz, S. B. Tuttle, S. L. Gibbs-Strauss, S. Jiang, H. Dehghani, and K. D. Paulsen, "Magnetic resonance-coupled fluorescence tomography scanner for molecular imaging of tissue," *Rev. Sci. Instr.* 79 (2008): 064302.

CHAPTER 13
Intraoperative Near-Infrared Fluorescent Imaging Exogenous Fluorescence Contrast Agents

Stephen J. Lomnes, Andrew J. Healey, and Pavel A. Fomitchov

13.1 Introduction

Interest in the field of intraoperative fluorescent imaging has grown rapidly over the last decade. This has been spurred on by innovative uses of commercially available fluorescent contrast agents like indocyanine green [1–14] as well as by the intense interest in the development of novel targeted fluorescent reporters for intraoperative guidance [15–29]. In this vein, the first molecularly targeted fluorescent contrast agent, hexaminolevulinate, recently came available in European markets with the promise to assist in the diagnosis of bladder cancer [30, 31]. In response to this trend, imaging technologies are being developed worldwide to address the unique and challenging requirements for making these contrast-agent-based innovations clinically successful [32–34].

This chapter provides a sampling of clinical indications that can be addressed by these technologies and then highlights some of the unique challenges and considerations in some particular aspects of contrast-agent and imaging-system design.

13.2 Unmet Medical Needs Addressed by Intraoperative NIR Fluorescence Imaging

When developing new technologies, it is critical to have a detailed understanding of the unmet medical needs being addressed. To measure the likelihood of adoption of a technology, one should consider carefully how the technology, if successful, would change patient management.

The unmet needs that are suitably addressed by interventional optical imaging technologies fall into two broad categories that contain: (1) aided screening, diagnostics, and staging, and (2) surgery guidance, complication reduction, and treatment verification. The first category applies predominantly to diseases impacting the eye, skin, endoluminal mucosa, and vasculature, which leverage the growth of minimally invasive, traditional light endoscopes and catheters.

Technologies focusing on screening, diagnostics, and staging indications should focus on areas in which established protocols are less effective. Hindrances to effectiveness can arise for a number of reasons, including the following: (1) the at-risk population is insufficiently defined; (2) screening compliance is low; (3) access to health care is limited; (4) screening sensitivity is low, and disease progression is rapid; and (5) screening specificity is low, resulting in expensive and burdensome follow-up. These can be, and are being, addressed in a number of ways by optical technologies.

On the other hand, technologies focusing on the intraoperative setting are poised to address other kinds of unmet medical needs, such as: (1) improving the long-term efficacy of primary treatments, (2) reducing the rate of complications, and (3) reducing the institution-to-institution variability in measures of efficacy and complication.

13.2.1 Improving Long-Term Efficacy of Primary Treatment

Surgical oncology represents one area in which the improvement of long-term efficacy can be highlighted. The majority of patients diagnosed with solid tumor cancers will undergo surgery in the course of their treatment. Of those diagnosed at a sufficiently early stage, surgery will play a critical role in the curative arm of therapy. In breast cancer, for example, the prognostic factors that impact the likelihood of disease progression at the time of surgery are defined by the VNPI, which scores patients according to: (1) the primary tumor size, (2) the presence of metastasis in lymph nodes, and (3) the width of the surgical margin [35].

A positive margin is generally defined to be a surgical specimen with less than 1 mm from the edge of the sample to the nearest tumor cell [35]. The role of the surgical margin width in determining the likelihood of the success of the curative surgery in breast cancer should not be understated.

The primary tumor size is generally well understood preoperatively through diagnostic imaging procedures and is not a candidate variable to control intraoperatively. Lymphatic staging, however, has been proposed as addressable intraoperatively. In breast cancer, sentinel lymph node biopsy (SLNB) has been implemented as the standard of care [36]. This is a procedure developed based on the validated hypothesis that if none of the lymph nodes sentinel to a solitary primary tumor are positive, then the likelihood that the patient is overall node negative is very high [37, 38]. From a workflow perspective, this means that after identification, dissection, and detailed evaluation of the sentinel nodes is complete with negative findings, the surgical team may forgo complete axilary lymph node biopsy (CLNB). This in turn reduces the likelihood of complications like lymphadema in a patient with otherwise normal lymphatics [39]. Typically, a visible dye, such as methylene blue or isolsulfan blue, radioisotopes, or both are injected peritumorally, and the tracers flow through the lymphatics and fill the sentinel nodes. These are identified either by visible tracing of the blue dye, by radiotracing using a handheld radiosensitive probe, or by lymphoscintigraphy [40]. Failures can occur in the procedure due to either incorrect identification of all nodes that are sentinel to the tumor or inaccurate evaluation of the lymph nodes that are resected [41]. Additionally, correct injection of the dye and correct interpretation of the lymphoscintigraphy images can be a source of variability from surgeon to surgeon [42]. Methods that both improve the accuracy and reduce the surgeon-to-surgeon variability in sentinel lymph node detection should improve the sensitivity of sentinel node biopsy. Improving the rate and accuracy of sentinel node detection provides the opportunity to upstage patients who would otherwise be falsely staged as node negative and receive less aggressive postoperative therapy than their condition warranted. Several groups have demonstrated lymphatic imaging with ICG [2, 3, 10, 11, 22], and others have explored novel fluorescent markers to fill this function [20, 22].

The third element of the VNPI is the width of surgical margins. The selection of dissection boundaries in lumpectomy is currently an imprecise science. The surgeon relies on visual assessment of gross pathology, palpation of the mass, and recall from X-ray, ultrasound, and MRI images of the mass to guide resection. In some cases, surgical clips and wires are preoperatively fixed into the breast around the mass under stereotactic imaging guidance [43]. In a 1,262 patient clinical study at Fox Chase Cancer Center in Philadelphia, lumpectomy of stage I to II patients after the first surgery was 59%; after re-excision in patients with positive margins, the positive and close-margin population was 23% [44]. Reduction in both the overall rate and the variability from center to center of positive margin status in patients undergoing lumpectomy could simplify the treatment of breast cancer for providers, payers, and patients.

13.2.2 Reducing the Rate of Complications

Most avoidable surgical complications are rare but exist with finite incidence. Nonetheless, in the United States, complications as a result of surgery constitute a substantial volume of malpractice lawsuits [45]. Recently, Medicare announced that treatments arising from avoidable medical errors would not be reimbursed [46, 47]. These facts together state the importance of increasing the tools available to surgeons to avoid medical errors and to verify that medical errors were not made at the time of surgery.

The highest unmet needs will be in areas with the highest number of complications arising from surgery. In 2006, more than 800,000 cholecystecomies, the surgical removal of the gallbladder, were performed in the United States [48]. This constitutes the most frequent single surgical procedure performed by general surgeons. The most frequent, albeit rare, complication resulting from this procedure is injury to the bile ducts. The rate of injury is difficult to determine precisely but is estimated to be between 0.35% and 1.3% by some authors [49–51]. Of the cases of iatrogenic injury, most that are not detected intraoperatively develop postoperative complications such as sepsis and infection [50]. Affected patients must be worked up diagnostically to confirm biliary injury as the reason for complication and, in many cases, undergo additional corrective surgery.

A retrospective review of more than 250 cases of iatrogenic laparoscopic bile duct injury found that: (1) injuries resulted from errors of perception and not of skill, knowledge, or judgment; (2) when errors occurred, surgeons typically did not recognize them; and (3) consequently, corrective action did not occur intraoperatively [52]. Most injuries that occur stem from the misidentification of the common bile duct (a duct that should remain in tact) as the cystic duct [52]. This can be exacerbated by patient-to-patient variability in anatomy and poor visualization of the entire biliary tree. Tools that can help surgeons intraoperatively confirm the relevant biliary anatomy and sensitively detect the presence of bile leak may help reduce the number of iatrogenic biliary injuries as a result of upper abdominal surgery and may improve the diagnostic workup of patients who develop postoperative complications that may mimic bile leak.

Complications in coronary artery bypass graft (CABG) procedures include stricture at the anastamosis of the graft to the native vessels [53]. The SPY system from Novadaq has been designed for use with ICG as a means for imaging blood flow through the anastamosis to verify graft patency. Validation clinical trials demonstrated that in 120 patients undergoing CABG with intraoperative fluorescent assessment of graft patency, 4.2% of patients required revision [54]. A clinical study of the ability of the ICG method to predict 50% stenoses postoperatively by X-ray angiography demonstrated a sensitivity of 83.3% and a specificity of 100%. Out of 106 patients, 12 presented with postoperative stenoses greater than 50%. In this study, the technique was compared to transit-time ultrasonography and found to be statistically superior [55].

Emerging applications in the reduction of postoperative complications include applications in prostate surgery, plastic reconstructive surgery, and organ transplant procedures. Recent conference presentations suggest that ICG can also be used in intraoperative visualizations of the cavernous nerves in rats [56] with the promise of reducing the rate of postoperative erectile dysfunction and urinary incontinence in patients following radical prostatectomy. It has been proposed that complications from plastic surgery may be addressed by assessing skin-graft perfusion after perforator flap surgery [57], and complications in organ transplantation can be addressed by assessing vessel patency in organ transplant [58].

13.3 Imaging Considerations

13.3.1 Contrast Media

Indocyanine green (e.g., IC-GREEN, Akorn) and fluorescein are among the dyes that are approved for human diagnostic use in major medical markets. Several groups are pursuing the development of alternative dyes and reporter conjugates that may provide benefits in intraoperative fluorescent imaging.

Indocyanine green is currently approved for use in humans for intravenous administration to determine cardiac output, hepatic function, and liver blood flow, as well as for ophthalmic angiography. It has in vivo absorption and emission in the near-infrared portion of the spectrum (ex. ~785 nm/em. ~815 nm).

Fluorescein (e.g., Fluorescite, Alcon Laboratories) is currently approved for use in humans for intravenous administration for diagnostic angiography or including the retina and iris vasculature. It has an in vivo absorption band in the blue portion of the spectrum between 465 and 490 nm and an emission peak in the yellow-green portion of the spectrum between 520 and 530 nm. Fluorescein is metabolized in vivo, and the base compound and metabolites are cleared predominantly through the kidneys. The short wavelength of fluorescein and subsequent short optical penetration depth in tissue make it suitable for ocular applications and not for imaging features more than 1 mm below tissue.

For novel NIR fluorescent contrast agents, a number of optical considerations are important. These include the emission and absorption wavelength, the molar extinction coefficient, and quantum yield. In general, higher molar extinction coefficients and higher quantum efficiencies are preferred. Several researchers and organizations are developing novel targeted fluorescent reporters in the extended red and near-infrared portions of the spectrum. The agent-dependent parameters are the biological performance of the agent with respect to target concentration at the desired imaging time point and the degree of nonspecific binding. Detailed discussion of considerations in the development of these agents can be found in Chapter 16.

From an imaging-system and application perspective, wavelength considerations can be substantially more subtle and have design influences that are highly application dependent. A detailed discussion of the tissue-dependant optical properties can be found in Chapter 1. The application-dependent parameters include the desired penetration depth and the contribution of autofluorescence in particular tissue types.

13.3.2 Tissue Penetration Depth

The imaging problem being addressed defines the desired wavelength from the perspective of the desired penetration depth. Reflectance-based fluorescence imaging systems are typically not depth-resolving devices; as such, they integrate the signal emanating from a range of tissue depths. This may lead to partial volume effects that depend on the size and depth of the target and the relative penetration depth of the light used in the tissue being considered [59].

In the diffuse optics regime, the penetration depth, δ, of a tissue is a function of wavelength and the particular tissue being imaged. The parameters used to derive the penetration depth are the absorption coefficient (μ_a), the scattering coefficient (μ_s), the anisotropy factor (g), and the wavelength of interest and is generally given by

$$\delta = \frac{1}{\sqrt{3\mu_a(\mu_a + \mu_s(1-g))}} = \frac{1}{\mu_{eff}} \qquad (13.1)$$

The penetration depth physically represents the distance into tissue at which light decreases in power density by $1/e$. In the wavelength range of 600 to 1,300 nm in soft tissues, μ_a typically varies between 0.01 and 1 mm^{-1}, μ_s varies between 10 and 100 mm^{-1} and falls slowly with increasing wavelength, and g varies between 0.8 and 0.95 for most tissues and is essentially wavelength independent [60].

Figure 13.1 shows a qualitative example of penetration depth as a function of wavelength based on published absorption and scatter properties of tissue for a hypothetical tissue constituency, but it is useful for general discussion.

Consider, for example, fluorescent labeling in a ureter at an expected depth of 5 mm with a dimension of 2 mm within that tissue versus the identification of a submucosal flat lesion 2 mm beneath the surface of tissue that is 5 mm thick.

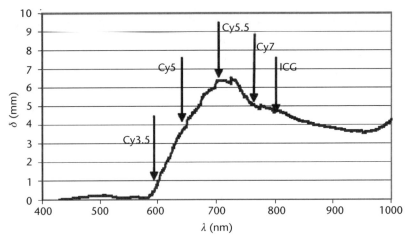

Figure 13.1 Penetration depth (δ) as a function of light wavelength (λ) for a hypothetical tissue based on literature values for absorption coefficient (μ_a), isotropy (g), and scattering coefficient (μ_s).

Assuming in both cases that a concentration ratio of 10:1 is achievable, the imaging-target-to-background ratio will be less than this. In the first case, a penetration depth greater than 5 mm would be desirable; in the latter, a penetration depth of 2 to 3 mm would be more adequate.

Figure 13.2 shows a schematic demonstrating the impact of the partial volume effect on imaging-target-to-background ratio.

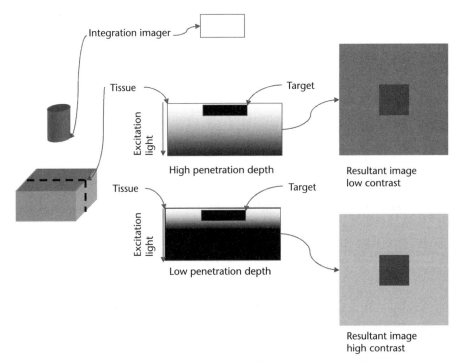

Figure 13.2 A schematic demonstrating the impact of the partial volume effect on imaging target-to-background ratio.

Table 13.1 shows experimental results of a porcine-tissue phantom study evaluating the imaging-target-to-background ratio of a 13 mm thick section of porcine tissue with an 5 mm thick inclusion embedded 2 mm below the surface. The concentration of dye in the target was 5 nM, and in the background material, it was 0.5 nM, providing a concentration ratio of 10:1.

In many applications, predictive modeling using light transport theories can be performed to estimate the performance of particular reporters [59], but this should also be done using detailed characterization of the optical properties of the particular tissues under study.

13.3.3 Autofluorescence

Naturally occurring fluorescence has been studied extensively in the visible wavelengths [61] and used clinically as a diagnostic biomarker in several commercially available systems [62]. In the context of using exogenously administered fluorescent probes, this can be a significant source of background that limits the imaging-target-to-background ratio.

It is generally accepted that autofluorescence decreases as the excitation wavelength increases; however, its contribution to imaging background, even in the NIR, should be taken into consideration [63].

Autofluorescence varies widely by tissue type and wavelength and is difficult to quantify in meaningful ways that are useful in designing imaging systems and setting agent targeting requirements. In this regard, Degrand et al. established a procedure for characterizing autofluorescence in terms of equivalent concentrations of a dye of interest in surgical imaging applications [64]. In this case, they report autofluorescence of different tissue types in terms of ICG equivalents and define the term as the fluorescence-intensity equivalent to a 1 mm thick dye inclusion per unit of excitation power density.

Figure 13.3 shows data collected reporting methylene blue equivalents of autofluorescence of different tissues in adult pigs.

13.3.4 Optical Design Considerations

Reflectance-based fluorescence imaging systems are typically quite simple in concept, but detailed design requires keen understanding of critical performance requirements, including imaging sensitivity, ambient lighting conditions, frame rate, imaging resolution, cost, and size.

Table 13.1 Estimated Penetration Depth and Measured Imaging Target-to-Background Ratio for Various Cy Dyes from a Porcine Tissue Phantom

Reporter (10:1)	Excitation Max (nm)	Estimated Penetration Depth (mm)	Image TBR
Cy3B	548	0.2	1.7:1
Cy5	646	4.4	3.0:1
Cy7	739	4.9	2.0:1

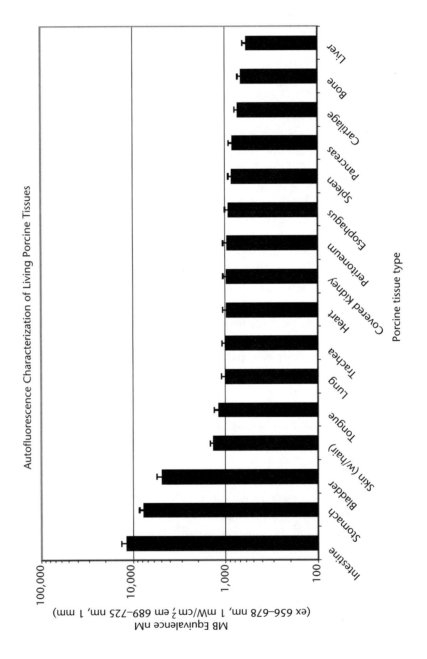

Figure 13.3 Methylene blue equivalence of autofluorescence by tissue type from living porcine tissues.

The challenge of the design of such systems should not be underestimated as, by analogy, fluorescence surgical systems must have comparable imaging sensitivity for fluorescence microscopes but from a working distance of 50 cm and at video frame rates in bright ambient lighting.

The high-level components of any reflectance-based fluorescence imaging system include excitation sources and filters, collection optics, emission filters, and detectors. To the benefit of this field, rapid advancements from adjacent and even unrelated industries are being made in all of these areas, which should drive innovation in this space.

13.3.5 Excitation

The excitation power density is linearly proportional to the emission power density and is a critical system component with respect to overall imaging sensitivity. In standoff surgical imaging applications, suitable surface power densities are 1 to 50 mW/cm^2 and are application and wavelength dependent. Near-surface imaging applications of bright dyes with high concentrations, such as fluorescence angiography, may be suitably imaged at 1 to 5 mW/cm^2, whereas receptor targeting and imaging of features at a significant depth in tissue may require substantially higher-power densities.

The upper bound of useful excitation power density may be defined by the photobleaching threshold of the dye under consideration or by the relative contribution of endogenous fluorescence. The latter comes into consideration when the amount of autofluorescence signal in an uninjected subject results in a substantial portion of the dynamic range of the detector at the desired imaging frame rate.

Excitation sources used are typically expanded laser diodes or light-emitting diode arrays. Filtration of these sources is also important given the presence of the light emission from these sources within the detection band of the system. Typically, interference-based filters are used in these applications.

Figure 13.4 shows an example of a high-powered illumination system based on arrays of LEDs, with means for placing interference filters in front of the LED modules. This system is designed to provide uniform filtered illumination of power densities up to 50 mW/cm^2. The modular design and back-end electronics allow for the introduction of multiple illumination channels.

13.3.6 Collection Optics and Emission Filtering

The goal of the optical system should be to maximize detection sensitivity, providing appropriate focus while minimizing imaging artifacts. In single-detector systems (e.g., fluorescence only), this is readily achievable by choosing a lens and filter with an appropriate entrance pupil diameter to maximize collection efficiency, while providing the required depth of field, field of view, filter cone half-angle specifications, and working distance.

Emission filters should be chosen that sufficiently block excitation and other lighting and sufficiently match the emission spectrum of the fluorophore being imaged. For high-dye-concentration applications, the crossover between the excitation filter and the emission filter should typically be five or higher. In-band trans-

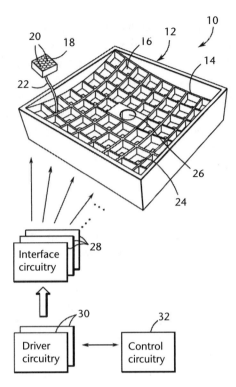

Figure 13.4 Schematic representation of a high-powered modular reconfigurable illumination system for a fluorescence-guided surgery system.

mission directly impacts imaging sensitivity and should be conserved. Typically, interference filters are used for this level of light-blocking performance. Interference filters degrade in performance as the angle of incidence of light increases from normal. The optical design and filter selection should be performed so as to minimize artifacts due to high-angle light transmission.

13.3.7 Detectors

CCD and CMOS detector technologies are advancing rapidly, spurred on by increased demand for small yet high-quality cameras in photonics applications, cell phones, webcams, and security markets. With all these advances, the variety of detector-technology options is very high. Some important considerations for fluorescence-guided-surgery applications are the sensor size, pixel size, number of pixels, well capacity, binning modes, camera electronic noise, and quantum efficiency in the emission band, to name just a few.

13.4 Future Outlook

Three driving factors are likely to increase the use of intraoperative fluorescence imaging technologies: increasing cost and complexity in delivering quality health care, the rapid advancement of high-quality, low-cost components integral to these systems, and the development and availability of specialized fluorescent contrast agents.

Intraoperative fluorescence imaging has the potential to provide cost-effective tools to potentially improve the efficacy of primary treatments and reduce the rates of intraoperatively undetected factors that will result in recovery complications across a wide range of surgical disciplines and locations. Improved primary outcomes will allow patients to avoid otherwise-required expensive chronic care and repeat procedures. Reducing the rates of complications detected postoperatively eliminates the need for diagnostic imaging and tests to determine the root cause of the complication, as well as the need for corrective intervention. In the event of postoperative complications, with the use of these tools, physicians will be able to quickly rule out these surgical complications as potential causes and focus on other possible root causes.

Additionally, the core technologies used in these imaging systems will benefit from widespread investment from adjacent industries. LED and laser technologies are increasingly of higher quality and lower cost with higher power output. Sensor development has been spurred on by digital and cell phone cameras, webcams, and the security and military markets, and it will continue to improve.

The development of novel targeted fluorescent contrast agents and high-sensitivity fluorescence imaging systems is a research area that is getting substantial investment from both the academic and industrial research arenas. The addition of even a few of these contrast agents to clinical practice will bolster the use and utility of these technologies.

References

[1] Soltesz, E. G., R. G. Laurence, A. M. De Grand, L. H. Cohn, T. Mihaljevic, and J. V. Frangioni. "Image-guided quantification of cardioplegia delivery during cardiac surgery." *Heart. Surg. Forum* 10(5) (2007): E381–E386.

[2] Ogata, F., M. Narushima, M. Mihara, R. Azuma, Y. Morimoto, and I. Koshima. "Intraoperative lymphography using indocyanine green dye for near-infrared fluorescence labeling in lymphedema." *Ann. Plast. Surg.* 59(2) (2007): 180–184.

[3] Ogata, F., M. Narushima, M. Mihara, R. Azuma, Y. Morimoto, and I. Koshima. "Intraoperative lymphography using indocyanine green dye for near-infrared fluorescence labeling in lymphedema." *Ann. Plast. Surg.* 59(2) (2007): 180–184.

[4] Kimura, T., N. Muguruma, S. Ito, S. Okamura, Y. Imoto, H. Miyamoto, M. Kaji, and E. Kudo. "Infrared fluorescence endoscopy for the diagnosis of superficial gastric tumors." *Gastrointest. Endosc.* 66(1) (2007): 37–43.

[5] Toens, C., C. J. Krones, U. Blum, V. Fernandez, J. Grommes, F. Hoelzl, M. Stumpf, U. Klinge, and V. Schumpelick. "Validation of IC-VIEW fluorescence videography in a rabbit model of mesenteric ischaemia and reperfusion." *Int. J. Colorec. Dis.* 21(4) (2006): 332–338.

[6] Holm, C., M. Mayr, E. Höfter, A. Becker, U. J. Pfeiffer, and W. Mühlbauer. "Intraoperative evaluation of skin-flap viability using laser-induced fluorescence of indocyanine green." *Br. J. Plast. Surg.* 55(8) (2002): 635–644.

[7] Holm, C., J. Tegeler, M. Mayr, A. Becker, U. J. Pfeiffer, and W. Mühlbauer. "Monitoring free flaps using laser-induced fluorescence of indocyanine green: A preliminary experience." *Microsurgery* 22(7) (2002): 278–287.

[8] Brancato, R., G. Trabucchi, U. Introini, and P. Avanza. "Hyperfluorescent plaque lesions in the late phases of indocyanine green angiography: A possible contraindication to the laser treatment of drusen." *Am. J. Ophthalmol.* 124(4) (1997): 554–557.

[9] Mordon, S., T. Desmettre, J. M. Devoisselle, and S. Soulie. "Thermal damage assessment of blood vessels in a hamster skin flap model by fluorescence measurement of a liposome-dye system." *Lasers Surg. Med.* 20(2) (1997): 131–141.

[10] Sevick-Muraca, E. M., R. Sharma, J. C. Rasmussen, M. V. Marshall, J. A. Wendt, H. Q. Pham, E. Bonefas, J. P. Houston, L. Sampath, K. E. Adams, D. K. Blanchard, R. E. Fisher, S. B. Chiang, R. Elledge, and M. E. Mawad. "Imaging of lymph flow in breast cancer patients after microdose administration of a near-infrared fluorophore: Feasibility study." *Radiology* 246(3) (2008): 734–741.

[11] Sharma, R., W. Wang, J. C. Rasmussen, A. Joshi, J. P. Houston, K. E. Adams, A. Cameron, S. Ke, S. Kwon, M. E. Mawad, and E. M. Sevick-Muraca. "Quantitative imaging of lymph function." *Am. J. Physiol. Heart Circ. Physiol.* 292(6) (2007): H3109–H3118.

[12] Reuthebuch, O., A. Häussler, M. Genoni, R. Tavakoli, D. Odavic, A. Kadner, and M. Turina. "Novadaq SPY: Intraoperative quality assessment in off-pump coronary artery bypass grafting." *Chest* 125(2) (2004): 418–424.

[13] Sekijima, M., T. Tojimbara, S. Sato, M. Nakamura, T. Kawase, K. Kai, Y. Urashima, I. Nakajima, S. Fuchinoue, and S. Teraoka. "An intraoperative fluorescent imaging system in organ transplantation." *Transpl. Proc.* 36(7) (2004): 2188–2190.

[14] Desai, N. D., S. Miwa, D. Kodama, T. Koyama, G. Cohen, M. P. Pelletier, E. A. Cohen, G. T. Christakis, B. S. Goldman, and S. E. Fremes. "A randomized comparison of intraoperative indocyanine green angiography and transit-time flow measurement to detect technical errors in coronary bypass grafts." *J. Thorac. Cardiovasc. Surg.* 132(3) (2006): 585–594.

[15] Sampath, L., S. Kwon, S. Ke, W. Wang, R. Schiff, M. E. Mawad, and E. M. Sevick-Muraca. "Dual-labeled trastuzumab-based imaging agent for the detection of human epidermal growth factor receptor 2 overexpression in breast cancer." *J. Nucl. Med.* 48(9) (2007): 1501–1510.

[16] Wang, W., S. Ke, S. Kwon, S. Yallampalli, A. G. Cameron, K. E. Adams, M. E. Mawad, and E. M. Sevick-Muraca. "A new optical and nuclear dual-labeled imaging agent targeting interleukin 11 receptor alpha-chain." *Bioconjug. Chem.* 18(2) (2007): 397–402. Epub February 22, 2007.

[17] Wang, W., S. Ke, Q. Wu, C. Charnsangavej, M. Gurfinkel, J. G. Gelovani, J. L. Abbruzzese, E. M. Sevick-Muraca, and C. Li. "Near-infrared optical imaging of integrin alphavbeta3 in human tumor xenografts." *Mol. Imag.* 3(4) (2004): 343–351.

[18] Ke, S., X. Wen, M. Gurfinkel, C. Charnsangavej, S. Wallace, E. M. Sevick-Muraca, and C. Li. "Near-infrared optical imaging of epidermal growth factor receptor in breast cancer xenografts." *Canc. Res.* 63(22) (2003): 7870–7875.

[19] Hoshino, K., H. Q. Ly, J. V. Frangioni, and R. J. Hajjar. "In vivo tracking in cardiac stem cell-based therapy." *Prog. Cardiovasc. Dis.* 49(6) (2007): 414–420.

[20] Frangioni, J. V., S. W. Kim, S. Ohnishi, S. Kim, and M. G. Bawendi. "Sentinel lymph node mapping with type-II quantum dots." *Methods Mol. Biol.* 374 (2007): 147–159.

[21] Ohnishi, S., J. L. Vanderheyden, E. Tanaka, B. Patel, and A. De. M. Grand, R. G. Laurence, K. Yamashita, and J. V. Frangioni. "Intraoperative detection of cell injury and cell death with an 800 nm near-infrared fluorescent annexin V derivative." *Am. J. Transplant.* 6(10) (2006): 2321–2331. Epub July 25, 2006.

[22] Ohnishi, S., S. J. Lomnes, R. G. Laurence, A. Gogbashian, G. Mariani, and J. V. Frangioni. "Organic alternatives to quantum dots for intraoperative near-infrared fluorescent sentinel lymph node mapping." *Mol. Imag.* 4(3) (2005): 172–181.

[23] Ye, Y., S. Bloch, B. Xu, and S. Achilefu. "Design, synthesis, and evaluation of near infrared fluorescent multimeric RGD peptides for targeting tumors." *J. Med. Chem.* 49(7) (2006): 2268–2275.

[24] Cai, W., K. Chen, Z. B. Li, S. S. Gambhir, and X. Chen. "Dual-function probe for PET and near-infrared fluorescence imaging of tumor vasculature." *J. Nucl. Med.* 48(11) (2007): 1862–1870.

[25] Cheng, Z., Y. Wu, Z. Xiong, S. S. Gambhir, and X. Chen. "Near-infrared fluorescent RGD peptides for optical imaging of integrin alphavbeta3 expression in living mice." *Bioconjug. Chem.* 6(6) (20051): 1433–1441.

[26] Lu, Y., H. Dang, B. Middleton, Z. Zhang, L. Washburn, M. Campbell-Thompson, M. A. Atkinson, S. S. Gambhir, J. Tian, and D. L. Kaufman. "Bioluminescent monitoring of islet graft survival after transplantation." *Mol. Ther.* 9(3) (2004): 428–435.

[27] McAlinden, T. P., J. B. Hynes, S. A. Patil, G. R. Westerhof, G. Jansen, J. H. Schornagel, S. S. Kerwar, and J. H. Freisheim. "Synthesis and biological evaluation of a fluorescent analogue of folic acid." *Biochemistry.* 30(23) (1991): 5674–5681.

[28] Zaheer, A., M. Murshed, A. M. De Grand, T. G. Morgan, G. Karsenty, and J. V. Frangioni. "Optical imaging of hydroxyapatite in the calcified vasculature of transgenic animals." *Arterioscler. Thromb. Vasc. Biol.* 26(5) (2006): 1132–1136.

[29] Humblet, V., R. Lapidus, L. R. Williams, T. Tsukamoto, C. Rojas, P. Majer, B. Hin, S. Ohnishi, A. M. De Grand, A. Zaheer, J. T. Renze, A. Nakayama, B. S. Slusher, and J. V. Frangioni. "High-affinity near-infrared fluorescent small-molecule contrast agents for in vivo imaging of prostate-specific membrane antigen." *Mol. Imag.* 4(4) (2005): 448–462.

[30] Witjes, J. A., and J. Douglass. "The role of hexaminolevulinate fluorescence cystoscopy in bladder cancer." *Nat. Clin. Pract. Urol.* 4(10) (2007): 542–549.

[31] Hexyl aminolevulinate: 5-ALA hexylester, 5-ALA hexylesther, aminolevulinic acid hexyl ester, hexaminolevulinate, hexyl 5-aminolevulinate, P 1206. *Drugs R. D.* 6(4) (2005): 235–238.

[32] De Grand, A. M., and J. V. Frangioni. "An operational near-infrared fluorescence imaging system prototype for large animal surgery." *Technol. Canc. Res. Treat.* 2(6) (2003): 553–562.

[33] Vogt, P. R., E. P. Bauer, and K. Graves. "Novadaq Spy Intraoperative Imaging System—current status." *Thorac. Cardiovasc. Surg.* 51(1) (2003): 49–51.

[34] Sevick-Muraca, E. M., J. P. Houston, and M. Gurfinkel. "Fluorescence-enhanced, near infrared diagnostic imaging with contrast agents." *Curr. Opin. Chem. Biol.* 6(5) (2002): 642–650.

[35] Silverstein, M. J., M. D. Lagios, P. H. Craig, J. R. Waisman, B. S. Lewinsky, W. J. Colburn, and D. N. Poller. "A prognostic index for ductal carcinoma in situ of the breast." *Cancer* 77(11) (1996): 2267–2274.

[36] Faries, M. B., and D. L. Morton. "Surgery and sentinel lymph node biopsy." *Semin. Oncol.* 34(6) (2007): 498–508.

[37] Casalegno, P. S., S. Sandrucci, M. Bellò, A. Durando, S. Danese, L. Silvestro, R. Pellerito, O. Testori, R. Roagna, M. Giai, R. Giani, R. Bussone, A. Favero, G. Bisi, M. Massobrio, G. Giardina, G. C. Mussa, P. Sismondi, and A. Mussa. "Sentinel lymph node and breast cancer staging: Final results of the Turin Multicenter Study." *Tumori* 86(4) (2000): 300–303.

[38] Noguchi, M., K. Motomura, S. Imoto, M. Miyauchi, K. Sato, H. Iwata, M. Ohta, M. Kurosumi, and K. Tsugawa. "A multicenter validation study of sentinel lymph node biopsy by the Japanese Breast Cancer Society." *Breast Canc. Res. Treat.* 63(1) (2000): 31–40.

[39] Purushotham, A. D., S. Upponi, M. B. Klevesath, L. Bobrow, K. Millar, J. P. Myles, and S. W. Duffy. "Morbidity after sentinel lymph node biopsy in primary breast cancer: Results from a randomized controlled trial." *J. Clin. Oncol.* 23(19) (2005): 4312–4321.

[40] Sutton, R., J. Kollias, V. Prasad, B. Chatterton, and P. Grantley Gill. "Same-day lymphoscintigraphy and sentinel node biopsy for early breast cancer." *ANZ J. Surg.* 72(8) (2002): 542–546.

[41] de Kanter, A. Y., M. B. Menke-Pluijmers, S. C. Henzen-Logmans, A. N. van Geel, C. J. van. Eijck, T. Wiggers, and A. M. Eggermont. "Reasons for failure to identify positive sentinel

[42] Dupont, E., C. Cox, S. Shivers, C. Salud, K. Nguyen, A. Cantor, and D. Reintgen. "Learning curves and breast cancer lymphatic mapping: Institutional volume index." *J. Surg. Res.* 97(1) (2001): 92–96.

[43] Burkholder, H. C., L. E. Witherspoon, R. P. Burns, J. S. Horn, and M. D. Biderman. "Breast surgery techniques: preoperative bracketing wire localization by surgeons." *Am. Surg.* 73(6) (2007): 574–578; see discussion 578–579.

[44] Renton, S. C., J. C. Gazet, H. T. Ford, C. Corbishley, and R. Sutcliffe. "The importance of the resection margin in conservative surgery for breast cancer." *Eur. J. Surg. Oncol.* 22(1) (1996): 17–22.

[45] Kern, K. A., "An overview of 711 general surgery liability cases. The anatomy of surgical malpractice claims." *Bull. Am. Coll. Surg.* 80(8) (1995): 34–49.

[46] Averill, R. F., J. C. Vertrees, E. C. McCullough, J. S. Hughes, and N. I. Goldfield. "Redesigning Medicare inpatient PPS to adjust payment for post-admission complications." *Health Care Financ. Rev.* 27(3) (2006): 83–93.

[47] Pear, R. "Medicare says it won't cover hospital errors," *New York Times*, August 19, 2007.

[48] "US Surgical Procedure Volumes," *Medtech Insight*, February 2007, www.medtechinsight.com/ReportA606.html.

[49] Karvonen, J., R. Gullichsen, S. Laine, P. Salminen, and J. M. Grönroos. "Bile duct injuries during laparoscopic cholecystectomy: Primary and long-term results from a single institution." *Surg. Endosc.* 21(7) (2007): 1069–1073.

[50] Richardson, M. C., G. Bell, and G. M. Fullarton. "Incidence and nature of bile duct injuries following laparoscopic cholecystectomy: An audit of 5913 cases." West of Scotland Laparoscopic Cholecystectomy Audit Group. *Br. J. Surg.* 83(10) (1996): 1356–1360.

[51] Gigot, J., J. Etienne, R. Aerts, E. Wibin, B. Dallemagne, F. Deweer, D. Fortunati, M. Legrand, L. Vereecken, J. Doumont, P. Van Reepinghen, and C. Beguin. "The dramatic reality of biliary tract injury during laparoscopic cholecystectomy. An anonymous multicenter Belgian survey of 65 patients." *Surg. Endosc.* 11(12) (1997): 1171–1178.

[52] Way, L. W., L. Stewart, W. Gantert, K. Liu, C. M. Lee, K. Whang, and J. G. Hunter. "Causes and prevention of laparoscopic bile duct injuries: analysis of 252 cases from a human factors and cognitive psychology perspective." *Ann. Surg.* 237(4) (2003): 460–469.

[53] D'Ancona, G., et al. "Graft revision after transit time flow measurement in off-pump coronary artery bypass grafting." *Eur. J. Cardiothorac. Surg.* 17 (2000): 287–293.

[54] Desai, N. D., S. Miwa, D. Kodama, G. Cohen, G. T. Christakis, B. S. Goldman, M. O. Baerlocher, M. P. Pelletier, and S. E. Fremes. "Improving the quality of coronary bypass surgery with intraoperative angiography: Validation of a new technique." *J. Am. Coll. Cardiol.* 46(8) (2005): 1521–1525.

[55] Desai, N. D., S. Miwa, D. Kodama, T. Koyama, G. Cohen, M. P. Pelletier, E. A. Cohen, G. T. Christakis, B. S. Goldman, and S. E. Fremes. "A randomized comparison of intraoperative indocyanine green angiography and transit-time flow measurement to detect technical errors in coronary bypass grafts." *J. Thorac. Cardiovasc. Surg.* 132(3) (2006): 585–594.

[56] Golijanin, D., et al. "Intraoperative visualization of cavernous nerves using near infrared fluorescence of indocyanine green in the rat." Presented at the World Congress of Endourology 2006. Abstract #1149, http://www.novadaq.com/content/view/202/125.

[57] Samson, Michel C., and Martin L. Newman, "Laser-assisted ICG angiography: Applications in perforator flap surgery." Presented at the American Society for Reconstructive Microsurgery 2008, http://www.novadaq.com/images/stories/pdf/laicga_asrm_abstract.pdf?phptlyAdmin=71jjN3SH7p1WsoZtmPkFgpJVhc3.

[58] Kubota, K., J. Kita, M. Shimoda, K. Rokkaku, M. Kato, Y. Iso, and T. Sawada. "Intraoperative assessment of reconstructed vessels in living-donor liver transplantation,

using a novel fluorescence imaging technique." *J. Hepatobil. Pancreat. Surg.* 13(2) (2006): 100–104.

[59] Krishnan, Kajoli B., Stephen J. Lomnes, Manohar Kollegal, Amey Joshi, and Andrew Healey. "Photon transport models for predictive assessment of imageability." *Proc. SPIE* 6009 (2005): 600900.

[60] Wilson, B. C., and S. L. Jacques. "Optical reflectance and transmittance of tissues: Principles and applications." *IEEE J. Quant. Electron.* 26(12) (1990): 2186–2199.

[61] Richards-Kortum, R., and E. M. Sevick-Muraca. "Quantitative optical spectroscopy for tissue diagnosis." *Annu. Rev. Phys. Chem.* 47 (1996): 555–606.

[62] Herth, F. J., A. Ernst, and H. D. Becker. "Autofluorescence bronchoscopy—a comparison of two systems (LIFE and D-Light)." *Respiration* 70(4) (2003): 395–398.

[63] Frangioni, J. V. "In vivo near-infrared fluorescence imaging." *Curr. Opin. Chem. Biol.* 7(5) (2003): 626–634.

[64] De Grand, A. M., S. J. Lomnes, D. S. Lee, M. Pietrzykowski, S. Ohnishi, T. G. Morgan, A. Gogbashian, R. G. Laurence, and J. V. Frangioni. "Tissue-like phantoms for near-infrared fluorescence imaging system assessment and the training of surgeons." *J. Biomed. Opt.* 11(1) (2006): 014007.

CHAPTER 14
Clinical Studies in Optical Imaging: An Industry Perspective*

Mario Khayat

14.1 Introduction

The commercialization of a medical device in any significant world market will normally call for regulatory clearance before distribution and sale will be allowed. The approval of a medical device will typically be based on an assessment of its "safety" and "efficacy" as defined by a regulatory body [1–3].

The road toward such approval will entail a formal process spanning all development steps and the conduct of clinical trials, which, aside from being country specific, will be more or less challenging and costly, depending on the technology of the particular device and mostly upon the clinical indication(s) sought for that device. As a reflection of that complexity, characteristically proportional to the level of risk, of the 8,000 medical devices allowed on the market in the United States, only 50 to 80 classed as high risk (class III) received market clearance in 2003 [4], while in 2006 the number of approved medical devices within that class totaled 36 [5].

The difficulty in developing a high-risk medical device will come initially from the outlay of significant effort and resources to move the concept from theory through the appropriate engineering development cycle. That technical development phase can take between 1 and 3 years, depending on the nature of the device, after which the system is ready for clinical testing. The clinical-trials phase, which can also span 1 to 2 years if long-term medical outcomes are required, is a key milestone as, in most cases, it will require an even greater outlay of company resources and will become the critical path toward commercialization or failure.

As optical technology continues to make significant strides in a growing number of clinical sectors, several in vivo medical devices using optical platforms have been commercialized in the last decade [6]. The intended use for these optical medical devices is becoming quite broad and ranges from instruments for the measurement of metabolic indices, such as pulse oximeters, to endoscopic imaging systems for cancer detection and diagnoses [7, 8]. Due to the novel nature of optical technology, these products naturally stem from internally conceived solutions or from

---

* This chapter reflects solely the opinion of the author based on his professional experience. It is not intended to be representative of actual events or to provide formal guidance on medical device development and regulatory approval.

outlicensed patents generated by academia. Consequently, early-stage start-ups develop a large number of optical medical devices as large, established companies will frequently market incremental releases of existing products.

As a result, developers of optical medical devices, particularly those classified as high risk, will face not only the conventional regulatory hurdles but also the need to validate uncharted science with limited resources to succeed in getting their products on the market.

This chapter gives a perspective on the processes that must be implemented for the development and approval of a high-risk optical medical device. Through the actual development of a novel NIR-laser breast-imaging device to be used initially for breast cancer diagnosis (SoftScan, ART Advanced Research Technologies, Saint-Laurent, Quebec), a presentation of the technical development processes leading toward the production of a clinical prototype within the constraints of market regulatory environments is provided. The focus then shifts to the major parameters to consider in the proper design and conduct of multicenter clinical trials and the analysis of clinical results thereafter.

14.2 Breast Cancer

According to the American Cancer Society, about 1.3 million women will be diagnosed with breast cancer annually worldwide, and about 465,000 will die from the disease [9]. X-ray mammography is the screening method of choice [10], and it is now generally established that early detection decreases mortality in women aged 40 years and over who follow an organized screening program [11, 12]. Aside from issues associated with "overdiagnosis" [13], the effectiveness of X-ray mammography remains considerably dependent on age [14] as well as other physiological parameters, such as breast density, body mass index (BMI), hormone-replacement therapy (HRT) status, or availability of complementary clinical information [15].

Other imaging modalities, such as magnetic resonance imaging (MRI) and ultrasound, have been found to be useful individually or in combination with mammography to increase sensitivity and specificity in some of these population segments [16]. Positron emission tomography (PET) also provides functional assessment based on metabolic uptake but requires injection of radiolabeled compounds, and its role in the preoperative context remains unclear [17]. All of these other technologies suffer from limitations, such as low specificity (MRI), low sensitivity (ultrasound, PET), and high cost (PET, MRI) [18]. Therefore, many needs remain unmet within the current breast-cancer-patient workflow, which comprises screening, diagnosis, staging, and treatment monitoring. Optical mammography, a nascent imaging modality that uses near-infrared (NIR) light to probe tissue, may play a significant role in addressing some of these limitations for breast cancer patients.

The field of optical imaging has experienced rapid evolution in the last decade as NIR diffuse optical spectroscopy (DOS) and diffuse optical tomography (DOT) have provided novel clinical insights through the imaging of unique optical and functional parameters of tissue [19]. NIR optical technology uses nonionizing radiation and can be applied noninvasively and repeatedly. With proper recovery of the optical properties of tissue [i.e., absorption (μ_a) and scatter (μ'_s) components], physiological parameters of the breast, such as deoxyhemoglobin (Hb) and oxyhemoglobin (HbO$_2$) indices, can be accurately derived. Several research groups demonstrated that the contrast in optical and physiological indices associated with metabolic changes, angiogenesis, and dysplasia can provide unique information that allows for better characterization and diagnosis of the lesions identified on standard X-ray mammograms [20–24].

14.3 Optical Breast-Imaging Technology

Several academic institutions in North America [25] and the European Union [26] have ongoing projects targeting breast cancer imaging in their research labs, but to date only a handful of companies have attempted to market an optical breast-imaging device. The additional difficulty inherent to imaging modalities beyond the regulatory framework and the challenges of optical science is the added complexity associated with the variability of additional user parameters to be accounted for during the design and the clinical-trials phases. This extra variability stems from the fact that an imaging technician typically operates most imaging devices, while a medical doctor must interpret results [27]. Added effort is thus required in the form of training and controls during both the design and the trial phases to insure the highest repeatability and consistency in the gathering of data and interpretation of results. This calls for greater product-development efforts in order to incorporate the interfaces that will ensure straightforward and unambiguous use of the technology. More particularly, in the U.S. regulatory environment, this also translates into larger statistical samples, while simultaneously imposing greater restrictions on the available population of patients, clinical operators, and clinical readers.

As a result of these difficulties, aside from Philips Healthcare (Best, Netherlands), which of late combines an optical breast imager with a fluorescent contrast agent [28], only three start-ups have undertaken a significant effort toward marketing optical devices for these indications. Notably, IDSI (Plantation, Florida), which was the first manufacturer to actually put an optical breast-imaging device on the market based on 3D tomographic imaging using 808 nm continuous-wave lasers, was followed by DOBI Medical International's (Mahwah, New Jersey) Comfortscan, which uses dynamic functional imaging to visualize deoxyhemoglobin changes. The third company is ART, which develops the SoftScan platform used in this case to illustrate the development and clinical-trials processes in this field.

14.4 Development Process

The requirements imposed for design controls and documentation by medical-device standards, such as ISO Standard 13485:2003 [29], or regulatory bodies [1–3] will establish an effective development process within an organization. The challenge for any medical device company will be to put into place a development process that is as straightforward as possible while including enough detail to ensure consistency and traceability (i.e., the ideal process should enable the organization to meet the applicable regulatory demands concurrently with its commercial ambitions in an effortless development environment).

As can be presumed from the preceding paragraphs, it is essential that within this process clinical development be tightly synchronized with product development. Continuous feedback between the R&D and clinical teams throughout the respective development phases will be crucial in ensuring that the final result is optimized for the clinical indication. The diagram in Figure 14.1 depicts a simplified illustration of such a model, loosely based on the FDA's "waterfall" model [30]. While insuring compliance with regulatory requirements, the medical device development process must be designed so as to allow coordinated steps between the engineering (Figure 14.1, white flowchart) and clinical phases (Figure 14.1, gray flowchart). Imbedded change-control and risk-assessment procedures are tenets of both processes that allow documentation of all modifications to the requirements and design. The following sections describe the major steps in the process illustrated by the flowcharts in Figure 14.1.

14.4.1 Product Definition

Companies usually perform a strategic review of prospective projects to ensure that they want to invest their resources in developing what is, in this case, a medical device. After the company's endorsement of the business case, the product-definition (PD) specification, referred to in FDA terminology as the "design input," becomes the key element in the successful development of that medical device [31]. The product definition will contain the marketing and necessary product-design information, including the clinical indication, which will form the foundation for all development activities. Not only will it become the basis upon which the resources are assigned, but it will also be the reference document against which all validation

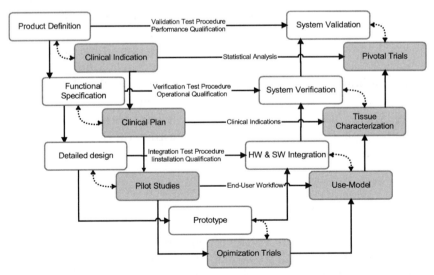

Figure 14.1 The proposed steps that must be integrated in the development process of a medical device in order to insure proper definition of the product specifications and their subsequent verification and validation. The proposed process allows for continuous feedback engineering (white) and clinical (gray) processes in order to ensure that the intended clinical goals are reached.

activities are based. Alas, organizations' medical devices frequently skim through this fundamental part of the process and move directly into the development phase due to either lack of experience or market pressures. The consequences of a deficient product specification are typically major development delays due to repeated redesigns and/or unacceptable performances, which in the worst case will lead to project termination.

The contents of a PD will address in detail three major aspects of the product:

1. *The clinical indication:* a description of the expected use-mode (role and positioning within the targeted clinical workflow) and a characterization of the clinical end users;
2. *The target markets and their applicable regulatory requirements:* those markets and requirements specific to the medical device as well as the standards that the product shall meet (e.g., Underwriters Laboratories, laser safety, biocompatibility);
3. The description of the device and each of its components and their salient features, as well as a specific indication of the expected performance for each feature.

The following sections provide an overview of each of these aspects. The PD becomes the reference for all ensuing top-level documents called for within the development process, and all validations will be traced back to it in order to insure the product meets its intended use and performance goals.

14.4.2 Clinical Indication

In the case of breast cancer imaging, the manufacturer can seek five key indications (i.e., screening, diagnosis, staging, treatment monitoring, and surgical guidance). The primary intended use for the device serving as a case example is defined as follows:

> The device is to be used as an adjunct to diagnostic mammography and clinical breast examination in patients who have equivocal mammographic findings. When interpreted by a trained physician, SoftScan images and indices provide physiological information, which may be associated with cancer development.

The clinical indication not only determines the design parameters of the clinical trials but also the positioning of the device within the existing patient workflow (Figure 14.2, points "A"). Accordingly, it identifies the device's clinical-use model and the type of health-care professional who will interact with it. In the present case, it is understood that, in the device's role as an adjunct to mammography, a medical imaging technologist will perform the acquisition on the SoftScan after an equivocal finding during the screening exam. A breast radiologist with access to the patient's screening mammograms performs the reading of the reconstructed images with the objective of improving diagnosis.

A potential secondary indication for the device is treatment monitoring. Tumors are often treated systemically with pharmacological or hormonal therapy prior to surgical excision. The objective is to shrink the tumor and render it hypoxic,

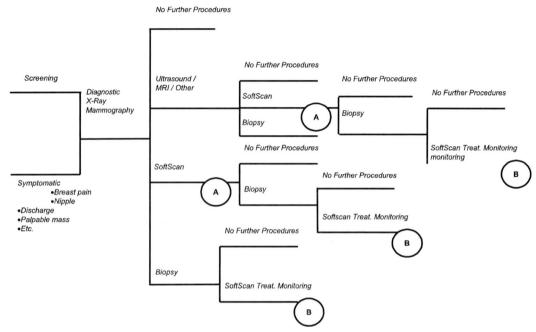

Figure 14.2 Intended positioning of the SoftScan optical breast-imaging device within the patient workflow: points A for diagnostic indication and points B for treatment-monitoring indication.

while simultaneously controlling spread. Measurement of tumor response is important to determine the adequacy of the selected treatment and the appropriate timing of surgical intervention (Figure 14.2, points "B"). Tumor response is often unpredictable and difficult to assess using structural imaging alone. Currently, X-ray, MRI, and PET are used for this purpose. These modalities are still limited to relatively slow structural assessments of change in tumor size or, for PET, exposure to further radiation at high cost. Optical devices offer a noninvasive alternative that can potentially provide functional information indicative of response at earlier stages than the preceding modalities.

One can infer that for the treatment-monitoring indication, the features developed within the product and the clinical-study design initially targeting the primary indication will have to be adapted to account for a new patient workflow and statistical outcome. Although considerably less significant because of the work performed with respect to the market clearance of the primary indication, an amendment and new clinical results would have to be produced in order to allow commercialization of the device for use in a treatment-monitoring function.

14.4.3 Target Markets

A company seriously pursuing the development of a medical device must select its target market(s) and its clinical indication(s) prior to starting the design of the product, as its development environment and approval path will be intimately linked to the sought market clearance, its specific regulatory requirements, and the expected revenue (reimbursement) potential that must be weighted against the required investment in resources.

Although the most demanding from a regulatory perspective, the U.S. marketplace represents about 40% of global medical device revenues [32]; thus, most manufacturers will strive to have their devices approved in that country. The European Union represents 30% of the world market, with England, France, Germany, and Italy together garnering 72% of that share [33]. Other "Tier 1" countries that offer significant market potential, such as Canada, Japan, or Australia, will typically impose similar requirements to those requested by the United States but demand a less complex clinical-trial design and conduct in their approval process. Most unregulated countries in the rest of the world will allow distribution of medical devices on the basis of their approval in either the United States or Tier 1 countries [34].

SoftScan was therefore anticipated to be initially sold in three specific markets (i.e., Canada, for geographical reasons, the European Union, and the United States, in that order). Once the markets and their respective regulations have been identified, the best means to ensure compliance with the requirements of these three regulatory bodies is to implement the necessary quality system within the development processes of the manufacturer.

ISO 13485:2003 certification [29] is required to satisfy Canadian requirements under the Canadian Medical Devices Regulations (CMDR), EU requirements under the Medical Devices Directive (MDD), and other international market requirements as applicable. The U.S. requirements, although closely linked to the ISO standards, rely on that country's own quality regulations as defined by the FDA Quality System Regulations (QSR) [3].

The quality practices, resources, and activities, as required by the Canadian, European, U.S., and ISO 13485:2003 quality-system requirements applicable to operations, must include medical device design, development, production, labeling, packaging, storage, distribution, installation, and the servicing and obsolescence of finished medical devices. These activities are regulated by:

- Health Canada as described in the Canadian Medical Devices Regulations SOR/DORS/98-282 [1];
- The European Commission as described in Council Directive 93/42/EEC [2];
- The FDA as described in the Federal Food, Drug, and Cosmetic Act and in the Code of Federal Regulations, 21 CFR Part 820, Quality System Regulation [3].

To support the human testing required to demonstrate the safety and effectiveness of a medical device, the quality-management system must comply with:

- ISO 14155 [29];
- ICH Guidelines for Good Clinical Practice [35];
- Code of Federal Regulations, 21 CFR Parts 50, 54, and 812 [3].

The requirements set forth in the applicable regulations and standards are intended to ensure that finished devices will be safe, effective, and otherwise in compliance with the applicable regulatory and statutory requirements.

If properly integrated, the manufacturer is obligated to comply with quality-system requirements from these regulations upon commencement of medical device design and development activities. Devices manufactured for use in U.S. clinical studies under an investigational device exemption (IDE) will be exempt only from the production section of the FDA Quality System Regulation.

14.4.4 Regulatory Risk Classification

Once the clinical indications and targeted markets have been established, the level of the requirements imposed by regulatory and statutory bodies must be determined by classifying the device within the parameters set by each regulatory organization. The risk classification is obtained through application to and consultation with the respective regulatory authority and, once established, will determine the appropriate levels of documentation, testing, and validation required from the development and clinical organizations in order to proceed with a request for market clearance.

To that effect, the following risk classification was determined for the breast-imaging device discussed in this chapter in accordance with the applicable regulations [1–3]:

- *Canada:* Class III in accordance with rule 10 (Medical Devices Regulations SOR/DORS/98-282, Section 6 and Schedule 1), medium-risk device;
- *European Union:* Class IIa in accordance with rule 10 (Council Directive 93/42/EEC, Article 9 and Annex IX), medium-low-risk device;
- *United States:* Class III—General Controls and Premarket Approval (Code of Federal Regulation, Title 21, Parts 860 through 892), high-risk device.

More specifically, the Canadian and EU classifications will require proof of compliance with quality and clinical good practices through appropriate clinical results to demonstrate the device's stated performance expectations.

The U.S. class III risk classification for the diagnostic indication of the optical breast imager is mostly due to lack of precedence from an existing device on the market. Had the latter not been the case, the device could have applied through a less demanding 510(k) premarket notification for market clearance. The optical breast-imaging device will instead be required to proceed through a premarket approval (PMA) process, the most stringent type of marketing application required by a regulatory agency. The PMA process will entail substantially more effort in the clinical-study design, conduct, and analysis beyond that required by other regulatory agencies in order to establish product "effectiveness" [36].

14.4.5 General Device Description

We will not go into the details of how to craft a product definition (PD) for brevity's sake. Suffice it to say that, as a general rule, the description of the components and features in the product definition is deemed adequate if an appropriate system-specification and -validation test plan can be produced using it as a basis (Figure 14.1).

SoftScan is a second-generation, prone, time-resolved, laser optical imaging device that measures photon migration through the breast at several near-infrared (NIR) optical wavelengths [37]. The wavelengths are selected to be sensitive to clinically significant physiologic parameters in breast tissue. The technique consists of launching brief pulses of NIR energy into the breast and measuring the temporal distribution of the emerging photons on the opposite side of the breast. The temporal point spread function (TPSF) is used to mathematically derive optical parameters, namely, absorption and scattering coefficients. From these coefficients, the breast's main chromophore concentrations, consisting of oxy- and deoxyhemoglobin, water, and lipid, are derived. Variations in hemoglobin concentrations and scatter provide a mechanism to diagnose breast lesions based on the angiogenic nature of cancer development.

As with most imaging systems, the device comprises two basic components: (1) an acquisition system (AS) composed of a scanning unit, an operator's console, and the optical compensation medium (OCM), and (2) a review workstation (RW) (Figure 14.3).

14.4.5.1 Acquisition System

The acquisition system is used to put the patient in the prone position on the patient table, placing the patient's breast in the scanning unit's aquarium cavity, and to control the scanning process in order to collect the raw optical data. To immobilize the patient's breast during the scanning process, it is gently compressed between two glass breast-stabilization plates. A breast-contour-imaging (BCI) prescan is then performed to acquire a spatial reference of the breast's contour. A proprietary oil-in-water emulsion, the optical compensation medium, then surrounds the breast in order to produce an optically homogeneous interface across the scanning area. Multiplexed laser pulses are launched through fibered couplers on one side of the breast and are collected at the other side by a coaligned detection head.

The laser emission assembly is composed of four individual pulsed semiconductor diode lasers operating at 690, 730, 780, and 830 nm with an average power output of 0.5 mW. The photons are collected through five optical fibers positioned on a mobile detector head in an M constellation on the collection side of the breast and detected by photomultiplier detection devices. Following a fast-intensity scan to allow laser optimization within the breast area selected by the operator, the breast is

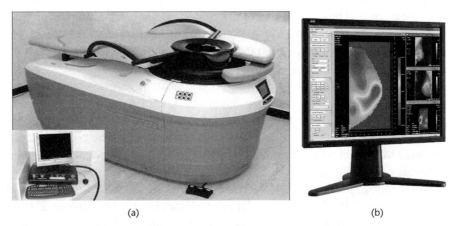

(a) (b)

Figure 14.3 (a) Scanning unit and operator console, and (b) review workstation displaying slice 6 of 9 of the optical scattering coefficient in a mediolateral oblique (MLO) view of the left breast with contiguous display of DICOM mammograms (upper right) for that patient.

scanned in a raster pattern at a selected step interval. The data is then transferred via DVD or network to the review workstation.

14.4.5.2 Review Workstation

Using a proprietary diffuse optical spectroscopy and tomography software package, the review workstation uses optimized algorithms to perform a reconstruction that provides the clinician a 3D image of the spatial distribution of absorption and scattering coefficients at all operative wavelengths (Figure 14.3).

The spectral dependence of the absorption may be combined with known values of molecular extinction coefficients [38] to calculate physiologically relevant parameters. A spectrally constrained reconstruction algorithm [39] is implemented to reconstruct 3D images of Hb and HbO_2 concentration indices (in μM). Using this information, derived images of total hemoglobin (HbT) content and blood saturation (S_tO_2) are produced, where $HbT = Hb + HbO_2$ (in μM) and $S_tO_2 = HbO_2/HbT \times 100\%$ (expressed as a percentage). The scattering amplitude A (arbitrary units) and the scattering power b (dimensionless) are estimated from the following relationship, which approximates Mie scattering in tissue in the NIR range [40, 41], where λ is the light's wavelength (in nanometers):

$$\mu'_s(\lambda) = A\lambda^{-b} \tag{14.1}$$

Because the spectral range of the system does not extend to regions where water and lipid concentrations are significant contributors to absorption [38], estimation of the water (H_2O) and lipid (Li) percentages was based on the empirical linear relationship with the estimated scattering power b [42].

In order to facilitate the adaptation of the radiologist to reading optical images, the mammograms are displayed in DICOM [43] format contiguously to their optical counterparts on the workstation.

An example of a clinical indication's driving the design of the device is given by the development of the X-ray-optical coregistration feature in the review workstation. The need emerged during the first attempted readings by clinicians during pilot clinical trials. The feature was required because X-ray mammography induces great deformation of the breast due to compression and produces two 2D views. The clinician needs to spatially reconcile the mammogram with the 3D optical image generated only with light compression. In order to facilitate this correlation, an automated colocalization tool was integrated into the review workstation software.

The colocalization tool computes the spatial mapping of the scanned optical area with respect to the mammogram through the use of the breast contours on the respective images (Color Plate 30). The deformation of the breast by compression is assumed to be elastic. The contour of the breast on the optical images is given by the breast-contour-imaging (BCI) prescan, and on the mammograms it is computed using endogenous fiducials identified by the clinician. The result allows direct mapping of a region of interest (ROI) in one modality to the other in 2D. The clinician can then easily select the slice that best represents the depth location of the lesion as inferred from the mammograms.

The addition of this feature is conducive to a reduction in the prospective training of clinical readers in diagnostic reading. It also minimizes the probability of intra- and interreader variability due to mislocalization of the lesion because of the initial lack of familiarity with optical image reading. Thereby, the feature insures greater consistency in the data collected through the clinical trials.

14.4.6 Design Control

As illustrated in Figure 14.1, once the system specification is established from the product definition, the process leading to a building a prototype and its transfer to manufacturing will require several steps that involve one or several iterations of verification and validation. These steps must be conducted in a manner that provides visibility to both the manufacturer and to regulatory bodies that the results obtained are clearly demonstrated and reproduced. For that purpose, it is necessary to integrate design controls throughout the device-development cycle. The remainder of this section presents a short description of these concepts.

All issues, whether clinical or technical, reported during the verification (against the system specifications) or validation (against the product definition) processes, must be addressed and accurately documented. If design changes are implemented as a consequence, the appropriate documentation and tests (regression testing) of the original verification and validation work must be updated. If design changes are not made for some issues, or if issues are not totally corrected, risk management must be applied to ensure that any remaining risk is acceptable. A risk-management process will be essential for regulatory approval, even if not specifically called for.

For the device in this example, the scope of the SoftScan risk analysis covers both design and clinical elements. Risk identification and the implementation of mitigation measures are conducted on a continuous basis to ensure that all potential hazards are controlled as the product evolves in its life cycle. A failure-mode effects and criticality analysis (FMECA) [31] was conducted to identify potential failure modes of system components and to rank each mode according to the combined influence of its probability of occurrence and the severity of its consequences, as shown in Table 14.1.

Furthermore, potential device hazards were identified for all reasonably foreseeable circumstances. Device hazards were considered for their effect on patients, operators, bystanders, service personnel, and the environment. Finally, for each identified risk, a solution or mitigation was determined either to eliminate the risk

Table 14.1 Risk Classification Scheme [44]

Probability	*Consequence*			
	Catastrophic–1	*Major–2*	*Moderate–3*	*Minor–4*
A–Frequent	High risk	High risk	High risk	Intermediate risk
B–Probable	High risk	High risk	Intermediate risk	Low risk
C–Occasional	High risk	Intermediate risk	Low risk	Low risk
D–Remote	Intermediate risk	Low risk	Low risk	Trivial risk
E–Improbable	Low risk	Low risk	Trivial risk	Trivial risk

or reduce it to an "as low as reasonably possible" (ALARP) [45] level. The resulting preapproval analysis for the SoftScan acquisition system component of the device is given as an example in Table 14.2.

Once the prototype has been shown to meet the intended use and performance requirements, it is ready for transfer to manufacturing. Actual design transfer is not a single event in time but a continuous exchange between manufacturing and engineering throughout the development of the medical device. This approach ensures that the manufacturing process can replicate the design successfully and repetitively without introducing unacceptable risk. At this point, the prototype will have undergone many iterations, taking it through significant changes and several pilot clinical trials, and it is ready to undergo pivotal studies.

14.5 Clinical Trials and Results

14.5.1 Clinical Plan

For medical devices, especially those classified in the high-risk category, a clinical plan is crucial to the realization and approval of the device. For proper verification and validation of a medical device, every step in the engineering development process should be confirmed through the appropriate clinical trials (Figure 14.1). Clinical trials can be classified into three categories: pilot studies, pivotal studies, and postmarketing studies.

Pivotal trials allow a medical device manufacturer to establish the "safety" and "effectiveness" of its system for the purpose of getting regulatory approval.

After regulatory approval is obtained, the postmarketing studies are performed in order to change the indication for the device or to validate what would be considered significant design changes. The next two sections cover the types of clinical trials necessary to get the product initially to market.

14.5.2 Pilot Studies

Pilot studies are preliminary clinical trials that aim to assess the design, feasibility, use model, performance, or features of a device. Used to gather additional information as needed during the initial phases of product development, they are typically conducted at a single clinical center and involve a limited number of subjects.

Table 14.2 SoftScan Acquisition System Risk Analysis Results [44]

Risk Level	Risk Type	Number of risks	Action
High	Unacceptable	0	Action or correction required
Intermediate	Undesirable	1	Tolerable only when risk reduction is unrealistic or when cost-to-benefit ratio does not justify the investment
Low	Acceptable with review	84	Tolerable when the costs of risk reduction would outweigh results obtained
Trivial	Acceptable, negligible	161	Tolerable, but should be stated in risk-analysis report

14.5 Clinical Trials and Results

Table 14.3 Evolution of the SoftScan Breast-Imaging Device and Salient Characteristics of the Different Generations over 7 Years of Development Up to the Point Where 3D, Diode Lasers, Recovery of Scatter, and Level 1 Laser Class Were Integrated in the "AR" Model

	Research Model	Upright	Tx	Ty	AR
Patient Position	Prone	Upright	Prone	Prone	Prone
Matching Medium	Liquid	Gel	Liquid	Liquid	Liquid
Number of Wavelengths	Single wavelength	Four-wavelength	Four-wavelength	Four-wavelength	Four-wavelength
Detection Geometry	Coaxial scan	Coaxial scan	Off-axis/X	Off-axis /X	Off-axis/M
Laser Source	Ti:Saph	Ti:Saph	Ti:Saph	Diodes	Diodes
Time-Domain Detector	Streak camera	Streak camera	Streak camera	Photon counting	Photon counting
Image Reconstruction	Homogeneous 2D	Homogeneous 2D	Inhomogeneous absorption 3D	Inhomogeneous absorption 3D	Inhomogeneous absorption and scattering 3D
Laser Class	3B	3B	3B	1	1

The first pilot safety and design trial of the optical breast-imaging system (Protocol 990286, "Assessment of the Safety and Ability of SoftScan Mammography to Detect an Anomaly Visible in X-ray Mammography") was performed in 2000. It was completed at one clinical center using a single-wavelength (800 nm), time-domain SoftScan prone system. The study demonstrated that the device was safe, produced no laser-related adverse experiences, and showed greater subject comfort compared to X-ray mammography. Concurrently, the initial findings also generated major modifications in the indication, which was changed from "screening" to "diagnosis," and in the device, which was modified from a single- to a multiwavelength system.

Several versions and pilot trials followed, driven by research, engineering, and clinical verification and validations tests with the ultimate objective of meeting the safety and effectiveness requirements for its intended use (see Table 14.3).

Throughout these trials, the design of the optical breast-imaging system evolved from its original single-wavelength coaxial scanning geometry to its current multiwavelength off-axis M-scan configuration. In parallel, optical image-reconstruction algorithms evolved from a homogeneous 2D version to a heterogeneous absorption and scattering 3D model. A first prototype of the current "AR" version was produced in late 2004, and clinical trials began in 2005.

This seemingly long delay between the initial prototype and the current version is in major part due to the novel nature of the optical-science field and the rapid advances in laser technology and mathematical models for optical diffusion during that period.

14.5.3 Tissue-Characterization Trials

Due to the lack of established standard optical technology for breast imaging, it was necessary to perform a "tissue-characterization" study. The objective was to determine a baseline reference for the reading rules of optical images within the targeted indication and to validate the performance of the device with the intent of obtaining Canadian and EU market clearances.

To that effect, the primary objectives of this study were to:

- Evaluate the system accuracy of optical-parameter measurements of normal, benign, and malignant breast tissue;
- Screen for potential safety issues.

The secondary objectives of this study were to:

- Evaluate system image quality;
- Evaluate system accuracy of physiologic index measurements of normal, benign, and malignant breast tissue;
- Evaluate system operating performance and reliability;
- Evaluate system review workstation usability, image quality, output quality, and review tools quality.

Establishing the clinical significance of an outcome measure was a key issue in the design of the trial because it not only led to the definition of effectiveness and trial success criteria but also influenced the sample size, study rationale, and control-group choice in the subsequent pivotal trial required for U.S. market approval. When outcomes are being selected for use as endpoints in a clinical study, whether for a pivotal trial or for postmarketing research, those outcomes must have clinical significance if the FDA is to give clearance. Therefore, the "tissue-characterization protocol" was used to test the methodology that pivotal trials would require without integrating the complexity and costs of randomized, blinded, multicenter readings.

For the purpose of Tier 1 approval, measurement of effectiveness was based on the following definition of primary and secondary efficacy variables:

> System accuracy, as measured by the differences between calculated reduced scattering, absorption, perfusion, saturation, oxyhemoglobin, deoxyhemoglobin and standard deviation thereof of normal, benign, and malignant breast tissue, calculated for the scanned area of the breast and historical reference comparators from contemporary academic literature.

The methods and results presented in this section were published at different stages of analysis in several scientific venues [46] and internal reports.

14.5.3.1 Population Demographics

The tissue-characterization trial recruited 108 pre- and postmenopausal women aged between 31 and 74 from a group of healthy volunteer subjects and/or patients who were scheduled to undergo a tissue biopsy or surgical excision of a suspicious breast lesion identified by X-ray mammographic evaluation. Among this population, 30 women were healthy volunteers with negative mammograms and 78 women were patients with abnormal findings. Table 14.4 presents the general

Table 14.4 Average and Standard Deviation for the Main Demographic Parameters of the Studied Population

	Age (yrs.)	BMI Index (kg/m^2)	Thickness (mm)		Scanning Area (cm^2)	
			Right	Left	Right	Left
Malignant (n = 17)	55.3 ± 8.6	24.5 ± 3.9	57.7 ± 9.3	58.1 ± 9.4	73.5 ± 22.9	74.9 ± 18.2
Benign (n = 25)	55.7 ± 9.1	26.2 ± 4.2	60.2 ± 9.2	59.9 ± 9.9	66.0 ± 29.1	66.9 ± 31.6
Healthy (n = 29)	53.8 ± 9.6	25.7 ± 5.5	61.9 ± 12.1	62.2 ± 11.3	67.6 ± 26.7	68.1 ± 27.5
All (n = 71)	54.6 ± 9.3	25.7 ± 4.9	60.5 ± 10.7	60.7 ± 10.5	68.2 ± 26.6	69.0 ± 27.3

demographics of the population. No significant differences were found between the healthy subjects and populations with lesion (malignant and benign) with respect to age or body mass index (BMI). The fact that no differences were found in terms of breast thickness and scanned area ensures that no bias is introduced by acquisition-related parameters. The patients with a suspicious region outside the scanned area and the patients with incomplete records were excluded from the statistical analysis leading to 15 patients with a malignant lesion (17 lesions), 25 with benign disease, and 29 with normal tissue.

Table 14.5 summarizes the types and number of lesions used for analysis purposes. In order to avoid interpretation errors, the lesion size was taken from the postsurgical reports, although it is reported on the mammography report. For several patients, the surgical report was not available because they were following neoadjuvant-chemotherapy treatment before surgery. In cases of multiple foci or components, the largest focal size was considered as the lesion size. Although all three lesions smaller than 0.5 cm were detected, due to the limited sample size, these results must be validated with a larger number of cases.

14.5.3.2 Optical Properties

For reference purposes, descriptive statistics for the optical and physiological parameters were calculated for all subjects under study (Table 14.6).

An initial evaluation based on the averages in Table 14.6 shows some validation of the underlying principles explaining cancer metabolism, but in some instances, results contradict findings reported by other groups. The HbT increases in malignant lesions as expected due to angiogenesis accompanying tumor growth [47]. We also observe changes in scattering as expected due to modifications in nuclear size and increase in organelles, such as mitochondria and other cellular structures [47]. Higher HbT and H_2O were reported as major contrast factors [48], but H_2O is not a noteworthy parameter in Table 14.6; nor is the predicted decrease in oxygen saturation observed [49].

14.5.3.3 Preliminary Sensitivity and Specificity Analysis

To assess the value of optical imaging in an adjunctive role, identification of the approach and parameters that provide best discrimination between the suspicious region (ROI) defined by the radiologist and what can be considered "healthy" tissue was sought.

Table 14.5 Types of Lesions Included in the Analysis Based on the Postbiopsy Histopathology Reports; Malignant Lesions Presented a Combination of Pathologies (DCIS = ductal carcinoma in situ, IDC = invasive ductal carcinoma, LCIS = lobular carcinoma in situ, ILC = invasive lobular carcinoma)

Malignant Lesion Types	Number of Cases
DCIS	9
IDC	3
IDC + DCIS	1
IDC + DCIS + LCIS	3
ILC + LCIS	1

Lesion Types	Number of cases [n, (%)]
Healthy tissue	29 (41%)
Fibroadenomas (other)	4 (6%)
Fibrocystic changes	6 (8%)
Sclerocystic modifications	9 (13%)
Usual ductal hyperplasia without atypia	1 (1%)
Atypical hyperplasia	1 (1%)
Fibrosis	2 (3%)
Other benign lesions	2 (3%)
Ductal carcinoma in situ (DCIS)	11 (16%)
Infiltrating ductal carcinoma	6 (8%)

Malignant Lesion Sizes (cm)	Number of Cases
≤0.5	3
≤1	4
≤2	3
≤4	1

To avoid introduction of a bias due to temporal (e.g., menstrual cycle) or demographic factors [48], a within-subject comparison of suspicious to healthy was required.

Three approaches for selecting the background region representative of "healthy" breast tissue versus the suspicious ROI were compared.

- *Method 1:* comparing the suspicious ROI of the diseased breast to its corresponding contralateral ROI;
- *Method 2:* considering the remaining breast tissue as the healthy area;
- *Method 3:* using a region (donut shaped) of equivalent size (in pixels) surrounding the lesion.

Preliminary analysis of the data demonstrated that the parameter values (pixel values) do not follow a normal distribution within a breast scan. Therefore, simple and multiple logistic regressions, which are not based on a normal distribution assumption, were used.

Table 14.6 Mean and Standard Deviation of the Breast Optical Properties and the Main Endogenous Chromophores for the Malignant (M), Benign (B), and Healthy (H) Populations Computed Using the Values of Each ROI Defined by the Clinician or Randomly Selected ROIs (Healthy Population)

Breast Optical Properties

Lesion Type	μ_a (mm^{-1}) (690 nm)	μ_a (mm^{-1}) (730 nm)	μ_a (mm^{-1}) (780 nm)	μ_a (mm^{-1}) (830 nm)	μ_s' (mm^{-1}) (690 nm)	μ_s' (mm^{-1}) (730 nm)	μ_s' (mm^{-1}) (780 nm)	μ_s' (mm^{-1}) (830 nm)
M	0.0052 ± 0.0015	0.0054 ± 0.0017	0.0060 ± 0.0020	0.0073 ± 0.0024	1.36 ± 0.35	1.35 ± 0.33	1.41 ± 0.43	1.41 ± 0.45
B	0.0038 ± 0.0013	0.0039 ± 0.0012	0.0039 ± 0.0011	0.0049 ± 0.0013	1.40 ± 0.37	1.29 ± 0.25	1.21 ± 0.20	1.13 ± 0.19
H	0.0036 ± 0.0014	0.0036 ± 0.0013	0.0038 ± 0.0012	0.0047 ± 0.0012	1.05 ± 0.16	1.01 ± 0.14	0.98 ± 0.13	0.94 ± 0.10

Main Endogenous Chromphores

Lesion Type	Hb (µMol)	HbO$_2$ (µMol)	H$_2$O (%)	Lipids (%)	HbT (µMol)	S$_t$O$_2$ (%)	A	b
M	7.92 ± 2.07	27.54 ± 12.05	0.10 ± 0.23	0.97 ± 0.33	35.46 ± 13.96	0.76 ± 0.05	1.53 ± 0.69	−0.15 ± 0.67
B	6.01 ± 2.43	13.02 ± 6.42	0.32 ± 0.47	0.37 ± 0.68	19.03 ± 7.23	0.64 ± 0.20	0.96 ± 0.25	1.06 ± 1.35
H	5.64 ± 2.68	14.23 ± 3.56	0.13 ± 0.12	0.64 ± 0.17	19.87 ± 5.71	0.72 ± 0.06	0.86 ± 0.09	0.51 ± 0.34

For each woman (malignant tumor, benign tumor, healthy), a series of *p*-values was obtained, each coming from a logistic regression applied to a given parameter (simple regression) for a given method of background selection. Following assumptions based on the observed behavior (Table 14.6) of optical and physiological parameters in malignant lesions (e.g., higher absorption related to blood content due to angiogenesis), a one-sided approach was used to obtain *p*-values. For results in the right direction, *p*-value/2 was used, and for results in the wrong direction, 1 − *p*-value/2. The goodness-of-fit was evaluated using the Hosmer-Lemeshow statistic.

Mean and standard deviations were calculated for these *p*-values for each group of women for each of the three background selection methods, and receiver-operating-characteristic (ROC) curves, as well as sensitivity and specificity, were computed from the series of *p*-values using different cutoff pairs. All analyses were performed using either MATLAB functions (MathWorks, Natick, Massachusetts) or SPSS statistical software (SPSS, Chicago, Illinois).

For proper statistical evaluation, correlation between parameters had to be accounted for since most parameters are derived from the same basic optical or physiological parameters. The Pearson's linear correlation between optical and physiological indices was considered for each category of malignant, benign, and healthy population.

For each patient of a category, a correlation matrix was computed, and then an average correlation matrix was computed for that category. It was determined that HbO$_2$, H$_2$O, μ_s' (830 nm), and S$_t$O$_2$ were the least correlated parameters.

Using the results of the correlation analysis in conjunction with the conclusions reached in the statistical analysis, it was determined that method 2, which uses the remaining area of the breast with lesion as comparator for contrast, provided the highest discrimination based on area under the ROC curve (e.g., see Figure 14.4 for oxyhemoglobin).

In general, method 2 gave the best discrimination in most parameters. The results may reflect the lack of precision in translating the ROI to the contralateral breast (method 1) and the presence of vasculature in the contralateral breast area for a large number of cases. For method 3 (surrounding donut-shaped background), the delineation of the ROI by the radiologist introduces significant variability in what is considered malignant and healthy tissue, especially when a limited number of pixels is selected.

Table 14.7 provides a statistical comparison of the sensitivity and specificity of malignant and benign lesions for some of the most uncorrelated parameters. The area under the ROC curve (Az) and the corresponding standard deviation and p-value are reported as well. The same statistical evaluations were performed for all available optically derived parameters. Although it is always possible to increase either parameter at the expense of the other, overall oxyhemoglobin achieves the best combination of specificity and sensitivity.

The results demonstrate the ability of optical mammography to noninvasively characterize breast lesions in a statistically significant manner when used adjunctively with X-ray screening. The high sensitivity and specificity, combined with the high system repeatability, validate the potential usefulness of the technology in clinical settings for diagnosis. These results for sensitivity and specificity compare favorably with most other imaging modalities used in a diagnostic capacity after a screening mammography, including positron emission tomography (82.2%,

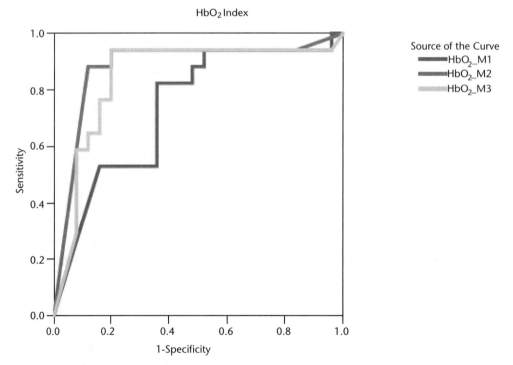

Figure 14.4 ROC curve for oxyhemoglobin using the three methods for healthy background definition. Method 2 (HbO_2_M2) gives the best area under the curve and, in this case, the highest cutoff (sensitivity, specificity) as well.

Table 14.7 Statistical Data Using Method 2 to Establish Contrast Between the Malignant and Healthy Tissue; Cutoff Points Based on *p*-Values Were Selected Around the Inflexion Point of the ROC Curves

Optical Index	Area Under Curve (Az)	Standard Error	*p-value*	Asymptotic 95% Confidence Interval		Sensitivity (%)	Specificity (%)
				Lower Bound	Upper Bound		
HbO_2	0.881	0.063	0.000006	0.758	1.004	88.20	88
S_rO_2	0.786	0.074	0.0016	0.64	0.932	64.70	88
H_2O	0.818	0.066	0.000006	0.759	0.998	88.20	88
μ'_s(830 nm)	0.672	0.085	0.061	0.505	0.838	88.20	48

78.3%), scintimammography (68.7%, 84.8%), magnetic resonance imaging (92.5%, 72.4%), and ultrasound (86.1%, 66.4%) [50].

14.5.3.4 Safety and Effectiveness

Effectiveness was assessed through historical comparators using technology equivalent to that of the predicated device [42, 51–53]. No clinical readings were performed to gather data other than the initial determination of the tumor location on the mammograms for the purpose of establishing the area to be scanned prior to imaging the patient.

Descriptive statistics (e.g., arithmetic mean, standard deviation) were used to analyze the primary-efficacy variable, system accuracy, as measured by the differences between calculated mean reduced scattering and standard deviation thereof of normal, benign, and malignant breast tissue, calculated for the scanned area and historical reference comparators from contemporary academic literature.

System accuracy, as calculated for the primary-efficacy variables for the normal population, demonstrated a calculated mean reduced scattering coefficient and a mean perfusion index for the scanned area of the breast consistent with the historical comparator.

Diagnostic efficacy of the device as determined through the use of exploratory efficacy variables was also established through descriptive statistics.

For the malignant-lesion population, the mean value of the reduced scattering coefficient found for the scanned lesion ROI at 780 to 784 nm was approximately 1.5 to 1.7 times that observed in the normal volunteer population of this study and the historical comparator. The mean perfusion index found for the scanned lesion ROI was approximately 1.8 to 1.9 times that observed in the normal volunteer population of this study. Finally, the historical comparator and the mean oxyhemoglobin index found for the scanned lesion ROI was approximately two times that found in the normal volunteer population of this study ($14.7 \pm 3.40 \mu M$).

Therefore, the system provides structural (i.e., reduced scattering coefficient) and physiologic (i.e., perfusion, oxyhemoglobin indices) information that can be useful during lesion characterization to discriminate malignant from normal breast tissue.

The device's safety assessment was based on the analysis of adverse events as reported by the entire population of patients scanned within this trial and summarized next.

Of the 47 adverse experiences (AEs) reported, the most frequent were musculoskeletal (predominantly neck pain). The severity of the reported AEs was predominantly "mild," and none were "severe." No AEs were attributable to system malfunctions.

Based partially on these findings (and the remainder of the required technical filings), approval for commercialization was obtained for both Canada and the European Union in 2006 and 2007, respectively.

14.6 Conclusions

The key steps and caveats that must be taken into account when launching a medical device were presented and illustrated through the actual development and regulatory approval of an NIR optical breast-imaging device. With proper processes and validation through clinical trials, the resulting device, even with optical technology, can be shown to be safe and effective so as to obtain regulatory approval.

Approval will be more or less exacting upon a manufacturer, depending on the clinical indication sought and the risk classification of the device. Until there is a precedent, optical devices that target diagnostic indications in the imaging field will be classified in the high-risk category. These market-clearance difficulties will be amplified if the manufacturer does not establish at the project's outset the appropriate development process integrating the required design controls and a clear product-definition specification.

Added difficulty arises when regulatory effectiveness requires showing statistically significant added value of the technology within the current breast-patient workflow. For the instrument used in this case, that added value was informally demonstrated through the reported results on sensitivity and specificity in the tissue-characterization study [46]. The preliminary internal analysis in this case shows that NIR optical imaging can potentially provide equal, and in some cases greater, diagnostic value than some existing modalities. The methods and results presented must still be taken into consideration in order to effectively integrate them into the clinical workflow. In the United States, formal validation will be obtained when the device meets the requirements imposed by the U.S. Food and Drug Administration through the completion of the ongoing pivotal trial on that device.

Clinical devices based on optical imaging technology face the typical developmental and regulatory hurdles imposed on all similar types of apparatus. These can be surmounted through rigorous development and clinical processes. Beyond these issues, the clinical optical-device manufacturer must also overcome barriers faced by all novel modalities that try to establish a new patient workflow paradigm within the existing clinical environment, a daunting task for any organization.

Acknowledgments

I gratefully acknowledge the contribution of the present and past ART team, which, over the last 4 years, has contributed to the formalization of this perspective.

References

[1] Council Directive 93/42/EEC of June 13, 1998, concerning medical devices (medical devices directive) (MDD).

[2] *Canada Gazette*, Part II, 132(11), Food and Drug Act, Medical Devices Regulations.

[3] U.S. FDA, Code of Federal Regulations, Title 21, Part 800–1200.

[4] Feigal, D. W., S. N. Gardner, and M. McClellan. "Ensuring safe and effective medical devices." *NEJM* 348 (2003): 191–192.

[5] www.fda.gov/cdrh/annual/fy2005/ode/part1.html.

[6] Red Herring Research, Life sciences report, "Near Infrared Spectroscopy," May 2007.

[7] Alfano, R. R., S. G. Demos, P. Galland, S. K. Gayen, Y. Guo, P. P. Ho, X. Liang, F. Liu, L. Wang, Q. Z. Wang, and W. B. Wang. "Time-resolved and nonlinear optical imaging for medical applications." *Ann. N.Y. Acad. Sci.* 838 (1998): 14–28.

[8] Gibson, A. P., J. C. Hebden, and S. R. Arridge. "Recent advances in diffuse optical imaging." *Phys. Med. Biol.* 50 (2005): R1–R43.

[9] www.imaginis.com/breasthealth/statistics.asp.

[10] Elmore, J. G., K. Armstrong, C. D. Lehman, and S. W Fletcher. "Screening for breast cancer." *JAMA* 293 (2005): 1245–1256.

[11] Humphrey, L. L., M. Helfand, B. K. Chan, and S. H. Woolf. "Breast cancer screening: A summary of the evidence for the U.S. Preventive Services Task Force." *Ann. Intern. Med.* 137(5) Part 1 (2002): 347–360.

[12] Duffy, S. W., et al. "Reduction in breast cancer mortality from organized service screening with mammography: 1. Further confirmation with extended data." *Canc. Epidemiol. Biomark. Prev.* 15(1) (2006): 45–51.

[13] Zackrisson, S., I. Andersson, L. Janzon, J. Manjer, and J. P. Garne. "Rate of over-diagnosis of breast cancer 15 years after end of Malmö mammographic screening trial: Follow-up study." *BMJ* 332 (2006): 689–691.

[14] Lucassen, A., E. Watson, and D. Eccles. "Advice about mammography for a young woman with a family history of breast cancer." *Br. Med. J.* 322 (2004): 1040–1042.

[15] Irwig, L., P. Macaskill, S. Walter, and N. Houssami. "New methods give better estimates of changes in diagnostic accuracy when prior information is provided." *J. Clin. Epidemiol.* 59 (2006): 299–307.

[16] Warner, E., et al. "Surveillance of BRCA1 and BRCA2 mutation carriers with magnetic resonance imaging, ultrasound, mammography, and clinical breast examination." *JAMA* 292 (2004): 1317–1325.

[17] Eubank, W. B., and D. A. Mankoff. "Evolving role of positron emission tomography in breast cancer imaging." *Semin. Nucl. Med.* 35 (2005): 84–99.

[18] Walter, C., et al. "Clinical diagnostic value of preoperative MR mammography and FDG-PET in suspicious breast lesions." *Eur. Radiol.* 13(7) (2003): 1651–1666.

[19] Ntziachristos, V., and B. Chance. "Probing physiology and molecular function using optical imaging: Applications to breast cancer." *Breast Canc. Res.* 3 (2001): 41–46.

[20] Rice, A., and C. M. Quinn. "Angiogenesis, thrombospodin, and ductal carcinoma in situ of the breast." *J. Clin. Pathol.* 55 (2002): 569–574.

[21] Vaupel, P., A. Mayer, S. Briest, and M. Hockel. "Oxygenation gain factor: A novel parameter characterizing the association between hemoglobin level and the oxygenation status of breast cancers." *Canc. Res.* 63 (2003): 7634–7637.

[22] Grosenick, D., et al. "Time-domain optical mammography: Initial clinical results on detection and characterization of breast tumors." *Appl. Opt.* 42 (2003): 3170–3186.

[23] Grosenick, D., et al. "Concentration and oxygen saturation of haemoglobin of 50 breast tumors determined by time-domain optical mammography." *Phys. Med. Biol.* 49 (2004): 1165–1181.

[24] Pogue, B., et al. "Quantitative hemoglobin tomography with diffuse near-infrared spectroscopy: Pilot results in the breast." *Radiology* 218 (2001): 261–266.
[25] http://imaging.cancer.gov/programsandresources/specializedinitiatives/ntroi.
[26] See www.medphys.ucl.ac.uk/research/borl/research.htm.
[27] Miglioretti, D. L., et al. "Radiologists characteristics associated with interpretative performance of diagnostic mammography," *J. Natl. Canc. Inst.* 99 (2007): 1854–1863.
[28] Bakker, L., et al. "Optical fluorescence imaging of breast cancer." International Symposium on Biophotonics, Nanophotonics and Metamaterials, Hangzhou, PRC, October 16–18, 2006, 23–25.
[29] www.iso.org/iso/home.htm.
[30] FDA, "Design control guidance for medical device manufacturers devices," March 11, 1997.
[31] Fries, R. C., *Handbook of medical device design*. Boca Raton, FL: CRC Press, 2001.
[32] Frost & Sullivan, "2003 industry outlook on medical devices," Whelan Charles.
[33] Frost & Sullivan, "Devices/technology," March 1, 2005.
[34] Pacific Bridge Medical, *Asian Med. Newslett.* 7(10) (October 5, 2007), www.pacificbridgemedical.com.
[35] www.ich.org.
[36] King, P. H., and R. C. Fries. *Design of biomedical devices and systems*. New York: Marcel Dekker, 2003.
[37] Intes, X., et al. "Time-domain optical mammography SoftScan: Initial results." *Acad. Radiol.* 12 (2005): 934–947.
[38] http://omlc.ogi.edu/spectra.
[39] Srinivasan, S., et al. "Near-infrared characterization of breast tumors in vivo using spectrally constrained reconstruction." *Technol. Canc. Res. Treat.* 4 (2005): 513–526.
[40] Van Staveren, H. J., C. J. M. Moes, J. van Marle, S. A. Prahl, and J. C. van Germet. "Light scattering in Intralipid-10% in the wavelength range of 400–1100 nm." *Appl. Opt.* 30 (1991): 4507–4514.
[41] Mourant, J. R., T. Fuselier, J. Boyer, T. M. Johnson, and I. J. Bigio. "Predictions and measurements of scattering and absorption over broad wavelength ranges in tissue phantoms." *Appl. Opt.* 39 (1997): 949–957.
[42] Cerussi, A., A. Berger, F. Bevilacqua, N. Shah, D. Jakubowski, J. Butler, F. R. Holcombe, and B. Tromberg. "Sources of absorption and scattering contrast for near-infrared optical mammography." *Acad. Radiol.* 8 (2001): 211–218.
[43] http://medical.nema.org.
[44] Advanced Research Technologies, Inc., internal document PCE-RT023-E SoftScan, *AR risk assessment report*.
[45] Health and Safety Executive. *Reducing risks, protecting people: HSE's decision-making process*. Crown, 2001.
[46] Khayat, M., et al. "Optical tomography as adjunct to X-ray mammography: Methods and results." *Proc. SPIE* 6431(2007).
[47] Taroni, P., A. Pifferi, A. Torricelli, D. Comelli, and R. Cubeddu. "In vivo absorption and scattering spectroscopy of biological tissues." *Photochem. Photobiol. Sci.* 2(2) (2003): 124–129.
[48] Pogue, B., et al. "Characterization of hemoglobin, water, and NIR scattering in breast tissue: Analysis of intersubject variability and menstrual cycle changes." *J. Biomed. Opt.* 9(3) (2004): 541–552.
[49] Tromberg, B. J., N. Shah, R. Lanning, A. Cerussi, J. Espinoza, T. Pham, L. Svaasand, and J. Butler, "Non-invasive in vivo characterization of breast tumors using photon migration spectroscopy." *Neoplasia* 2(1–2) (2000): 26–40.

[50] AHRQ, "Effectiveness of noninvasive diagnostic tests for breast abnormalities: Executive summary." No. 2 (Pub. No. 06-EHC005-1), February 2006, AHRQ, http://effectivehealthcare.ahrq.gov/healthInfo.cfm?infotype=rr&DocID=37&ProcessID=3.

[51] Durduran, T., et al. "Bulk optical properties of healthy female breast tissue." *Phys. Med. Biol.* 47 (2002): 2847–2861.

[52] Shah, N., et al. "Noninvasive functional optical spectroscopy of human breast tissue." *PNAS* 98 (2001): 4420–4425.

[53] Srinivasan, S., et al. "Interpreting hemoglobin and water concentration, oxygen saturation, and scattering measured in vivo by near-infrared breast tomography." *PNAS* 100 (2003): 12349–12354.

CHAPTER 15
Regulation and Regulatory Science for Optical Imaging*

T. Joshua Pfefer and Bruce A. Drum

15.1 Introduction

Increasing numbers of medical devices based on advanced optical imaging techniques have entered the marketplace in recent years. These devices are making a significant impact on disease diagnosis, surveillance, and monitoring in a variety of medical fields, such as ophthalmology, oncology, and pathology. Optical imaging systems provide diagnostic information impacting patient health and are therefore subject to governmental regulatory oversight.

The regulation of medical devices takes different forms in different countries, but the common purpose is to promote public health and welfare by setting and enforcing minimal criteria for device safety and effectiveness. Due to the proliferation of technologically advanced biomedical instruments with equally great potential for benefit or harm, this is an area of interest to national governments and governmental consortia as well as investors, businesspeople, scientists, clinicians, and patients throughout the world.

The need for patient protection is affirmed in the first requirement of the "Essential Principles of Safety and Performance of Medical Devices" drafted by the Global Harmonization Task Force and reaffirmed by the World Health Organization (WHO) [1, 2]:

> Medical devices should be designed and manufactured in such a way that, when used under the conditions and for the purposes intended and, where applicable, by virtue of the technical knowledge, experience, education or training of intended users, they will not compromise the clinical condition or the safety of patients, or the safety and health of users or, where applicable, other persons, provided that any risks which may be associated with their use constitute acceptable risks when

---

* This chapter represents the professional opinion of the authors. It is not intended to contain a complete discussion of FDA regulations, and it is not an official document, guidance, or policy of the U.S. government, the Department of Health and Human Services, or the Food and Drug Administration, nor should any official endorsement be inferred. The mention of commercial products, their sources, or their use in connection with material reported herein is not to be construed as either an actual or implied endorsement of such products by the Department of Health and Human Services.

weighed against the benefits to the patient and are compatible with a high level of protection of health and safety.

In addition to its safety, a device's effectiveness is typically a vital concern as well. As stated by the WHO, "Performance is closely linked to safety. . . . A patient monitor that does not perform well could pose serious clinical safety problems to the patient. Thus, the safety and performance of medical devices are normally considered together" [2]. Device effectiveness is also important because devices that do not produce significant therapeutic or diagnostic effects may cause a critical delay in the administration of appropriate medical care.

In developing strategies to evaluate safety and effectiveness, regulatory agencies must negotiate an often fine line between overly burdensome regulation that hinders medical advances and overly lax regulation that allows unsafe products to reach the market. The true complexity of this task becomes more evident when one considers the enormous quantity and diversity of medical devices. More than 20,000 firms worldwide produce over 80,000 brands and models of medical devices for the U.S. market [3]. Each year, 8,000 new medical devices are marketed in the United States [4]. According to the WHO, 1.5 million different medical devices are currently available in a rapidly growing global market of approximately $260 billion [5], a level that surpasses the gross domestic product of all but 26 individual countries [6]. The quantity and diversity of medical devices in the United States is so great that even the U.S. Food and Drug Administration's (FDA) classification system, designed to simplify the regulation process, contains approximately 1,700 different generic types of devices. In spite of FDA efforts to ensure safety and effectiveness, researchers have estimated that the number of injuries in the United States from medical devices was approximately 454,000 in a 12 month period between 1999 and 2000 [7] and greater than 489,000 for the corresponding period in 2004 and 2005 [Brockton J. Hefflin, MD, personal communication, December 13, 2007].

Worldwide efforts to implement an appropriate level of medical device regulation have increased dramatically in recent years. These regulations cover a large part of the product development cycle, from preclinical and clinical studies to market introduction, real-world clinical use, device modification, and product disposal. Given the maturation of the optical imaging field, there is a growing need to understand these regulatory issues and how they impact the development of marketable clinical products. Therefore, this chapter addresses general medical device regulation issues and regulatory procedures specific to the U.S. FDA as well as regulatory-science topics of direct relevance to optical imaging. Our intent is to provide a brief summary that can also serve as a jumping-off point for those interested in exploring specific issues in greater depth.

15.2 Fundamental Concepts in Medical Device Regulation

As an introduction to medical device regulation, this section provides a brief description of several general issues and terms, including *premarket* and *postmarket, safety, effectiveness, risk evaluation, labeling,* and *standards.*

15.2 Fundamental Concepts in Medical Device Regulation

15.2.1 Premarket and Postmarket

The term *premarket* refers to the product phase from conception to official clearance or approval to advertise and sell the product. The majority of regulatory issues fall into this category, including those related to the conduct of preclinical and clinical studies, adherence to performance and safety standards, and requirements for obtaining clearance or approval for marketing. The term *postmarket* refers to issues that are considered after a device has been cleared or approved for marketing, such as postmarket clinical studies, adverse event reporting, and postmarket enforcement.

15.2.2 Safety

A device can be defined as safe to the extent that its use does not cause illness and injury. There are myriad mechanisms by which a medical device can adversely affect patient health. Hazards can be subdivided into categories, such as biocompatibility, sterility, electromagnetic interference, electrical, thermal, mechanical, radiation (ionizing or nonionizing), and software. Light sources used in optical imaging present risks such as thermal injury, mechanical ablation, mutagenic DNA alterations, photochemical retinal injury, or hazardous interactions with photosensitive drugs (see Section 15.6). Unsafe devices can result from improper manufacturing processes, failure of individual components or the connections between components, degradation over time, wear resulting from repeated or continual use, or damage to a device. Additionally, use-related hazards and human factors engineering must also be considered when assessing device safety [8].

15.2.3 Effectiveness

In the context of medical device regulation, effectiveness can be defined as the device's ability to produce the intended medical result in a real-world environment. The establishment of effectiveness requires valid scientific evidence from well-designed and controlled preclinical and/or clinical trials, including appropriate statistical analyses of patient subpopulations. Device effectiveness is strongly linked to safety as the performance of the device can have a direct or indirect impact on patient health. An ineffective diagnostic device might generate an excessive number of false negatives, leading to unchecked disease progression, or false positives, leading to further tests that carry greater risks or to inappropriate treatment. Evaluating device effectiveness also reduces the potential for marketing of sham devices that might result in a waste of limited health care funds and a delay in the receipt of appropriate medical care.

15.2.4 Risk Evaluation

While patient safety is paramount in device regulation, absolute safety is not only practically impossible but an inappropriate goal. Any medical device, even a tongue depressor, carries some risk for injury. Furthermore, if a uniform level of safety were mandated for all devices, very limited options might be available to patients in the greatest need, since medical care for severe conditions often requires the highest risk treatments (e.g., the implantation of a cardiac defibrillator). Device safety, therefore, must be analyzed in conjunction with effectiveness using a risk-management approach based on scientific evidence. For the safety level of a device to be acceptable, the benefits to health from its use must at least outweigh the risks to patient health [9].

The analysis of risk involves the identification and description of all potential hazards and how they occur, as well as an assessment of their likelihood and the severity of their consequences. Some of the criteria used in such an analysis include level of invasiveness, duration of contact, physiological systems involved, and short- and long-term effects to the local tissue region and the entire body. Evaluation of risk may occur at multiple points in the premarket process, such as during the clinical trial approval process, during classification of a device to determine the appropriate level of regulation required, and during the evaluation of devices in higher risk categories, where a thorough assessment is performed of the risks and benefits relative to the success and complication rates of the current standard of care.

15.2.5 Labeling

The safety and effectiveness of a device often depend as much on the manner in which it is used as on its technological features. In order to ensure proper application of the device, labeling is provided with the device. Labeling includes both the description of the product and its instructions for use. This includes any warnings and exclusion criteria of which the clinician and patient should be aware. Any advertising provided by the manufacturer is also considered to be part of the labeling. Due to its clinical importance, labeling evaluation is a key part of the regulatory process.

15.2.6 Standards

According to the International Organization for Standardization (ISO), "Standards are documented agreements containing technical specifications or other precise criteria to be used consistently as rules, guidelines or definitions of characteristics, to ensure that materials, products, process and services are fit for their purpose" [10]. Standards are developed by consensus among clinical, academic, industrial, and governmental entities and cover both safety and performance. Regulatory agencies often use conformance with medical device standards developed by national or international organizations as a way to facilitate the regulatory process while ensuring the safety and effectiveness of a device. Furthermore, the use of standards minimizes confusion regarding the technical definition and specification of similar devices. Other standards organizations besides the ISO that address optical imaging issues include the International Electrotechnical Commission (IEC) and the American National Standards Institute (ANSI). Information on standards issues relevant to the U.S. FDA is provided in Section 15.5.6.2.

15.3 Medical Device Regulation Throughout the World

Many governments throughout the world recognize the need to regulate medical devices. While the exact approach taken varies from country to country, almost all countries with well-developed regulatory procedures recognize the need for regulatory controls, such as premarket device evaluation, postmarket surveillance, and recognition of performance and safety standards. Table 15.1 provides a brief overview of some of the regulatory bodies and their primary regulatory mechanisms. In order to reduce government and industry workload and to standardize procedures from country to country, the European Union has adopted common procedures for medical device regulation. Standardization of regulatory practices is now being taken to a worldwide scale, as described in the following section.

15.3.1 International Harmonization of Medical Device Regulation

The Global Harmonization Task Force (GHTF; www.ghtf.org) is a voluntary group of representatives from medical device regulatory authorities, including the U.S. FDA, and industry from various countries. The purpose of the GHTF is to encourage convergence in the regulation of medical devices and provide a forum for information exchange between countries with varying levels of experience in medical device regulation. Harmonization is accomplished through the publication of guidance documents on a variety of regulatory issues. The GHTF comprises representatives from dozens of member countries grouped into three geographical areas, Europe, Asia-Pacific, and North America, each of which regulates medical devices using its own unique regulatory framework. The GHTF contains five study groups: SG1 compares regulatory systems around the world, isolates the elements that are suitable or unsuitable for harmonization, and develops standardized formats for premarket submissions as well as harmonized product labeling requirements; SG2 reviews current adverse event reporting and postmarket surveillance and analyses of data collection and reporting systems; SG3 examines existing quality system requirements; SG4 examines quality-system auditing practices; and SG5 promotes convergence of requirements for evidence of clinical safety and performance, the

Table 15.1 Selected Regulatory Agencies Around the World

Country	Regulatory Agency	Control Mechanism	Web Site
Australia	Therapeutic Goods Administration	"Listing" and "registration" on Australian Register of Therapeutic Goods	www.tga.gov.au
Canada	Health Canada	Device license	www.hc-sc.gc.ca
China	State Food and Drug Administration	Registration certificate	www.sfda.gov.cn
European Union (e.g., United Kingdom)	Member-country agency (e.g., Medicines and Healthcare Products Regulatory Agency)	Compliance label (CE mark) based on EU medical device directives	ec.europa.eu/enterprise/medical_devices (e.g., www.mhra.gov.uk)
Israel	Ministry of Health, Medical-Device Department	Marketing authorization license	www.health.gov.il
Japan	Ministry of Health, Labor, and Welfare, Pharmaceuticals and Medical Devices	Approval and notification	www.pmda.go.jp
Russia	Ministry of Health of the Russian Federation	Registration	www.mednet.ru
United States	Food and Drug Administration	Premarket Notification [510(k)] and Premarket Approval (PMA)	www.fda.gov

content and format for clinical study reports, and the conduct and documentation of clinical evaluations. The guidance documents generated by individual study groups are made available for implementation by member nation regulatory agencies.

15.4 FDA Background

This section provides background on the FDA, including its history, the laws upon which its authority is based, and its organizational structure. As a federal government agency within the Department of Health and Human Services, the FDA is under the authority of the executive branch of the U.S. government.

15.4.1 FDA Mission

The Federal Food, Drug, and Cosmetic Act [11] and Title 21 of the Code of Federal Regulations (CFR) [12] lay out the FDA's mission. In addition to food and drugs, the FDA is responsible for a variety of products, as delineated in its mission statement [13]:

> The FDA is responsible for protecting the public health by assuring the safety, efficacy, and security of human and veterinary drugs, biological products, medical devices, our nation's food supply, cosmetics, and products that emit radiation. The FDA is also responsible for advancing the public health by helping to speed innovations that make medicines and foods more effective, safer, and more affordable; and helping the public get the accurate, science-based information they need to use medicines and foods to improve their health.

15.4.2 FDA History and Authorizing Legislation

The history of food, drug, and medical device regulation in the United States contains numerous public health crises, from revelations about ineffective vaccines, unethical product testing, and unsanitary food production facilities in the 1800s to the Elixir Sulfanilamide and the Dalkon Shield tragedies in the 1900s. Many of these episodes resulted in the enacting of new laws, such as the Vaccine Act of 1813, the 1906 Food and Drugs Act, the Food, Drug, and Cosmetic Act of 1938, and the 1976 Medical Device Amendments. The development of an effective system for the regulation of medical devices has taken many years, and given the continual rapid progress of medical technology, this process will likely continue well into the future.

The current regulations under which medical devices are cleared for marketing are primarily derived from the 1976 Medical Device Amendments to the Food, Drug, and Cosmetic Act, the Safe Medical Devices Amendments of 1990, and the FDA Modernization Act of 1997. The Medical Device User Fee and Modernization Act (MDUFMA) of 2002 amended the Federal Food, Drug, and Cosmetic (FFD&C) Act to provide user fees for premarket reviews, to enable establishment inspections to be conducted by accredited third parties, and to establish new regulatory requirements for reprocessed single use devices. Most recently, the Medical Device User Fee Act (MDUFA) of 2007 renewed and updated the device user fee legislation.

15.4.3 Organizational Structure of the FDA

Figure 15.1 presents a diagram that illustrates the FDA organizational elements most important to optical imaging and lists relevant acronyms. Of the six centers that perform the primary functions of the agency, the Center for Devices and Radiological Health (CDRH) is most relevant to optical imaging regulation as it regulates medical devices. However, the Center for Drug Evaluation and Research (CDER) has authority to regulate contrast agents for all imaging modalities through the New Drug Application (NDA) mechanism. The Office of Combination Products within the Office of the Commissioner works to resolve issues that are unique to products subject to regulation by more than one center (e.g., optical devices used with contrast agents).

The CDRH offices most directly relevant to premarket regulation of optical imaging systems are the Office of Device Evaluation (ODE) and the Office of In Vitro Diagnostic Device Evaluation and Safety (OIVD). While ODE regulates almost all optical devices used on patients, OIVD has jurisdiction over benchtop, microscopy-based systems as well as a limited range of in vivo devices, including diabetes-related diagnostics. The Office of Compliance (OC) and Office of Surveillance and Biometrics (OSB) perform postmarket regulatory activities that apply to devices cleared by CDRH. The Office of Communication, Education, and Radiation Programs (OCER) works to ensure the safety of all radiation emitting products (based on Title 21, CFR, Parts 1,000 to 1,050); however, these activities are beyond the scope of this chapter. The Office of Science and Engineering Laboratories (OSEL) performs regulatory science research and provides ODE, OIVD, and OSB with additional scientific expertise for regulatory reviews and product testing. Within ODE, divisions are organized by clinical specialty. Therefore, reviews performed on optical devices in general, or even on devices based on the same optical approach, are not all routed to the same division. For example, optical coherence tomography (OCT) devices for retinal examination would be reviewed by the Division of Ophthalmic and Ear, Nose, and Throat Devices (DOED), whereas intravascular OCT systems would be reviewed by the Division of Cardiovascular Devices (DCD). Within ODE, divisions are organized into branches, many of which have significant experience with optical diagnostic systems, including the Urology and Lithotripsy Devices Branch (ULDB) and Obstetrics/Gynecology Devices Branch (OGDB) in the Division of Reproductive, Abdominal, and Radiological Devices (DRARD), the Ear, Nose, and Throat Branch (ENTB) and Diagnostic and Surgical Devices Branch (DSDB) in DOED, and the Cardiac Electrophysiology and Monitoring Devices Branch (CEMB) in DCD. Device developers can obtain assistance via the Internet [14] by contacting the Division of Small Manufacturers, International and Consumer Assistance (DSMICA) or the relevant CDRH division or branch.

15.5 Overview of FDA Regulations

This section provides an overview of the FDA medical device regulatory process. Much of this information is derived from the Federal Food, Drug, and Cosmetic Act

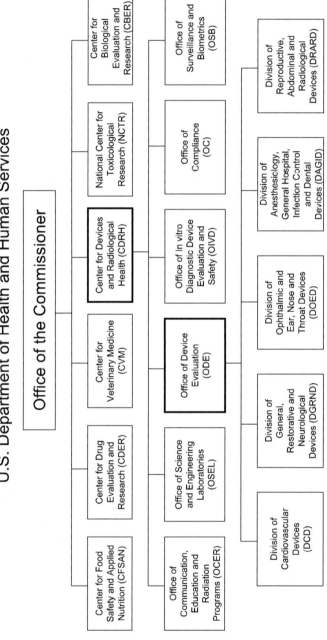

Figure 15.1 Abbreviated organization chart for the FDA focusing on entities relevant to optical imaging devices (December 2007).

[11] and Title 21 of the Code of Federal Regulations (CFR) [12]. Furthermore, extensive information on these regulations and their implementation is available on CDRH's Web site [15]. Figure 15.2 provides a diagrammatic summary of the regulatory process throughout a product's life cycle, which can be used as a reference for topics addressed in this section.

15.5.1 Classification

The FDA uses a three-tier classification system to categorize medical devices based on risk. Devices are classified as Class I, Class II, or Class III, from lowest to highest risk, with the class level determining the degree of regulatory oversight required. The FDA has also implemented a three-letter product code system to enable uniform indexing of all devices, as well as to distinguish similar devices that require different levels of regulatory oversight. For example, ac- and dc-powered versions of the same device typically receive different product codes. Also, new devices that have similar intended uses (device's general task or function) but different indications for use (specific target population and/or medical condition), or that may employ different a technology than currently regulated devices, are sometimes given a new product code. Table 15.2 provides a listing of codes and classifications for various types of optical devices.

CDRH's Product Classification Database, which can be found on the center's Web site [15], contains medical device names and associated information to assist sponsors (device developers) in identifying the appropriate regulatory procedures. This database contains device names and their corresponding product codes, which identify the device's generic category. The product code assigned to a device is based

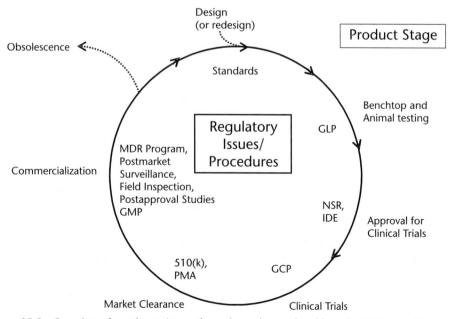

Figure 15.2 Overview of regulatory issues throughout the product life cycle. (GLP: good laboratory practices; NSR: nonsignificant risk; IDE: investigative device exemption; GCP: good clinical practices; PMA: premarket approval; MDR: medical device reporting; GMP: good manufacturing practices.)

Table 15.2 Information for Selected Optical Diagnostic and Photodynamic Therapy Devices, as Listed in the CDRH Product Classification Database (December 2007)

Device Name	Device Class	Product Code	Regulation Number
Aggregometer, platelet, photooptical scanning	2	JBY	864.6675
Aid, vision, optical, ac-powered	1	HPI	886.5915
Aid, vision, optical, dc-powered	1	HPE	886.5915
Analyzer, diagnostic, fiber-optic (colon)	3	MOA	—
Caries detector, laser light, transmission	2	NTK	872.175
Catheter, oximeter, fiber-optic, reprocessed	2	NMB	870.1230
Endoscope, accessories, narrowband spectrum	2	NWB	876.1500
Infrared spectroscopy measurement, urinary calculi	1	JNP	862.1780
Laser, fluorescence caries detection	2	NBL	872.1745
Microscope, automated, image analysis	2	NOT	864.186
Microscope, fluorescence/UV	1	IBK	864.36
Ophthalmoscope, laser, scanning	2	MYC	886.157
Orthosis, cranial, laser scan	2	OAN	882.597
Sensor, electro-optical (cervical cancer)	3	MWM	—
System, automated scanning microscope and image analysis for FISH assays	2	NTH	866.4700
System, imaging, fluorescence (ear, nose, and throat)	3	MRK	—
System, imaging, optical coherence tomography (general and plastic surgery)	2	NQQ	892.1560
System, immunomagnetic, circulating cancer cell, enumeration	2	NQI	866.602
System, laser, fiber-optic, photodynamic	3	MVG	—
System, laser, photodynamic therapy	3	MVF	—
Tomography, optical coherence (ophthalmic)	2	OBO	886.1570

on the medical device product classification and is tied to a specific regulation number, which can be used to identify information, such as special controls (regulatory requirements) for a specific device type. Note that a device is cleared [510(k)] or approved (PMA) with a primary product code and associated regulation number, but it may have secondary product codes listed as well.

15.5.1.1 Class I

Class I devices have a relatively low level of risk and are thus subject only to the following general controls: The device must be substantially equivalent to a legally marketed predicate device, that is, a previously marketed device with a similar intended use, principles of operation, and technological characteristics. The device should not introduce new types of safety or effectiveness questions, and it should perform its intended function at least as well as the predicate device. The device must not be adulterated (contaminated, poorly designed, or poorly manufactured so that it does not perform one or more of its intended functions) or misbranded (have labeling or claims that are false or misleading). The manufacturer and/or distributor of the device must register as a device establishment and list the device with the FDA.

The manufacturer must conform to the FDA's Good Manufacturing Practices (GMPs) and Quality System Regulations (QSR). A 510(k) Premarket Notification may be required, although most Class I devices are exempt from the 510(k) submission requirement, and some are also exempt from some GMP requirements. The exemption status of each device is included with its listing in the Code of Federal Regulations.

15.5.1.2 Class II

Class II devices are moderate-risk devices for which general controls are not sufficient to provide reasonable assurance of safety and effectiveness, but established testing methods can provide adequate performance data to do so. These devices typically require 510(k) premarket notification (described in Section 15.5.3.1) prior to marketing. In addition to the general controls listed above, Class II devices require device-specific requirements, called special controls, which may include special labeling or postmarket surveillance studies. Additionally, performance tests are typically required to verify conformance to applicable standards and/or comparability to a predicate device (i.e., an existing, legally marketed device of the same type). The performance tests may include engineering validation studies and/or clinical trials. The clinical trial may be a nonsignificant risk study or a significant risk study requiring Investigational Device Exemption (IDE) from the FDA.

15.5.1.3 Class III

Class III includes high-risk devices or those without a legitimate predicate for which the risks are not sufficiently understood to be adequately assessed by Class II special controls. For these devices, reasonable assurance of safety and effectiveness requires an IDE clinical trial or data from a foreign clinical trial that meets the same standards of study design and control as an IDE trial, followed by a Premarket Approval (PMA) application. Additionally, specific performance tests may be requested to verify conformance to applicable standards.

15.5.1.4 Unclassified Devices

A device is unclassified if its only predicate is an unclassified, preamendment device that was in commercial distribution prior to passage of the 1976 Medical Device Amendments to the Food, Drug, and Cosmetic Act. If a manufacturer believes that a new device has an unclassified device as its only predicate, or if it is not clear whether a device has a legally marketed predicate device, the manufacturer can submit a 513(g) Request for Classification Information. If the device is the first of its kind and the level of risk associated appears to be low, the manufacturer can submit a 510(K) and get a determination of not substantially equivalent and, therefore, class III. The manufacturer may then request that a risk-based classification determination be made for the device, a de novo classification, which may result in special controls guidance from the FDA. Such controls are intended for all subsequent devices of the same type as well.

15.5.2 Early Premarket Interactions

Perhaps the most important interactions between sponsors and the FDA are those that occur well before a PMA or 510(k) is submitted, as these discussions lay the groundwork for all interactions that follow. The primary regulatory mechanisms at this stage—the presubmission meeting, the nonsignificant risk (NSR) designation, and the IDE—all involve preparations for clinical studies.

15.5.2.1 Presubmission Meeting

The FDA encourages sponsors to begin discussions with the appropriate or OIVD ODE division well in advance of submitting an IDE or performing a clinical trial. This communication may take the form of a "presubmission" meeting, with either formal or informal guidance, and/or a written submission. These types of interactions enable CDRH to provide advice on potentially troublesome parts of the regulatory process, such as preclinical testing plans, development of the IDE application, clinical trial design, and protocols for foreign studies intended to support a marketing application. The sponsor may submit a written request for a formal guidance meeting to reach a written Agreement Meeting with the FDA on an investigational plan, including a clinical protocol under 520g(7) of the act.

15.5.2.2 Institutional Review Boards and the Nonsignificant Risk Designation

The FDA has established requirements regarding institutional review board (IRB) activities in order to protect the rights, safety, and welfare of human participants in research studies [16]. IRBs are groups formally designated to review and monitor biomedical studies involving human subjects. Since clinical trials are often required to complete a 510(k) or PMA, one of an IRB's primary tasks is to determine if proposed studies pose significant risk (SR) or nonsignificant risk (NSR) or if the study is exempt. A significant risk device "presents a potential for serious risk to the health, safety, or welfare of a subject." Devices that qualify as NSR can be used in a clinical study without further FDA approval. However, if an IRB finds that a study includes the use of a significant risk device, the study must get an NSR designation or an approved IDE from the FDA before the investigation can commence. Compliance with these procedures is assessed through inspections of IRB records.

15.5.2.3 Investigational Device Exemption

If the device does not qualify as NSR, the sponsor must then apply for an IDE designation from the FDA prior to commencing a U.S. clinical trial (the FDA has no jurisdiction over foreign clinical device trials but can accept data from foreign studies if they are scientifically valid and in accordance with IDE regulations) [17]. The IDE application has several required elements, including the following: a report of prior clinical, animal, and laboratory testing of the device; an investigational plan that includes a protocol, risk analysis, device description, and monitoring procedures; a description of the methods, facilities, and controls used for the manufacture, processing, packing, storage, and installation of the device; and copies of device labeling and of all informed consent forms and related materials provided to patients. It is essential that the device, preclinical testing, and investigational plan are described in the IDE application and that sufficient justification is provided for initiating the clinical trial. In order to make changes to the device and/or protocol after an IDE has been approved, a new application, a supplemental application, or a 5 day notice must be provided to the FDA, depending on the extent of the changes. The average FDA review time for original IDE applications is 29 days [18].

15.5.3 Premarket Submissions

This section provides an overview of the two primary marketing clearance mechanisms mentioned briefly in the prior sections: the 510(k) and the PMA. For the sake of brevity, discussion of a variety of other regulatory routes, such as the humanitarian device exemption, and details regarding the options available within each regulatory route (e.g., types of PMAs and PMA supplements) are not discussed here.

15.5.3.1 Premarket Notification

The Premarket Notification, or 510(k), is the primary mechanism used to regulate Class II devices, but it can apply to Class I and Class III devices as well. The goal of the 510(k) is to establish that the device is substantially equivalent to a legally marketed, or "predicate," device. An appropriate predicate device is a classified device that was marketed prior to passage of the 1976 Medical Device Amendments on May 28 of that year, reclassified from Class III to Class II or Class I, or cleared previously through the 510(k) process. The application [15] must include, in part, the following: registration and listing information; a concise statement of the proposed indications for use; a description of the device and its principles of operation; a description of any software components of the device with a statement of whether the software is of a low, moderate, or high level of concern, as well as a justification for the level proposed; evidence or certification that applicable safety standards are met (e.g., electrical safety, radiation safety, and sterility standards); a side-by-side comparison of specifications of the new device with those of the predicate device(s); a device summary or summary statement; labeling of the predicate device(s) and draft labeling of the new device. When a standard is used in support of any new 510(k), the submission must also be accompanied by a completed Standards Data Form for 510(k)'s (FDA Form 3654). In order for a device to be considered substantially equivalent to a predicate device, the sponsor must demonstrate that it: (1) has the same intended use and technological characteristics as the predicate device, or (2) has the same intended use as the predicate but different technological characteristics, yet does not raise new questions of safety or effectiveness and is at least as safe and effective as the predicate. When a 510(k) is cleared by the FDA, the device is declared to be substantially equivalent. The average FDA review time from receipt to final decision for original 510(k) applications is 49 days, whereas the average total review time is 69 days [18]. The discrepancy between these two figures is due to time taken by sponsors to respond to FDA requests for additional information.

15.5.3.2 Premarket Approval

The Premarket Approval (PMA) application is the most stringent device regulatory process required by the FDA. Since products requiring PMAs are Class III devices—high-risk devices that pose a significant risk of illness or injury—or devices found not substantially equivalent to Class I or Class II predicates through the 510(k) process, a PMA typically requires more extensive information and study than a 510(k). The PMA is an actual FDA approval of the device that requires submission of significant clinical data and statistical analysis sufficient to provide reasonable assurance that the device is safe and effective for its intended use and to support device claims made by the sponsor. Specifically, a PMA application must include, in part, manufacturing information; a complete description of the device and its principles of operation; a listing of all published and unpublished literature concerning the device; evidence of safety and effectiveness for intended use and indications for use; a description and the results of all preclinical performance and validation test procedures for functions related to safety and effectiveness; a description including the protocol, results, and interpretation of one or more controlled clinical trials (IDE studies or comparable foreign studies); a summary of safety and effectiveness data (SSED) document; and complete final labeling. If the FDA determines that the PMA contains sufficient valid scientific evidence for reasonable assurance of safety and effectiveness, the application is approved, allowing the sponsor to market the device legally in the United States.

If a device is the first of its kind, or if the FDA lacks the expertise needed to evaluate safety and effectiveness, the agency may refer a PMA to an advisory panel for review and recommendation. This panel comprises clinical practitioners and academic researchers as well as consumer, patient, and industry representatives. The panel must hold a public meeting to review the PMA and submit a final report that details its recommendation. The FDA takes into consideration the transcript of the meeting, the panel's recommendation(s), and its own internal review of the device in reaching a final decision. However, the agency is not obligated to comply with the recommendations of the panel.

For a PMA-approved device, any modifications that affect safety or effectiveness must be evaluated through a supplemental PMA application. These changes may include a new indication for use, altered labeling, and/or a revision to the performance or design specifications of the system. If a modification does not alter the safety or effectiveness of the device, a supplement is not required; rather, the change must be reported in a postapproval periodic (e.g., annual) report. Average FDA review time for original PMAs and panel-track PMA supplements is 271 days, whereas average total review time is 290 days [18].

15.5.4 Postmarket Issues

The FDA has numerous means of ensuring the safety and effectiveness of cleared or approved medical devices. Four key mechanisms include: adverse event reporting, postmarket studies, applied epidemiologic research, and field inspections of facilities. Adverse events are identified through the medical device reporting (MDR) system, which requires manufacturers to report any incident in which their device may have malfunctioned or caused or contributed to a death, serious injury, or illness. Furthermore, user facilities, including hospitals, nursing homes, and outpatient clinics, must report any serious injury, illness, or fatality caused or contributed to by a medical device to manufacturers, whereas medical device-related deaths must be reported directly to the FDA. The second postmarket tool is the postmarket surveillance study. The agency has the discretion to require sponsors to investigate certain aspects of a cleared device's safety and effectiveness. Third, FDA epidemiologists perform original research on germane device issues, typically using secondary data. These studies can be useful in identifying problems with a device or providing information regarding the way a device is used in practice. The fourth approach used by the FDA is the field inspection. Trained investigators visit manufacturing sites on a routine basis as well as "for cause." The primary goal of routine inspections is typically to determine whether the manufacturer has properly implemented the GMPs.

15.5.5 Combination Products and Contrast Agents

A combination product is defined as a system that contains two or more components that fall under the jurisdiction of different centers in the FDA and are required to achieve their intended uses, indications, or effects. For example, a photodynamic therapy system or contrast-enhanced optical imaging system would be a combination product, since both CDRH and CDER have jurisdiction. The Office of Combination Products is responsible for assigning review responsibility for combination products and designates the FDA center with primary jurisdiction for the premarket review. The lead center assignment is based on a determination of which component produces the primary mode of action of the combination product. The lead center then consults with the agencies that regulate other components, as necessary, to perform the review. Drug-device combination products that involve optics have typically resulted in separate approvals from CDRH and CDER, such as those for a photosensitizer and illumination system intended for combined use as a photodynamic therapy product. Optical imaging contrast agents that have been approved can be found on the CDER Web site (www.fda.gov/cder), along with guidance documents on the development of drug and biological products (contrast agents) for medical imaging [19].

15.5.6 Regulatory Submission Aids

Two types of materials are available to facilitate the preparation of regulatory submissions. Guidance documents are generated by the FDA for use by sponsors and other relevant parties, whereas consensus standards are developed by national or international organizations and can be recognized by the FDA as appropriate for use in supporting an application for device marketing.

15.5.6.1 Guidance Documents

CDRH has developed a series of Good Guidance Practice (GGP) documents, commonly referred to as "guidance documents." Guidance documents provide information related to the processing, content, and evaluation of regulatory submissions; the design production, manufacturing, and testing of regulated products; and inspection and enforcement procedures. While guidance documents provide a wide variety of information useful to sponsors, they are not a replacement for early presubmission discussions with FDA staff. Furthermore, they are not binding, and alternative approaches may be used as long as they satisfy the relevant statutory requirements.

Guidance documents are available through a searchable database on the CDRH Web site [15]. Currently available guidances for optical imaging focus on ophthalmoscopes, retinoscopes, ingestible telemetric imaging systems, and automated fluorescence in situ hybridization systems. Several other guidance documents are available that may also be useful in preparing optical imaging submissions, such as those pertaining to systems that incorporate laser sources and image management devices.

Sections on topics such as sterility, electromagnetic compatibility and interference, software, and wireless technology are often contained within guidance documents for individual device types. Separate guidance documents are also available that cover these subtopics in greater detail. Numerous other guidance documents available from the FDA provide general information of use to sponsors on a variety of topics, including many of the issues discussed in this chapter.

15.5.6.2 Standards

The FDA uses consensus standards to facilitate the regulatory process, while providing reasonable assurance of safety and/or effectiveness for many aspects of medical devices. Documentation of conformance to these standards can be used to support regulatory submissions, such as IDEs and PMAs. Furthermore, standards can be used to help establish the substantial equivalence of a new device to a legally marketed predicate device for 510(k)'s. However, not all standards are recognized by the FDA. Standards task groups in the CDRH evaluate device-relevant standards and revisions of standards as candidates for FDA recognition. At least annually, the current list of FDA-recognized standards is published in the Federal Register. Standards information can be found in databases on CDRH's Web site [15], including the Product Classification Database (see Section 15.5.1), which contains information on consensus standards that apply to specific device types, and a searchable database of consensus standards recognized by the agency. Additionally, this Web site contains guidance documents covering documentation of standards conformance [20].

15.5.7 Good Practices

In order to ensure that a medical device has been studied and constructed in a manner that is consistent with ensuring public health, the FDA has developed good practice guidelines for laboratory studies, clinical studies, and manufacturing procedures. These three sets of guidelines are entitled Good Laboratory Practice (GLP), Good Clinical Practice (GCP), and Good Manufacturing Practice (GMP).

GLP regulations apply to preclinical laboratory studies, primarily safety studies, that are performed in support of applications for research and marketing clearance, including IDEs and PMAs. These guidelines cover organization, personnel, facilities, equipment, operation of testing facilities, test and control articles, and the protocol for and conduct of a nonclinical laboratory study and records and reports. GLPs are intended to ensure the quality and integrity of safety data obtained from animal studies submitted to the FDA.

GCPs govern clinical studies and apply to the manufacturers, sponsors, clinical investigators, IRBs, and the medical device. They are divided into five sections that cover the following topics: investigational device exemptions, including the responsibilities of sponsors and investigators, labeling, records, and reports; the protection of human subjects, including the requirements and general elements of informed consent; the procedures for and responsibilities of IRBs that approve clinical investigation protocols; the disclosure of financial compensation to clinical investigators; and design controls of the QSR for ensuring that the specified device design requirements are met.

The current GMP regulations [21] require that manufacturers have a quality system for the design, manufacture, packaging, labeling, storage, installation, and servicing of medical devices intended for commercial distribution in the United States. The regulations also require that specifications and controls be established for devices and that devices be designed and manufactured under quality systems to meet these specifications; that devices be correctly installed, checked, and serviced; that quality data be analyzed to identify and correct quality problems; and that complaints be processed. The FDA monitors device-problem data and inspects the operations and records of device developers and manufacturers to determine compliance with the GMP requirements in the QSR. The QSR [21] covers quality management and organization, device design, buildings, equipment, purchase and handling of components, production and process controls, packaging and labeling control, device evaluation, distribution, installation, complaint handling, servicing, and records.

15.6 Regulatory Science: Optical Safety Hazards

Numerous scientific issues play significant roles in the regulatory process for optical imaging devices, from calibration and validation to the device's physical mechanism and clinical biostatistics. However, due to space constraints, this section will focus on the single most important area of regulatory science for biomedical optics: tissue-damage mechanisms for ultraviolet, visible, and infrared radiation.

As discussed previously, safety hazards that must be addressed during the regulatory process include tissue trauma, electrical shock, material toxicity, disease transmission, electromagnetic compatibility, and software malfunction, among others. While these issues are applicable to a variety of devices, optical devices represent unique hazards that stem from the interaction of light with biological tissue. The recommended exposure limits for protecting patients and device operators from these safety risks are listed in international standards (Section 15.5.6.2). In this section, we provide a technical review of fundamental optical damage processes. Following standard practice, these optical hazards have been broken down according to their primary mechanism into three general categories: photochemical, photothermal, and photomechanical.

15.6.1 Photochemical Damage

Photochemical damage pathways involve the direct absorption of light followed by chemical/biomolecular reaction, typically due to the high energy level of shorter wavelength (ultraviolet) photons. These hazards are unique when compared with other optical damage processes in that they depend on total dose, yet are relatively independent of dose rate. Repeated photochemical insult can result in significant damage, including carcinogenesis.

The phototoxicity of ultraviolet (UV) radiation in skin is well known, in particular due to the ability of solar UV radiation to generate DNA damage resulting in skin cancer. UV radiation is often classified into four bands: UVA1 (340 to 400 nm), UVA2 (320 to 340 nm), UVB (280 to 320 nm), and UVC (100 to 280 nm). There are two primary mechanisms for UV damage; one governs UVA1, and another governs UV2A, UVB, and UVC [22]. The latter mechanism involves the absorption of radiation by DNA and RNA, causing adjacent pyrimidine bases to bond and form DNA lesions such as cyclobutane pyrimidine dimers (CPDs) and 6-4 pyrimidine photoproducts. CPDs are considered to be the primary damage mechanism due to their greater frequency and slower repair rate. Lesions that are not repaired can cause "signature" mutations in DNA sequences, such as cytosine to thymine transitions [23]. In addition to DNA damage, these wavelengths can also produce erythema, melanogenesis, and thickening of skin layers. Several mechanisms act to prevent the progression from DNA damage to carcinogenesis. The first is DNA repair through mechanisms such as nucleotide excision repair. If DNA is not repaired, then the p53 protein, which is activated upon UV damage, acts to initiate two other mechanisms. The first of these is an arrest of the cell growth cycle, followed by DNA repair. If, however, DNA damage is too severe for repair, p53 acts to initiate apoptosis. Failing repair and apoptosis, transmission of mutations to daughter cells may occur, resulting in transformation and carcinogenesis.

The dominant mechanism of UVA1 radiation is not as well established as that of shorter UV wavelengths. It is believed that UVA1 produces reactive oxygen species through interaction with endogenous photosensitizers such as flavins and urocanic acid [24]. The ensuing production of free radicals leads to the mutagenic lesion 8-hydroxydeoxyguanine, which in turn produces DNA mutations as well as damage to membranes and other cellular constituents [25].

Prior studies have used skin erythema as a damage endpoint to develop an action spectrum for evaluating the potential of a UV-emitting device to cause photochemical damage in the skin [26, 27]. In turn, erythema has been correlated with DNA damage [28]. Using this data on erythemal action spectra, the American Conference of Governmental Industrial Hygienists (ACGIH) has developed guidelines for UV safety that "should not be regarded as fine lines between safe and dangerous levels" [29]. Figure 15.3 presents two sets of corresponding data published by ACGIH. One curve represents threshold limit values (TLVs), radiant exposure values from a monochromatic source that should not produce adverse health effects in humans. The second curve is the relative spectral effectiveness, or $S(\lambda)$, relative to a monochromatic source at 270 nm, or action spectrum. This quantity is of particular use when analyzing nonmonochromatic sources since it can be used as a weighting function to determine the effective irradiance (E_{eff}):

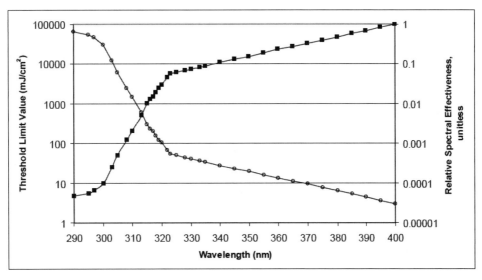

Figure 15.3 Threshold limit values (shaded squares) and relative spectral effectiveness (open circles) for UV-induced photochemical damage in skin [29].

$$E_{eff} = \sum E_\lambda S(\lambda) \Delta \lambda \tag{15.1}$$

where E_λ is the spectral irradiance, W/(cm^2·nm), and $\Delta \lambda$ is the bandwidth. ACGIH guidelines suggest that the product of E_{eff} and the exposure time should not exceed 3.0 mJ/cm^2.

There are three primary types of photochemical hazards unique to ophthalmic structures. These injury mechanisms in the cornea, lens, and retina can all be attributed to ultraviolet or short visible wavelengths. Injury to the cornea caused by UVB/C radiation is known as photokeratitis—epithelial cell damage that triggers corneal inflammation, clouding, and erythema, among other symptoms. Exposure thresholds for UVB-induced corneal damage are in the 10 to 100 J/cm^2 range [30]. A similar effect that is also produced in the conjunctiva, or eyelid membranes, is referred to as photoconjunctivitis [31]. This injury is essentially equivalent to a sunburn in highly sensitive tissues of the eye. While painful, these injuries tend to resolve within 24 hours and do not have long-term effects.

The lens is at greater risk for damage from UVA radiation due to the greater penetration depth in this wavelength range. A UVA injury to the lens triggers a process involving alterations in lens proteins, formation of fluorescent chromophores, pigmentation, and interference with the synthesis of lens proteins (catalyse-insoluble proteins) leading to cataract formation [32].

The third type of photochemical hazard is photoretinitis, or "blue-light" photochemical injury to the retina. Photoretinitis is produced by excessive irradiation in the 400- to 550-nm wavelength region, with the most harmful wavelengths being those near 440 nm. The injury involves a disruption in the recovery process of photoreceptors, leading to oxidative damage and scotoma formation [33]. Guidelines for preventing photochemical damage are described in several standards including IEC 60825-1.

15.6.2 Photosensitivity

Abnormal sensitivity to light, or photosensitization, is known to result from specific diseases and the administration of exogenous compounds, including numerous medications. For many optical devices, these conditions would represent a contraindication for use. Diseases that are known to cause photosensitivity include erythropoietic protoporphyria and lupus erythematosus [34]. While the former disease causes a buildup of the photosensitizer protoporphyrin in the skin, the mechanism of the latter is more complex, involving an abnormal and excessive physiological response to ultraviolet radiation damage.

Photodamage due to absorption by exogenous chromophores is well known from its use in photodynamic therapy procedures for a variety of applications, such as tumor ablation [35]. The photosensitizers used in photodynamic therapy procedures, such as porfimer sodium, generate singlet oxygen, which causes cellular and vascular damage, leading to tissue necrosis. Thus, even the use of common optical diagnostic devices, such as pulse oximeters, can be dangerous [36]. These medications can render a patient photosensitive for weeks after a procedure [37] and remain detectable in tissue for months [38]. In addition to photosensitizers, numerous medications can cause photosensitivity. These include antihistamines, coal-tar derivatives, psoralens, and tetracyclines [39]. Some patients taking these medications have extensive reactions when exposed to light, including sunburnlike rashes, hives, swelling, and blistering [40].

15.6.3 Photothermal Effects

A common safety hazard encountered in biomedical optics involves the absorption of radiant energy in tissue and/or conduction from heated surfaces, resulting in temperature rise and thermal injury or burn. Temperature distributions in tissue are determined through three heat transfer mechanisms: convection, conduction, and radiation. However, the problem rapidly becomes highly complex and nonlinear when physiological and biochemical factors are considered, such as perfusion, phase change, transient environmental conditions, tissue morphology, and optical and thermal properties, as well as dynamic changes in these properties.

The Pennes bioheat equation is typically used to describe heat transfer in biological tissue. It is identical to the standard Fourier heat transfer equation used to calculate heat transfer in a solid body, except that it includes the effect of a generalized heat source/sink due to perfusion:

$$\rho c \frac{\partial T}{\partial \tau} = \nabla \cdot (k \nabla T) + \omega_b c_b \rho_b (T_b - T) + Q \tag{15.2}$$

where ω_b is the volumetric perfusion rate (1/s) and the subscript b refers to blood, k is thermal conductivity, T is temperature, Q is the heat source term, ρ is density, c is specific heat capacity, and τ is time.

Optical radiation is refracted, reflected, scattered, and absorbed by tissue. These complex light-tissue interactions are highly dependent on tissue optical properties—refractive index, scattering, and absorption coefficients—which vary with wavelength and tissue constituent. Absorbed radiation is converted to thermal energy, which results in temperature rise. The rate of heat generation (Q in W/cm^3) produced by light propagating at any point in tissue is $Q = \mu_a \phi(x,y)$, where ϕ is fluence (W/cm^2). Diffusion of this heat within the tissue is typically dominated by conduction and convection, the latter primarily becoming significant in blood vessels and at the tissue surface.

Evaporation at the tissue surface can act as a significant heat sink. However, the loss of water in tissue can lead to desiccation, which can in turn alter fundamental tissue properties (e.g., thermal conductivity), thus making the problem a dynamic, nonlinear one. Other dynamic changes can be produced, such as optical property variations, as a function of temperature and thermal damage [41]. Elevated temperatures may also trigger a variety of physiological effects [42], including heat shock protein generation [43] and thermoregulatory perfusion changes [44].

Larger increases in temperature eventually lead to molecular changes, most notably the denaturation of proteins such as collagen, albumin, and hemoglobin. Denaturation can bring about changes in other fundamental tissue properties, such as specific heat capacity [45], and optical properties, such as increased scattering [46, 47]. Severe thermal injury can alter blood perfusion, with denaturation of vessel wall proteins or blood constituents causing temporary or permanent vessel occlusion [48]. The gold standard for identifying thermally induced tissue damage is histopathological examination. However, highly sensitive techniques for detecting thermal injury involve fluorescence and reflectance spectroscopy [49] and birefringence loss [50]. Polarization-sensitive OCT has also been shown to be useful for detecting thermal damage in tissue [51].

In 1947, Henriques and Moritz [52] introduced a method for quantifying and predicting the onset and extent of thermal injury based on the Arrhenius rate process equation:

$$\frac{d\Omega(t)}{dt} = A \exp\left[-\frac{E_a}{RT(t)}\right] \tag{15.3}$$

$$\Omega(t) = \ln\left(\frac{C(t)}{C(0)}\right) = A \int_0^\tau \exp\left[-\frac{E_a}{RT(t)}\right] dt \tag{15.4}$$

where C is the concentration of living cells or molecules in the native state, R is the universal gas constant (8.31 J/mole/K), and the two primary material properties are the frequency factor or molecular collision rate, A (1/second), and the activation energy, E_a (J/mole) [42]. This equation summarizes damage processes in a single, dimensionless parameter (Ω) based on the concept that thermal damage is an exponential function of temperature and a linear function of time (exposure duration). By convention, $\Omega = 1.0$ is the threshold for observable thermal coagulation or a first-degree burn, whereas $\Omega = 10$ and $\Omega = 100$ correspond to second- and third-degree burns, respectively. An Ω value of 1.0 also corresponds to a damage concentration of 63%.

Each set of thermal damage parameters (A, E_a) describes the relationship between exposure duration and threshold temperature (the temperature required for coagulation). Figure 15.4 illustrates the relationship between threshold temper-

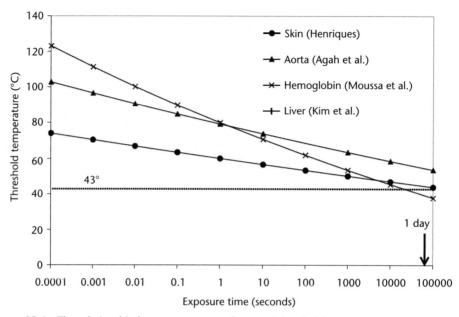

Figure 15.4 The relationship between exposure time and threshold temperature for thermal coagulation [41, 55–57].

atures and exposure time, as calculated directly from thermal damage parameters for various biological tissues. The data indicate that thermal damage can be produced by high-temperature exposures of less than 1 ms, such as during pulsed laser irradiation [53], or by low-temperature, long-term exposures [54]. The 43°C safety limit specified in IEC 60601-1:2005 (Medical Electrical Equipment—Part 1: General Requirements for Basic Safety and Essential Performance) is included in Figure 15.4 for comparison with the calculated threshold values at long exposure times. A more thorough discussion of rate process analyses of laser-induced thermal damage is provided by Pearce and Thomsen [42].

15.6.4 Photomechanical Damage

It is well established that laser irradiation can generate photomechanical effects, resulting in tissue ablation [58, 59]. This effect has been successfully exploited for numerous clinical applications, including laser lithotripsy and laser-assisted in situ keratomileusis (LASIK). In recent years, the use of pulsed lasers has become increasingly popular for imaging techniques, such as time-resolved fluorescence, multiphoton spectroscopy and optical coherence tomography. Therefore, the same mechanisms that have produced desirable effects during therapeutic procedures now have the potential to generate significant damage during diagnostic procedures. While pulsed-laser-induced ablation incorporates a variety of highly complex phenomenon that are well-delineated elsewhere [58, 59], this section provides an overview of fundamental processes and considerations.

Ablation mechanisms are determined by irradiation parameters such as pulse duration (τ_p), radiant exposure, and wavelength, as well as tissue material properties, such as thermal diffusivity (α), absorption coefficient (μ_a, which is a function of wavelength), and speed of sound (σ). These parameters determine whether the irradiation event satisfies one or both of the key ablation conditions: thermal and stress confinement. A laser pulse is thermally confined when the laser pulse duration is shorter than the thermal diffusion time (τ), defined as

$$\tau = \frac{1}{4\alpha\mu_a^2} \qquad (15.5)$$

Thermal confinement represents the condition in which heat diffusion from the irradiated region is minimal during the laser pulse. Stress confinement occurs when the following condition is satisfied:

$$\tau_p < \frac{1}{\sigma\mu_a} \qquad (15.6)$$

This represents an irradiation event in which the pulse duration is shorter than the time required for stress waves generated by thermoelastic expansion to exit the irradiated volume.

Ablation events can be placed in one of four categories: continuous-wave ablation, thermally confined ablation, stress-confined ablation, and plasma-mediated ablation. Each category can be defined in terms of both the parameters that cause the ablation process and the characteristic effects produced during the ablation event.

Continuous-wave (CW) ablation occurs for laser exposures that are neither stress nor thermally confined. Typically, this involves lasers that provide exposure durations of hundreds of milliseconds or greater (e.g., CO_2 lasers). However, CW ablation can occur for pulses as short as several microseconds when tissue absorption coefficients are high (e.g., Erbium:YAG lasers). CW ablation is typically characterized by subsurface superheating and steam formation that drives the explosive ejection of tissue, followed by tissue carbonization and ultimately an irregular ablation crater surrounded by a wide extent of thermal damage.

A number of common pulsed lasers (e.g., the free-running Ho:YAG laser with τ_p on the order of hundreds of microseconds) produce ablation events that are thermally but not stress confined. These lasers cause rapid, localized heating that leads to limited thermal damage in adjacent tissue, although the extent of damage can expand significantly with multiple pulses. Rapid heating leads to explosive vaporization, causing expanding vapor and gas to eject tissue material. Pressure waves are generated both at the onset and during the vaporization process. When such an event occurs in an enclosed environment, a vapor bubble can form that causes mechanical damage upon expansion as well as due to pressures generated upon bubble collapse.

Laser pulses that are both thermally and stress confined (e.g., Q-switched Nd:YAG) cause rapid thermoelastic expansion and tensile stresses. Negative stresses cause a decrease in the threshold required for cavitation, which in turn drives material ejection and formation of shock waves. When cavitation occurs in a liquid environment away from any interface, bubbles are generated that tend to be spherical in shape. On collapse of such a highly symmetric bubble, strong pressure or shock waves can be produced. This process tends to produce greater mechanical damage than nonstress-confined laser pulses but less thermal damage. For pulse durations of less than 1 ns down to 10 ps, self-focusing can concentrate radiation from a collimated beam and thus lower the ablation threshold.

Plasma-mediated ablation is produced by very short, high-intensity laser pulses (typically nano-, pico- or femtosecond lasers) that exceed threshold irradiance for laser-induced breakdown (10^9 to 10^{12} W/cm^2). This type of ablation is unique in that it can occur in nonabsorbing media, given sufficient irradiance levels. Plasma generation in absorbing media involves rapid temperature rise followed by thermionic emission of free electrons, whereas in transparent media multiphoton processes initiate ionization avalanche. In either case, the resulting plasma can reach temperatures well over 1,000K and generate hundreds of megapascals of pressure. Once formed, plasmas absorb incoming light, thus shielding deeper regions from further irradiation. While the ablation process for laser-induced plasmas is similar to that for stress-confined ablation events involving linear absorption, the mechanical effects produced are more intense (e.g., larger pressure transients, more forceful tissue ejection). Individual ablation events produced by plasma-mediated ablation tend to produce minimal collateral thermal injury; however, when an ultrafast pulsed laser is used in a high-repetition-rate mode, small increases in thermal energy can accumulate over time, resulting in a superpositioning effect and thermal damage.

15.7 Conclusions

Through this brief overview of regulation and regulatory science issues for optical imaging, we have attempted to provide the reader with a perspective not often present in the biomedical optics literature, yet one that is becoming increasingly important as the field matures. The information provided here represents a starting point for exploration of the regulatory process. While this process can be intimidating, by understanding the regulatory framework and relevant scientific issues, sponsors will be better equipped to accomplish key tasks. Among these are identifying and resolving safety hazards, implementing essential requirements, and establishing meaningful communication with regulatory agency staff. If these goals can be achieved, the result will likely be reduced sponsor frustration and more timely achievement of the common goal of clinical optical imaging systems that enhance public health.

Acknowledgments

We gratefully acknowledge the editorial contributions of Dr. Tony Durkin and Bob Faaland.

References

[1] Global Harmonization Task Force, "GHTF-SG1, Essential Principles of Safety and Performance of Medical Devices," 2005, http://www.ghtf.org.

[2] Cheng, M., "Medical device regulations: Global overview and guiding principles," World Health Organization, 2003, http://www.who.int.

[3] "Just the Facts: Better Health Care with Quality Medical Devices," Office of Public Affairs, Food, and Drug Administration, 2002, http://www.fda.gov.

[4] Feigal, D. W., S. N. Gardner, and M. McClellan, "Ensuring safe and effective medical devices," *NEJM* 348 (2003): 191–192.

[5] "Regulatory challenges," *WHO Drug Information* 17(4) (2003): 231–233.

[6] "Total GDP 2006," World Development Indicators Database, World Bank, 2007, http://www.worldbank.org.

[7] Hefflin, B., T. Gross, and T. Schroeder, "Estimates of medical device-associated adverse events from emergency departments," *Am. J. Prev. Med.* 27(3) (2004): 246–253.

[8] Sawyer, D., et al., "Do it by design: An introduction to human factors in medical devices," U.S. Department of Health and Human Services, 1996, http://www.fda.gov/cdrh/humfac/doit.html.

[9] Code of Federal Regulations, Food and Drugs, Title 21, Part 860, Washington, DC: U.S. Government Printing Office, 2001.

[10] International Organization for Standardization, http://www.iso.org.

[11] Federal Food, Drug, and Cosmetic Act—as Amended February, 1998, Washington, DC: U.S. Government Printing Office, 1999-454-701/83020.

[12] Code of Federal Regulations, Food and Drugs, Title 21, Parts 800–1299, Washington, DC: U.S. Government Printing Office, 2001.

[13] Food and Drug Administration, http://www.fda.gov/opacom/morechoices/mission.html.

[14] CDRH/FDA, CDRH Industry Support, http://www.fda.gov/cdrh/industry/support.

[15] Food and Drug Administration, http://www.fda.gov/cdrh/devadvice.

[16] "Information sheet guidance for IRBs, clinical investigators, and sponsors. Significant risk and nonsignificant risk medical device studies," Good Clinical Practice Program, Food and Drug Administration, U.S. Department of Health and Human Services, 2006, http://www.fda.gov/oc/gcp/guidance.html.

[17] Code of Federal Regulations, Food and Drugs, Title 21, Part 812, Washington, DC: U.S. Government Printing Office, 2001.

[18] "Office of device evaluation, annual report, fiscal year 2005," U.S. Department of Health and Human Services, http://www.fda.gov/cdrh/annual/fy2005/code.

[19] FDA (CBER and CDER), "Guidance for industry, developing medical imaging drug and biological products (parts 1–3)," U.S. Dept. of Health and Human Services, 2004, http://www.fda.gov/cber/guidelines.htm.

[20] FDA, "Recognition and use of consensus standards: Final guidance for industry and FDA staff," U.S. Dept. of Health and Human Services, 2007, http://www.fda.gov/cdrh/guidance.html.

[21] Code of Federal Regulations, Food and Drugs, Title 21, Part 820, Washington, DC: U.S. Government Printing Office, 2001.

[22] Drobetsky, E. A., J. Turcotte, and A. Chateauneuf, "A role for ultraviolet A in solar mutagenesis," *Proc. Natl. Acad. Sci.* 92 (1995): 2350–2354.

[23] Matsumura, Y., and H. N. Ananthaswamy, "Toxic effects of ultraviolet radiation on the skin," *Toxicol. Appl. Pharmacol.* 195(3) (2004): 298–308.

[24] Baier, J., et al., "Singlet oxygen generation by UVA light exposure of endogenous photosensitizers," *Biophys. J.* 91 (2006): 1452–1459.

[25] Kvam, E., and R. M. Tyrrell, "Induction of oxidative DNA base damage in human skin cells by UV and near visible radiation," *Carcinogenesis* 18(12) (1997): 2379–2384.

[26] Diffey, B. L., "Solar ultraviolet radiation effects on biological systems," *Phys. Med. Biol.* 36(3) (1991): 299–328.

[27] Anders, A., et al., "Action spectrum for erythema in humans investigated with dye lasers," *Photchem. Photobiol.* 61(2) (1995): 200–205.

[28] Young, A. R., et al., "The similarity of action spectra for thymine dimers in human epidermis and erythema suggests that DNA is the chromophore for erythema," *J. Invest. Derm.* 111 (1998): 982–988.

[29] "TLVs and BEIs. 2001," American Conference of Governmental Industrial Hygienists, Cincinnati, OH: ACGIH Worldwide, 2001.

[30] Zuclich, J. A., "Ultraviolet-induced photochemical damage in ocular tissues," *Health Phys.* 56(5) (1989): 671–682.

[31] Boyce, P. R., "Light and health," in *Human Factors in Lighting*, Macmillan: New York, 1981.

[32] Oliva, M. S., and H. A. C. Taylor, "Ultraviolet radiation and the eye," *Int. Ophth. Clin.* 45(1) (2005): 1–17.

[33] Ham, W. T. J., H. A. Mueller, and D. H. Sliney, "Retinal sensitivity to damage from short wavelength light," *Nature* 260(5547) (1976): 153–155.

[34] Poblete-Gutiérrez, P., et al., "The porphyrias: Clinical presentation, diagnosis and treatment," *Eur. J. Dermatol.* 16(3) (2006): 230–240.

[35] Dougherty, T. J., "An Update on photodynamic therapy applications," *J. Clin. Laser Med. Surg.* 20(1) (2002): 3–7.

[36] Radu, A., et al., "Pulse oximeter as a cause of skin burn during photodynamic therapy," *Endoscopy* 31(9) (1999): 831–833.

[37] Sibata, C. H., et al., "Photodynamic therapy in oncology," *Expert Opin. Pharmacother.* 2 (2001): 917–927.

[38] Pfefer, T. J., K. T. Schomacker, and N. S. Nishioka, "Long-term effects of photodynamic therapy on fluorescence spectroscopy in the human esophagus," *Photochem. Photobiol.* 73(6) (2001): 664–668.

[39] Levine, J., "Medications that increase sensitivity to light: A 1990 listing," U.S. Dept. of Health and Human Services, 1990, Washington DC: Government Printing Office (FDA91-8280).

[40] Reid, C. D., "Chemical photosensitivity: Another reason to be careful in the sun," *FDA Consumer*, May 1996, http://www.fda.gov/fdac/features/496_sun.html.

[41] Kim, B., S. L. Jacques, S. Rastegar, S. Thomsen, and M. Motamedi, "Nonlinear finite-element analysis of the role of dynamic changes in blood perfusion and optical properties in laser coagulation of tissue," *IEEE J. Sel. Topics Quant. Elect.* 2(4) (1996): 922–933.

[42] Pearce, J., and S. Thomsen, "Rate process analysis of thermal damage," in A. J. Welch and M. J. C. van Gemert (eds.), *Optical-thermal response of laser-irradiated tissue*, New York: Plenum Press, 1995.

[43] Park, H. G., et al., "Cellular responses to mild heat stress," *Cell. Mol. Life Sci.* 62(1) (2005): 10–23.

[44] Charkoudian, N., "Skin blood flow in adult human thermoregulation: How it works, when it does not, and why," *Mayo Clin. Proc.* 78(5) (2003): 603–612.

[45] Si, M. S., et al., "Dynamic heat capacity changes of laser-irradiated type I collagen films," *Lasers Surg. Med.* 19(1) (1996): 17–22.

[46] Pfefer, T. J., et al., "Pulsed laser-induced thermal damage in whole blood," *J. Biomech. Eng.* 122(2) (2000): 196–202.

[47] Ritz, J. P., et al., "Optical properties of native and coagulated porcine liver tissue between 400 and 2400 nm," *Lasers Surg. Med.* 29(3) (2001): 205–212.

[48] Barton, J. K., et al., "Simultaneous irradiation and imaging of blood vessels during pulsed laser delivery," *Lasers Surg. Med.* 24(3) (1999): 236–243.

[49] Buttemere, C. R., et al., "In vivo assessment of thermal damage in the liver using optical spectroscopy," *J. Biomed. Opt.* 9(5) (2004): 1018–1027.

[50] Thomsen, S., J. A. Pearce, and W. F. Cheong, "Changes in birefringence as markers of thermal damage in tissues," *IEEE Trans. Biomed. Eng.* 36(12) (1989): 1174–1170.

[51] Park, B. H., et al., "In vivo burn depth determination by high-speed fiber-based polarization sensitive optical coherence tomography," *J. Biomed. Opt.* 6(4) (2001): 474–479.

[52] Henriques, F. C., and A. R. Moritz, "Studies in thermal injury: I. The conduction of heat to and through skin and the temperature attained therein. A theoretical and experimental investigation," *Am. J. Pathol.* 23 (1947): 531–549.

[53] Pfefer, T. J., et al., "Dynamics of pulsed holmium: YAG laser photocoagulation of albumen," *Phys. Med. Biol.* 45(5) (2000): 1099–1114.

[54] Wille, J., et al., "Pulse oximeter-induced digital injury: Frequency rate and possible causative factors," *Crit. Care Med.* 28(10) (2000): 3555–3557.

[55] Henriques, F. C., "Studies in thermal injury: V. The predictability and significance of thermally induced rate processes leading to irreversible epidermal injury," *Arch. Pathol.* 43 (1947): 489–502.

[56] Agah, R., et al., "Rate process model for arterial tissue thermal damage: Implications on vessel photocoagulation," *Lasers Surg. Med.* 15 (1994): 176–184.

[57] Moussa, N. A., E. N. Tell, and E. G. Cravalho, "Time progression of hemolysis of erythrocyte populations exposed to supraphysiological temperatures," *ASME J. Biomech. Eng.* 101 (1979): 213–217.

[58] van Leeuwen, T. G., et al., "Pulsed laser ablation of soft tissue," in A. J. Welch and M. J. C. van Gemert, (eds.), *Optical-Thermal Response of Laser-Irradiated Tissue*, New York: Plenum Press, 1995.

[59] Vogel, A., and V. Venugopalan, "Mechanisms of pulsed laser ablation of biological tissues," *Chem. Rev.* 103(2) (2003): 577–644.

CHAPTER 16
Emerging Optical Imaging Technologies: Contrast Agents

Kai Licha, Michael Schirner, and Gavin Henry

16.1 Introduction

Diagnostic imaging continues to revolutionize medicine with increasing insight and detail into the function of the body. The imaging technologies available today make use of the wide spectrum of electromagnetic radiation, from radiowaves (magnetic resonance imaging), to visible and near-infrared light (optical imaging), to X-rays (X-ray computed tomography) and gamma rays (single photon emission computed tomography and positron emission tomography).

In some imaging techniques, contrast may arise from different properties of the tissue being measured (such as bone to soft tissue in CT) but often, for the generation of useful images, a contrast agent or reporter probe is required [1]. Here, a brief overview of contrast agents is provided for the main imaging modalities, except optical, which is covered in the next section. Approved contrast agents for X-ray can be divided into barium sulfate suspensions for imaging the gastrointestinal (GI) tract and other water-soluble agents that contain iodinated aromatic rings. Iodine-containing reagents have developed over time from ionic monomers to nonionic dimers with lower osmolality und viscosity [2]. The strength of MRI is its high spatial resolution compared to other imaging modalities, whereas its sensitivity to detection is low. This can, however, be enhanced, allowing the technique to be applied even to the imaging of molecular targets. Contrast agents for MRI can be divided into paramagnetic or superparamagnetic, for example, including ultrasmall supermagnetic iron oxide particles, used to enhance relaxivity or selectivity with detection levels around 10^{-8} M, and gadolinium complexes, mainly with DTPA and DOTA, used for longitudinal relaxation with a detection threshold around 10^{-4} M [1].

Imaging with radiolabeled probes has become a highly innovative and competitive field [3]. Radioactive isotopes fall into two classes: PET and SPECT, those that emit positrons (e.g., carbon-11, fluorine-18, gallium-68, copper-64, yittrium-86, iodine-124), which annihilate upon collision with protons in the body, generating gamma radiation, and those that emit gamma radiation directly (e.g., technetium-99m, indium-111, iodine-123/125), which is detected by a gamma camera and usually has a lower detection efficiency (the probe emits radioactivity constantly, giving rise to a higher background signal). Only trace amounts of these substances are needed, which makes them particularly interesting for the measurement of biological processes. The distribution of radioactivity within the body is detected and evaluated to give tomographic images. Chemically, the radiolabeled structures can be divided into those that are organic synthetic molecules with covalent bonds to the isotope (fluorine-18, carbon-11, iodine isotopes) and those that require complexing or chelating moieties, such as DOTA systems (e.g., for gallium-68 or indium-111) or N/S-chelates (e.g., for technetium-99m). Radiochemistry using chelator conjugates is easier to accomplish but limited to metal isotopes, while covalently labeled structures require organic synthetic pathways to be established, yielding molecules with only minor structural changes compared to a respective parent drug compound. Figure 16.1 depicts typical contrast-agent structures.

As pointed out in other parts in this book, most of the parameters of each of these imaging modalities are complimentary and serve a distinct role. While CT and MRI provide morphological and functional information based on their high spatial resolution, they have limited sensitivity for contrast agents. Radioimaging methods and optical imaging enable capture of molecular information due to their high detection sensitivity for emitting probes but provide little spatial information.

As a logical consequence of recently emerged multimodality imaging solutions, such as the already routinely established PET-CT, there is increasing demand for novel chemical or biochemical probes with multimodal capabilities. Many combinations are conceivable, and the objective of these efforts is to increase diagnostic value by creating synergies from the different parameters of the imaging modalities. These ideas will also lead to added product differentiation in the marketplace.

Biological background and possible clinical applications have already been reviewed (e.g., in [4]). This chapter focuses on the chemistry behind these approaches and gives an overview of the various design principles. According to the versatile nature of diagnostic imaging, the chemistries involved span a wide range, covering nanotechnology, organic synthesis, radiochemistry, metal coordination chemistry, and bioconjugation techniques.

16.2 Optical Probes

16.2.1 Fluorophores as Contrast Agents for Optical Imaging

Organic chemistry has created an enormous range of fluorescent dyes for life science applications. Perhaps the most versatile class of fluorophores in the area of biological in vivo imaging has been the cyanine dyes. They are available at practically each desired absorption wavelength from the visible to near-infrared spectral range, making them useful for both superficial and deep tissue imaging [5]. The latter is achieved by using light in the near-infrared spectrum (NIR, 650 to 950 nm) to maximize tissue penetrance and to minimize autofluorescence from nontarget tissue. In addition, fluorophores based on fluoresceins and rhodamines, both established as labels for bioanalytical methodology, have been used to design novel probes for in vivo imaging.

Clinical applications can illustrate the utility of each of these fluorphore types. Approved in the 1960s as a diagnostic drug for the assessment of hepatic function

16.2 Optical Probes

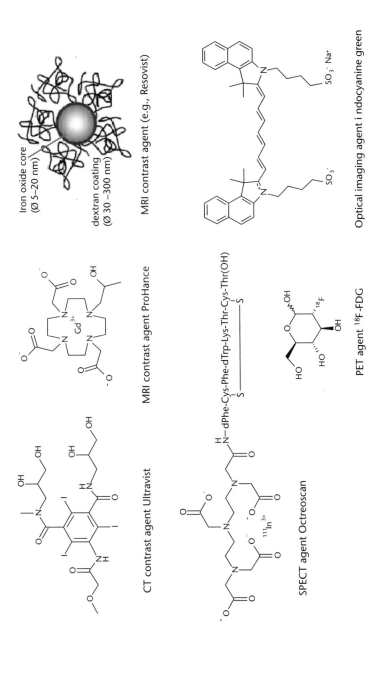

Figure 16.1 Examples of clinically approved contrast agents and imaging probes for X-ray/CT, MRI, PET, SPECT, and optical imaging to illustrate the diversity of chemical structures involved, featuring organic, inorganic, nano-, radio-, dye, and bioconjugate chemistry.

and rediscovered in the 1990s as an imaging agent, the carbocyanine dye indocyanine green (ICG, absorption approximately 780 to 800 nm) is today, together with fluorescein, frequently applied for fluorescence angiography of vascular disorders in ophthalmology [6]. Beyond ICG, various novel cyanine-dye derivatives have been created as passively targeted contrast agents of simple synthetic availability. Examples are the dye SIDAG [7, 8], TSC, a tetrasulfonated alternative [9], IRDye78-CA, and sugar-conjugated versions [10, 11]. These dyes have demonstrated successful visualization of different types of experimental tumors based on passive or nontargeted tissue uptake mechanisms and have also been applied in intraoperative imaging settings [12]. Many of these fluorophore structures have found entrance into targeted and fluorescence activation approaches (Section 16.2.3) as well as multimodality probe design (Section 16.3). Color Plate 31 illustrates the basic principles of probe design.

16.2.2 Fluorophore Conjugates for Targeting and Activation

Factors such as high instrumental sensitivity for detection, low required dosages, lack of radiation, and progress in the development of photonic technologies have made optical imaging the fastest growing field of imaging research besides PET. Targeted optical agents have been designed in broad variety by utilizing novel targeting ligands as vehicles for the delivery of fluorophores, which are coupled using well-established bioconjugation chemistry [5, 13].

Substantial efforts have been undertaken to synthesize and characterize targeted fluorophore conjugates based on peptide ligands to G-protein-coupled receptors (GPCRs), such as somatostatin (SST), vasoactive intestinal peptide (VIP), and bombesin. For example, the pharmacologically optimized SST analog octreotate was shown to internalize into tumor cells with a variety of different fluorophores [14–16]. Similarly, the conjugate Cybesin targeting the bombesin receptor [17] and a cyanine conjugate with a derivative of vasoactive intestinal peptide [18] have been described. Integrin targeting ($\alpha v\beta 3$ and $\alpha v\beta 5$) has been accomplished by adapting the well-known peptide ligands containing the RGD-motif to fluorescence imaging [19–22]. Originating from radiolabeled conjugates (e.g., the clinically approved OctreoScan), this research area has recently been redirected to multimodality probe design employing radiolabeled elements in addition to fluorophores (see Section 16.3.2).

Likewise, fluorophore labels have been used in broad variety to generate targeted conjugates with bioengineered proteins, antibodies, and antibody mimetics for in vivo imaging. First, in vivo images have been published by Folli et al. [23] and Ballou et al. [24], who used IgG antibodies. The angiogenesis-specific extracellular matrix protein ED-B fibronectin was targeted using highly affine single-chain antibodies, permitting visualization of this target in many disease models, such as tumors [25], atherosclerosis [26], and corneal neovascularization [27]. Other examples for antibody- and protein-based targeting probes are cyanine conjugates with annexin V [28, 29], epidermal growth factor (EGF) [30], low-density lipoprotein (LDL) [31], an IgM antibody to image lymph nodes [32], and peptosome constructs [33].

Metabolic optical imaging, employing small molecule ligands, can be regarded as a third field of imaging probe design, in part derived from approaches elucidated formerly at the radiodiagnostic level. Such probes include, for example, vitamin folic acid [34, 35], Vitamin B12 linked to Cy5 (CobalaFluor) [36], or fluorescent bisphosphonate probes targeting hydroxyapatite [37]. ^{18}F-radiolabeled 2-fluorodeoxyglucose (^{18}F-FDG) glucose served as the model for near-infrared fluorescent counterparts, but it does not act through the GLUT transporter pathway [38].

Color Plate 31 illustrates the different contrasting principles and depicts a selected assembly of chemical probe structures representing these principles.

Probes that alter their photophysical characteristics upon contacting a desired target have recently been developed and are often described as "activatable." Activatable NIRF agents exist in a baseline quenched state until cleavage or activation by the desired enzyme produces fragments of single fluorescing dyes. This subject has been reviewed extensively in the literature [39]. The major chemical entity has been the poly(L-lysine)/poly(ethylene gylcol) graft polymer labeled with a high number of cyanine dyes (in most cases, Cy5.5 [40]). Attachment of the fluorophores either directly or via cleavable peptide sequences to this polymer caused strong fluorescence quenching. These probes have meanwhile been commercialized as research probes for the quantification of enzyme activity in vivo and the validation of animal models and therapeutic protocols.

Attempts to design probes at a low molecular-weight level have been published by Zheng et al., who synthesized probes of dimeric character consisting of an effector, a cleavable linker peptide, and a quencher unit [41]. For instance, the photodynamic activity and fluorescence of a photosensitizer was quenched by BHQ-3 linked in close proximity to the photosensitizer via an MMP-7 cleavable peptide sequence [42].

16.2.3 Fluorescent Nanoparticles

Quantum dots (QDs) are perhaps the most prominent fluorescent nanoparticles in bioanalytics and life science imaging [43, 44]. These semiconductor nanocrystal materials consisting of atoms such as Cd, Se, Te, S, and Zn can today be controlled extremely well with respect to their optical properties and their chemical behavior, gaining interest primarily as fluorescent tags for biological molecules due to their high quantum yield and photostability [43, 44]. Surface modifications with hydrophilic groups, PEGs, and block polymers [45–47] as well as with targeting vectors, such as antibodies [44, 48] and peptides [49], have expanded their applications into many areas of imaging research, including approaches to multimodal imaging (see Section 16.3.1).

Likewise, materials that are either metal-free or consist of matrices doped with metal atoms have been studied as alternatives to QDs [50]. Interesting properties have been described for upconverting rare-earth nanophosphores [51] and particles based on silica materials with incorporated organic dye molecules [52]. A Rhodamin-doped, silica-coated nanoparticle has been used for apoptosis imaging by way of additional conjugation to Annexin V [53]. An organically modified silica matrix (PEBBLE technology) was applied to incorporate ICG and study photoacoustic imaging contrast [54]. The expansion of sophisticated nanomaterials into imaging continues even further, such as with surface-modified nanodiamonds, which are extremely photostable and have been used in cellular imaging [55], or semiconducting single-walled carbon nanotubes for near-infrared fluorescence imaging [56].

Nanoparticular structures based on micellar assemblies of amphiphilic molecules or tensidic components are particularly suited to incorporate multiple effector molecules since these components can be individually prepared and combined in different ways. More recent approaches have thus been mainly geared toward multimodality imaging and are therefore discussed in Section 16.3 (see Table 16.1).

16.3 Multimodality Probes for Optical Imaging

16.3.1 Probes for Optical Imaging and MRI

The field of multimodality imaging involving optical and MRI imaging has truly flourished in the past 5 years. Compared to other imaging modalities, MRI offers high spatial resolution but relatively low sensitivity to detection. Contrast can be

Table 16.1 Summary of Multimodality Design Approaches Employing a Fluorescent Component and a Second Detection Unit

Second Modality	Second Effector Unit	Fluorophore Unit	Diseases; Techniques	References
MRI	Iron oxide particle	Cyanine	Tumors, atherosclerosis, lymph nodes; Cell microscopy, in vivo imaging	● [59–61, 63, 106] ○ [28, 60–62, 73–75]
MRI	Iron oxide particle	Fluorescein, rhodamine, Alexa Fluor dye	Tumors; Cell microscopy, in vivo imaging	● [63, 69, 104] ○ [75, 105]
MRI	Gadolinium oxide particle	Fluorescein, rhodamine, cyanine	Tumors; In vivo imaging	● [79]
MRI	Gd complex	Cyanine	Tumors, lymph nodes; In vivo imaging	● [81, 86, 88]
MRI	Gd complex	Fluorescein, rhodamine, Ru-complex, phthalocyanine, NBD	Tumors, atherosclerosis; Cell imaging, in vivo imaging	● [74, 85, 93] ○ [82–84]
MRI	Gd complex	QD	Cell microscopy	● [90] ○ [67, 91]
MRI	Manganese	QD	Cell microscopy	● [92]
SPECT	In-111 chelate	Cyanine, Alexa Fluor dye	Physicochem. characterization, in vivo organ distribution, in vivo tumor imaging	● [94, 96] ○ [97–100]
PET	Ga-68 chelate, Cu-64 chelate	Cyanine	Physicochem. characterization	● [96] ○ [95]
PET	I-124	Chlorin (pheophorbide)	Physicochem. characterization, in vivo tumor imaging	○ [101]

Notes:
● Nontargeted probe design, conceptual chemical work.
○ Targeted probe design, bioconjugation with biological targeting molecules.

enhanced by either paramagnetic agents (e.g., Gd^{3+} complexes) or superparamagnetic particles (e.g., iron oxide particles), with the latter allowing the technique to image even molecular targets [57, 58].

The first multimodality probes with relevance to optical imaging had combined fluorescent dyes with imaging ability for MRI based on iron oxide nanoparticle techniques [59–64]. The rationale behind this combination derived from the need to validate the biological behavior of iron oxide particles by a second complimentary detection method and to facilitate correlation between in vivo and in vitro (microscopy) techniques. The synthetic chemistry has been reasonably straightforward, requiring the surface conjugation of commercially available fluorophores (e.g., Cy5.5, Alexa Fluor dyes) to different particle-coating materials [60, 65–68]. One application of such systems is the imaging of pancreatic islets, involved in type 1 diabetes, which has been performed both in vitro [69] and in vivo [70].

Both passively distributing iron oxide particles and targeted systems employing a targeting vehicle as third component have been synthesized. A feasible strategy applies the readily available dextran-coated particles (CLIOs) to generate a certain number of amino groups by reductive amination of the saccharide moieties and use them for reaction with amino-reactive dyes (e.g., Cy5.5-NHS ester) as well as for further modification to attach peptide and protein vehicles (e.g., E-selectin [65], TAT-peptide [62, 71], Annexin V [72, 73], and VCAM-1 peptide [74]). Specific accumulation of a VCAM-1 targeted construct in atherosclerotic lesions was demonstrated by comparative ex vivo MRI and fluorescence images of aortic vessels from ApoE–/– mice [74] as depicted in Color Plate 32.

A simple way to introduce fluorescence into an antibody-conjugated particle is to use the fluorescently labeled antibody per se, as shown with herceptin-FITC [63]. More sophisticated constructs have been made by the coupling of functionalized coating polymers, for instance, bifunctional PEGs, to the iron oxide surface, subsequently followed by the conjugation of both targeting vehicles and fluorophores to an exterior PEG functionality [64]. Accordingly, iron particles were functionalized with a fluorescent dye and TAT-peptide using a PEG-modified phospholipid micelle coating instead of dextran [75]. A different coating strategy involved lipid-based co-block-polymers, which allowed fluorophores to be noncovalently bound and proteins to be attached on the surface, as shown with Annexin V [76]. The Weissleder group has even created "smart" nanoparticles, which combine CLIO with many NIR dye units linked by a polyarginine backbone, which can be activated by certain enzymes to free the quenched dye units, causing them to fluorescence when excited [77].

The application of such probes for the noninvasive imaging of brain tumors (MRI) followed by the intraoperative delinearization of tumor margins during surgery (fluorescence) highlights the usefulness of one and the same probe along a diagnostic and therapeutic intervention [59].

Some MRI/optical multimodality contrast agents use light scattering instead of fluorescence to create an image (see Figure 16.2). An example with a gold-coated iron oxide core also offers the possibility of photothermal therapy, as shown for cancer cells in vitro [78]. Another example similar to iron oxide nanoparticles in its concept involves gadolinium oxide nanoparticles. The paper published by Riviere et al. [79] shows such a nanoparticle core embedded in a polysiloxane shell, the inner

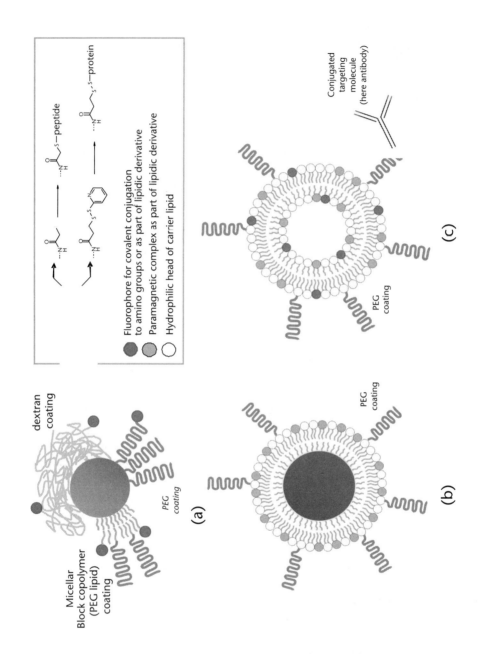

Figure 16.2 Illustration of MRI-optical probe design: (a) iron oxide particles with three different coating types for fluorophore labeling and bioconjugation, (b) quantum dots with paramagnetic coating entities based on lipidic components, and (c) multicomponent nanoparticles with paramagnetic and fluorescent lipidic components forming liposamal/micellar architectures.

surface of which was functionalized with organic dyes and the outer with PEG groups, that is well suited for MRI and optical imaging in vivo. One elegant approach is to use materials that can give contrast in both techniques, as demonstrated with gold nanorods [80]. They can be coated with transferrin to promote uptake in the Tf-receptor-positive cell line HeLa, and like QD, the absorption wavelength of these nanorods can be tuned.

The second approach toward multimodality probes for optical imaging and MRI involves the use of chelators for paramagnetic metal ions, mostly gadolinium. In combination either with particle carriers (e.g., LDL) or as lipidic derivatives forming micellar structures, a variety of novel constructs have been proposed as dual imaging probes. Examples include the imaging of low-density lipoprotein (LDL) receptors using a probe with a Gd-DTPA moiety for MRI and a cyanine dye for fluorescent confocal microscopy [81, 82]. LDL has also been labeled with Gd complex and a phthalocyanine dye for microscopy [83]. Immunomicelles have similarly been constructed based on phospholipidic moieties that are converted into targeted contrast agents by incubation with Gd-DTPA and incorporation of a fluorescent phospholipid, as well as linked to macrophage-specific antibody [84]. Furthermore, gadolinium complex and rhodamine were combined into a lipidic nanoparticle, which proved effective for in vivo MRI imaging and in vitro fluorescence microscopy for investigating angiogenesis in a murine model [85].

As an alternative to micelles or particles, macromolecular delivery can be accomplished by employing structures based on polymers or dendrimers, such as polylysine or PAMAMs. In that respect, cyanine dye or fluorescein/rhodamine labels were added to dendrimeric systems derived from macromolecular MRI dendrimers or polymers carrying multiple Gd-complex units [86, 87]. Color Plate 32 illustrates examples of their application in multimodal imaging of sentinel lymph nodes. Similarly, Gd-DTPA-polylysine was further modified by labeling a few of the free amino groups with cyanine dye NHS-esters (e.g., Cy5.5-NHS ester, Cy7-NHS ester, or IRDye800 NHS ester), yielding a dual imaging probe that was applied for the intraoperative delineation of tumor margins [88]. A similar approach was also followed by Bornhop et al. [89].

An interesting approach based on quantum dots has been accomplished by coating the QD with paramagnetic lipids (Gd complex–stearyl moieties), adding magnetic relaxivity to the fluorescent particle, followed by the conjugation of target-specific peptidic structures to the surface [76, 90]. Similarly, dendritic biotinylated Gd-complex structures were linked to the QD surface [91]. Alternatively, incorporation of MRI detectability into the QD core itself was achieved by the addition of manganese, which produced sufficient MR response at the cellular level [92]. More than 500 gadolinium chelate groups, together with fluorescein dye,were conjugated onto a viral capsid [93] to give a potent contrast agent with potential for vascular imaging.

16.3.2 Probes for Optical Imaging and SPECT/PET

The coregistration of optical probes with nuclear imaging methods provides the opportunity to enhance the diagnostic accuracy of optical methods. The quantification of fluorescence signals within deeper three-dimensional tissue segments remains difficult due both to light attenuation by absorption and scattering processes and to fluorescence quenching. Radioactive emission is quantifiable in tissues and would therefore allow probe concentrations to be more accurately determined. Thus, attempts have been undertaken to synthesize and characterize dual-labeled molecules involving both a fluorophore structure and a moiety for radiolabeling.

The most common combination for optical/radio imaging involves a cyanine dye conjugated to a DOTA/DTPA chelator (e.g., for indium [94], copper [95], or both [96]). These structures were named monomolecular multimodal imaging agents (MOMIAs) since they are designed to be readily applicable as dual-labeled molecules introducing a fluorophore and a radiochelate at once.

Examples of such agents comprising additional biomolecules conjugated for targeting include the herceptin antibody combined with cyanine and DTPA, permitting labeling with yttrium or indium for tumor imaging [97], or defined synthetic conjugates consisting of the (K)RGD peptide, cyanine dye, and DTPA [98, 99] for melanoma tumor imaging (see Color Plate 33). Alexa Fluor fluorphore has also been used in combination with indium nanoparticle micelles to combine SPECT imaging with fluorescence microscopy for the imaging of rabbit tumors [100].

Apparently, most of the radionuclides applied for multimodality design have been SPECT isotopes, mainly due to their easier availability. Extension to PET isotopes, such as Ga-68 or Cu-64, has been proposed but not much elucidated to date. The combination of PET probes involving fluorine-18 with fluorophores has not been part of this research landscape, obviously due to the more constrained synthetic options available with covalent fluorination chemistry. The advantage would be that fluorine introduction into existing probes represents a much lesser structural interference with any parent chemical structure than usually reached with large metal chelating moieties. There is an example, however, of covalently bound iodine-124 on a photosensitizer, which serves as an agent for PET and optical imaging and has additional therapeutic capabilities due to the photosensitizing chlorin entity employed as its core structure [101] (Color Plate 34).

Achilefu et al. elegantly stated an outlook for this kind of multimodality combination, suggesting that the nuclear component should be used to provide a whole-body image and the optical dye should guide tissue biopsy, giving high-resolution images of tissue boundaries. Alternatively, fused images could consist of a probe that uses PET to provide its localization and optical to show activity [102].

16.3.3 Probes for Optical Imaging and Therapy

Studies on activatable probes with quenched fluorescence have expanded into systems where, beside the fluorophore, a second optical structure is part of a dual-labeled molecule. For example, photosensitizers for photodynamic therapy (PDT) based on the well-known pheophorbide derivatives have been combined with a cyanine dye to dimer exhibiting PDT activity as well as strong near-infrared detectability [101, 103].

Iron oxide nanoparticles have even been conjugated through a dextran coating to organic dye and porphyrin [104] and tested in vitro for suitability in MRI, optical imaging, and photodynamic therapy. A similar example using Photofrin and iron oxide nanoparticles was shown by Ross et al. [105].

Combination with enzyme-cleavable peptide sequences was demonstrated to give effective "molecular beacons," which exhibit both quenched fluorescence and quenched phototoxic activity. Such constructs are composed of a photosensitzer (e.g., pyropheophorbide a), a peptide sequence cleavable by enzymes (e.g., MMP-7 or caspase-3), and a quenching chromophore. PDT-induced apoposis was shown to translate into caspase-3 induction, which can be ultimately visualized by fluorescence enhancement [41].

Photothermal treatment has been proposed by West et al. [106, 107] using a gold nanoshell that absorbs and scatters in the infrared region to provide optical contrast and photothermal ablation of tumors.

16.4 Summary and Conclusions

In this review, we have given an overview of the state of the art for contrast agents in multimodality imaging involving optical techniques. We gave a brief overview of the main techniques for diagnostic imaging from a chemical perspective and a more in-depth coverage of optical imaging, concentrating on fluorophores, their conjugates for targeting and activation, and fluorescent nanoparticles. The focus of the review was the overview of multimodal optical imaging probes that have been additionally functionalized as contrast agents for MRI, PET/SPECT, or therapy.

In the past few years, there has been a remarkable surge in the number of publications in the area of multimodal optical contrast agents, especially those including MRI nanoparticles. The development of this area is a symbiotic process driven by advances in many areas, including instrumentation, software, chemistry, and biology. The rising profile of this area and the increased awareness of the importance of codevelopment of such programs between several parties with complimentary expertise gives hope that these highly specialized probes will reach the marketplace and that patients will benefit from them.

References

[1] Sosnovik, D., and R. Weissleder, "Magnetic resonance and fluorescence based molecular imaging technologies," *Prog. Drug Res.* 62 (2005): 83–115.

[2] Yu, S. B., and A. D. Watson, "Metal-based X-ray contrast media," *Chem. Rev.* 99 (1999): 2353–2378.

[3] Peñuelas, I., and S. S. Gambhir, "Imaging studies for evaluating gene therapy in translational research," *Drug Disc. Today: Technol.* 2 (2005): 335–343.

[4] Moseley, M., and G. Donnan, "Multimodality imaging," *Stroke* 35, Suppl. 1 (2004): 2632–2634.

[5] Licha, K., and C. Olbrich, "Optical imaging in drug discovery and diagnostic applications," *Adv. Drug Deliv. Rev.* 57(8) (2005): 1087–1108.

[6] Richards, G., G. Soubrane, and L. Yanuzzi (eds.), *Fluorescein angiography: Textbook and atlas*, New York: Thieme, 1998.

[7] Licha, K., et al., "Hydrophilic cyanine dyes as contrast agents for near-infrared tumor imaging: Synthesis, photophysical properties and spectroscopic in vivo characterization," *Photochem. Photobiol.* 72(3) (2000): 392–398.

[8] Ebert, B., et al., "Near-infrared fluorescent dyes for enhanced contrast in optical mammography: Phantom experiments," *J. Biomed. Opt.* 6(2) (2001): 134–140.

[9] Perlitz, C., et al., "Comparison of two tricarbocyanine-based dyes for fluorescence optical imaging," *J. Fluorescence* 15(3) (2005): 443–454.

[10] Zhang, Z., and S. Achilefu, "Synthesis and evaluation of polyhydroxylated near-infrared carbocyanine molecular probes," *Organ. Lett.* 6(12) (2004): 2067–2070.

[11] Ye, Y., et al., "Multivalent carbocyanine molecular probes: Synthesis and applications," *Bioconj. Chem.* 16(1) (2005): 51–61.

[12] Nakayama, A., et al., "Functional near-infrared fluorescence imaging for cardiac surgery and targeted gene therapy," *Mol. Imag.* 1(4) (2002): 365–377.

[13] Tung, C. H., "Fluorescent peptide probes for in vivo diagnostic imaging," *Biopolymers* 76(5) (2004): 391–403.

[14] Becker, A., et al., "Receptor-targeted optical imaging of tumors with near-infrared fluorescent ligands," *Nat. Biotechnol.* 19(4) (2001): 327–231.

[15] Bugaj, J. E., et al., "Novel fluorescent contrast agents for optical imaging of in vivo tumors based on a receptor-targeted dye-peptide conjugate platform," *J. Biomed. Opt.* 6(2) (2001): 122–133.

[16] Mier, W., et al., "Fluorescent somatostatin receptor probes for the intraoperative detection of tumor tissue with long-wavelength visible light," *Bioorgan. Medicin. Chem.* 10(8) (2002): 2543–2552.

[17] Pu, Y., et al., "Spectral polarization imaging of human prostate cancer tissue using a near-infrared receptor-targeted contrast agent," *Technol. Canc. Res. Treat.* 4(4) (2005): 429–436.

[18] Bhargava, S., et al., "A complete substitutional analysis of VIP for better tumor imaging properties," *J. Mol. Recog.* 15(3) (2002): 145–153.

[19] Aina, O. H., et al., "Near-infrared optical imaging of ovarian cancer xenografts with novel alpha 3-integrin binding peptide OA02," *Mol. Imag.* 4(4) (2005): 439–447.

[20] Wang, W., et al., "Near-infrared optical imaging of integrin alphavbeta3 in human tumor xenografts," *Mol. Imag.* 3(4) (2004): 343–351.

[21] Achilefu, S., et al., "Synergistic effects of light-emitting probes and peptides for targeting and monitoring integrin expression." *Proc. Natl. Acad. Sci. USA* 102(22) (2005): 7976–7981.

[22] Chen, X., P. S. Conti, and R. A. Moats, "In vivo near-infrared fluorescence imaging of integrin alphavbeta3 in brain tumor xenografts," *Canc. Res.* 64(21) (2004): 8009–8014.

[23] Folli, S., et al., "Antibody-indocyanin conjugates for immunophotodetection of human squamous cell carcinoma in nude mice," *Canc. Res.* 54(10) (1994): 2643–2649.

[24] Ballou, B., et al., "Cyanine fluorochrome-labeled antibodies in vivo: Assessment of tumor imaging using Cy3, Cy5, Cy5.5, and Cy7," *Canc. Detect. Preven.* 22(3) (1998): 251–257.

[25] Neri, D., et al., "Touched by affinity-maturated antibody fragments of an angiogenesis associated fibronectin isoform," *Nat. Biotechnol.* 15(11) (1997): 1271–1275.

[26] Matter, C. M., et al. "Molecular imaging of atherosclerotic plaques using a human antibody against the extra-domain B of fibronectin," *Circ. Res.* 95(12) (2004): 1225–1233.

[27] Birchler, M., et al., "Selective targeting and photocoagulation of ocular angiogenesis mediated by a phage-derived human antibody fragment," *Nat. Biotechnol.* 17(10) (1999): 984–988.

[28] Schellenberger, E. A., et al., "Magneto/optical annexin V, a multimodal protein," *Bioconj. Chem.* 15(5) (2004): 1062–1064.

[29] Petrovsky, A., et al., "2 near-infrared fluorescent imaging of tumor apoptosis," *Canc. Res.* 63(8) (2003): 1936–1942.

[30] Ke, S., et al., "Near-infrared optical imaging of epidermal growth factor receptor in breast cancer xenografts," *Canc. Res.* 63(22) (2003): 7870–7875.

[31] Zheng, G., et al., "Rerouting lipoprotein nanoparticles to selected alternate receptors for the targeted delivery of cancer diagnostic and therapeutic agents," *Proc. Natl. Acad. Sci. USA* 102(49) (2005): 17757–17762.

[32] Licha, K., et al., "Optical molecular imaging of lymph nodes using a targeted vascular contrast agent," *J. Biomed. Opt.* 10(4) (2005): 41205.

[33] Tanisaka, H., et al., "Near-infrared fluorescent labeled peptosome for application to cancer imaging," *Bioconj. Chem.* 19(1) (2008): 109–117.

[34] Moon, W. K., et al., "2 enhanced tumor detection using a folate receptor-targeted near-infrared fluorochrome conjugate," *Bioconj. Chem.* 14(3) (2003): 539–545.

[35] Chen, W. T., et al., "Arthritis imaging using a near-infrared fluorescence folate-targeted probe," *Arthrit. Res. Ther.* 7(2) (2005): R310–R317.

[36] McGreevy, J. M., et al., "Minimally invasive lymphatic mapping using fluorescently labeled vitamin B12," *J. Surg. Res.* 111(1) (2003): 38–44.

[37] Lenkinski, R. E., et al., "Near-infrared fluorescence imaging of microcalcification in an animal model of breast cancer," *Acad. Radiol.* 10 (2003): 1159–1164.

[38] Cheng, Z., et al., "Near-infrared fluorescent deoxyglucose analogue for tumor optical imaging in cell culture and living mice," *Bioconj. Chem.* 17(3) (2006): 662–669.

[39] Rao, J., et al., "Fluorescence imaging in vivo: Recent advances," *Curr. Opin. Biotechnol.* 18(1) (2007): 17–25.

[40] Weissleder, R., et al., "In vivo imaging of tumors with protease-activated near-infrared fluorescent probes," *Nat. Biotechnol.* 17(4) (1999): 375–378.

[41] Stefflova, K., J. Chen, and G. Zheng, "Killer beacons for combined cancer imaging and therapy," *Curr. Medicin. Chem.* 14(20) (2007): 2110–2125.

[42] Zheng, G., et al., "Photodynamic molecular beacon as an activatable photosensitizer based on protease-controlled singlet oxygen quenching and activation," *Proc. Natl. Acad. Sci. USA* 104 (2007): 8989–8994.

[43] Chan, W. C., et al., "Luminescent quantum dots for multiplexed biological detection and imaging," *Curr. Opin. Biotechnol.* 13(1) (2002): 40–46.

[44] Michalet, X., et al., "Quantum dots for live cells, in vivo imaging, and diagnostics," *Science* 307(5709) (2005): 538–544.

[45] Ballou, B., et al., "Noninvasive imaging of quantum dots in mice," *Bioconj. Chem.* 15(1) (2004): 79–86.

[46] Kim, S., and M. G. Bawendi, "Oligomeric ligands for luminescent and stable nanocrystal quantum dots," *J. Am. Chem. Soc.* 12(48) (2003): 14652–14653.

[47] Gao, X., et al., "In vivo cancer targeting and imaging with semiconductor quantum dots." *Nat. Biotechnol.* 22(8) (2004): 969–976.

[48] Wu, X., et al., "Immunofluorescent labeling of cancer marker Her2 and other cellular targets with semiconductor quantum dots," *Nat. Biotechnol.* 21(1) (2003): 41–46.

[49] Akerman, M. E., et al., "Nanocrystal targeting in vivo," *Proc. Natl. Acad. Sci. USA* 99(20) (2002): 12617–12621.

[50] Santra, S., et al., "Luminescent nanoparticle probes for bioimaging," *Journal of Nanoscience and Nanotechnology*, Vol. 4, No. 6, 2004, pp. 590–599.

[51] Chen, Z., et al., "Versatile synthesis strategy for carboxylic acid-functionalized upconverting nanophosphors as biological labels," *Journal of the American Chemical Society*, Vol. 130, No. 10, 2008, pp. 3023–3029.

[52] Bringley, J. F., et al., "Silica nanoparticles encapsulating near-infrared emissive cyanine dyes," *Journal of Colloid and Interface Science*, Vol. 320, No. 1, 2008, pp. 132–139.

[53] Shi, H., et al., "Rhodamine B isothiocyanate doped silica-coated fluorescent nanoparticles (RBITC-DSFNPs)-based bioprobes conjugated to Annexin V for apoptosis detection and imaging," *Nanomedicine*, Vol. 3, No. 4, 2007, pp. 266–272.

[54] Kim, G., et al., "Indocyanine-green-embedded PEBBLEs as a contrast agent for photoacoustic imaging," *Journal of Biomedical Optics*, Vol. 12, No. 4, 2007, 044020.

[55] Yu, S. L., et al., "Bright fluorescent nanodiamonds: no photobleaching and low cytotoxicity," *Journal of the American Chemical Society*, Vol. 127, No. 50, 2008, pp. 17604–17605.

[56] Welsher, K., et al., "Selective probing and imaging of cells with single walled carbon nanotubes as near-infrared fluorescent molecules," *Nano Letters*, Vol. 8, No. 2, 2008, pp. 586–590.

[57] Mahmood, U., and L. Josephson, "Molecular MR imaging probes," *Proc. IEEE* 93(4) (2006): 800–808.

[58] Frullano, T., and T. J. Meade, "Multimodal MRI contrast agents," *J. Biolog. Inorgan. Chem.* 12(7) (2007): 939–949.

[59] Kircher, M. F., et al., "A multimodal nanoparticle for preoperative magnetic resonance imaging and intraoperative optical brain tumor delineation," *Canc. Res.* 63 (2003): 8122–8125.

[60] Weissleder, R., et al., "Cell-specific targeting of nanoparticles by multivalent attachment of small molecules," *Nat. Biotechnol.* 23(11) (2005): 1418–1423.

[61] Sosnovik, D. E., and R. Weissleder, "Magnetic resonance and fluorescence based molecular imaging technologies," *Prog. Drug Res.* 62 (2005): 83–115.

[62] Koch, A. M., et al., "Uptake and metabolism of a dual fluorochrome Tat-nanoparticle in HeLa Cells," *Bioconj. Chem.* 14(6) (2003): 1115–1121.

[63] Huh, Y. M., et al., "In vivo magnetic resonance detection of cancer by using multifunctional magnetic nanocrystals," *J. Am. Chem. Soc.* 127(35) (2005): 12387–12391.

[64] Veiseh, O., et al., "Optical and MRI multifunctional nanoprobe for targeting gliomas," *Nano Lett.* 5(6) (2005): 1003–1008.

[65] Funovics, M., et al., "Nanoparticles for the optical imaging of tumor E-selectin," *Neoplasia* 7(10) (2005): 904–911.

[66] Quinti, L., R. Weissleder, and C. H. Tung, "A fluorescent nanosensor for apoptotic cells," *Nano Lett.* 6(3) (2006): 488–490.

[67] Lee, H., et al., "Thermally cross-linked superparamagnetic iron oxide nanoparticles: Synthesis and application as a dual imaging probe for cancer in vivo," *J. Am. Chem. Soc.* 129 (2007): 12739–12745.

[68] Jaffer, F., A., et al., "Cellular imaging of inflammation in atherosclerosis using magnetofluorescent nanomaterials," *Mol. Imag.* 5 (2006): 85–92.

[69] Denis, M. C., et al., "Imaging inflammation of the pancreatic islets in type 1 diabetes," *Proc. Natl. Acad. Sci.* 101 (2004): 12634–12639.

[70] Medarova, Z., et al., "In vivo multimodal imaging of transplanted pancreatic islets," *Nat. Protoc.* 1 (2006): 429–435.

[71] Pittet, M. J., et al., "Labeling of immune cells for in vivo imaging using magnetofluorescent nanoparticles," *Nat. Protoc.* 1(1) (2006): 73–79.

[72] Schellenberger, E. A., et al., "Magneto/optical annexin V, a multimodal protein," *Bioconj. Chem.* 15(5) (2004): 1062–1064.

[73] Sosnovik, D. E., et al., "Magnetic resonance imaging of cardiomyocyte apoptosis with a novel magneto-optical nanoparticle," *Mag. Res. Med.* 54 (2005): 718–724.

[74] Kelly, K. A., et al., "Detection of vascular adhesion molecule-1 expression using a novel multimodal nanoparticle," *Circ. Res.* 96 (2005): 327–336.

[75] Josephson, L., et al., "Near-infrared fluorescent nanoparticles as combined MR/optical imaging probes," *Bioconj. Chem.* 13 (2002): 554–560.

[76] van Tilborg, G. A. F., et al., "Annexin A5-functionalized bimodal lipid-based contrast agents for the detection of apoptosis," *Bioconj. Chem.* 17(4) (2006): 741–749.

[77] Mulder, W. J. M., et al., "A liposomal system for contrast-enhanced magnetic resonance imaging of molecular targets," *Bioconj. Chem.* 15 (2004): 799–806.

[78] Larson, T. A., et al., "Hybrid plasmonic magnetic nanoparticles as molecular specific agents for MRI/optical imaging and photothermal therapy of cancer cells," *Nanotechnology* 18 (2007): 325101–325108.

[79] Bridot, J. L., et al., "Hybrid gadolinium oxide nanoparticles: Multimodal contrast agents for in vivo imaging," *J. Am. Chem. Soc.* 129(16) (2007): 5076–5084.

[80] Ding, H., et al., "Gold nanorods coated with multilayer polyelectrolyte as contrast agents for multimodal imaging," *J. Phys. Chem. C* 111 (2007): 12552–12557.

[81] Li, H., et al., "MR and fluorescent imaging of low-density lipoprotein receptors," *Acad. Radiol.* 11(11) (2004): 1251–1259.

[82] Frias, J. C., et al., "Properties of a versatile nanoparticle platform contrast agent to image and characterize atherosclerotic plaques by magnetic resonance imaging," *Nano Lett.* 6 (2006): 2220–2224.

[83] Corbin, I. R., et al., "Low-density lipoprotein nanoparticles as magnetic resonance imaging contrast agents," *Neoplasia* 8 (2006): 488–498.

[84] Lipinski, M. J., et al., "MRI to detect atherosclerosis with gadolinium-containing immunomicelles targeting the macrophage scavenger receptor," *Mag. Res. Med.* 56 (2006): 601–610.

[85] Mulder, W. J. M., et al., "MR molecular imaging and fluorescence microscopy for identification of activated tumor endothelium using a bimodal lipidic nanoparticle," *FASEB J.* 19 (2005): 2008–2010.

[86] Talanov, V. S., et al., "Dendrimer-based nanoprobe for dual modality magnetic resonance and fluorescence imaging," *Nano Lett.* 6 (2006): 1459–1463.

[87] Modo, M., et al., "Mapping transplanted stem cell migration after a stroke: A serial, in vivo magnetic resonance imaging study," *NeuroImage* 21 (2004): 311–317.

[88] Uzgiris, E. E., et al., "A multimodal contrast agent for preoperative MR imaging and intraoperative tumor margin delineation," *Technol. Canc. Res. Treat.* 5 (2006): 301–309.

[89] Manning, H. C., et al., "Targeted molecular imaging agents for cellular-scale bimodal imaging," *Bioconj. Chem.* 15 (2004): 1488–1495.

[90] Mulder, W. J. M., et al., "Quantum dots with a paramagnetic coating as a bimodal molecular imaging probe," *Nano Lett.* 6 (2006): 1–6.

[91] Prinzen, L., et al., "Optical and magnetic resonance imaging of cell death and platelet activation using annexin A5-functionalized quantum dots," *Nano Lett.* 7 (2007): 93–100.

[92] Shizhong, W., et al., "Core/shell quantum dots with high relaxivity and photoluminescence for multimodality imaging," *J. Am. Chem. Soc.* 129 (2007): 3848–3856.

[93] Anderson, E. A., et al., "Viral nanoparticles donning a paramagnetic coat: Conjugation of MRI contrast agents to the MS2 capsid," *Nano Lett.* 6 (2006): 1160–1164.

[94] Zhang, Z., et al., "Monomolecular multimodal fluorescence-radioisotope imaging agents," *Bioconj. Chem.* 16 (2005): 1232–1239.

[95] Edwards, W. B., et al., "Synthesis and radiolabeling of a somatostatin analog for multimodal imaging," *Proc. SPIE* 6097(3) (2006): 1–8.

[96] Zhang, Z., and S. Achilefu, "Spectral properties of pro-multimodal imaging agents derived from a NIR dye and a metal chelator," *Photochem. Photobiol.* 81 (2005): 1499–1504.

[97] Xu, H., et al., "Design, synthesis, and characterization of a dual modality positron emission tomography and fluorescence imaging agent for monoclonal antibody tumor-targeted imaging," *J. Medicin. Chem.* 50 (2007): 4759–4765.

[98] Houston, J. P., et al., "Quality analysis of in vivo near-infrared fluorescence and conventional gamma images acquired using a dual-labeled tumor-targeting probe," *J. Biomed. Opt.* 10(054010) (2005): 1–11.

[99] Li, C., et al., "Dual optical and nuclear imaging in human melanoma xenografts using a single targeted imaging probe," *Nucl. Med. Biol.* 33 (2006): 349–358.

[100] Hu, G., et al., "Imaging of Vx-2 rabbit tumors with $\alpha_v\beta_3$-integrin-targeted 111In nanoparticles," *Int. J. Canc.* 120 (2007): 1951–1957.

[101] Pandey, S. K., et al., "Multimodality agents for tumor imaging (PET, fluorescence) and photodynamic therapy: A possible 'see and treat' approach," *J. Medicin. Chem.* 48 (2005): 6286–6295.

[102] Culver, J., W. Akers, and S. Achilefu, "Multimodality molecular imaging with combined optical and SPECT/PET modalities," *J. Nucl. Med.* 49 (2008): 169–172.

[103] Chen, Y., et al., "A novel approach to a bifunctional photosensitizer for tumor imaging and phototherapy," *Bioconj. Chem.* 16 (2005): 1264–1274.

[104] McCarthy, J. R., F. A. Jaffer, and R. Weissleder, "A macrophage-targeted theranostic nanoparticle for biomedical applications," *Small* 2 (2006): 983–987.

[105] Reddy, G. R., et al., "Vascular targeted nanoparticles for imaging and treatment of brain tumors," *Clin. Canc. Res.* 12 (2006): 6677–6686.

[106] Tréhin, R., et al., "Fluorescent nanoparticle uptake for brain tumor visualization," *Neoplasia* 8 (2006): 302–311.

[107] Gobin, A. M., et al., "Near-infrared resonant nanoshells for combined optical imaging and photothermal cancer therapy," *Nano Lett.* 7 (2007): 1929–1934.

CHAPTER 17
Emerging Optical Imaging Techniques: Fluorescence Molecular Tomography and Beyond

Ralf B. Schulz and Vasilis Ntziachristos

17.1 Introduction

Imaging the spatial distribution of specific biomarkers inside tissue is an essential requirement for the advancement of biological sciences. The interest to employ optical imaging methods for that purpose has been sparked by the development of a large number of fluorescence-emitting molecular probes that allow tagging an optical signal to specific biochemical processes or molecules [1]. Optical imaging research originally focused on ex vivo methods studying thin tissue sections in which photon scattering remained negligible, so simple microscopy or photographic imaging techniques proved sufficient. However, such studies were not capable of tracking the development and treatment of a disease in living specimen over time or dynamic interactions of tissue components.

To enable biological study in unperturbed environments and over time, efforts initially concentrated on physically eliminating signal from scattered photons to enable imaging in thick tissues [2–4]. Such methods, including optical coherence tomography and confocal or two-photon microscopy, can resolve tissue structures or the presence of fluorophores with a spatial resolution on the order of a few microns to a few hundred nanometers. Penetration depth in this case, however, is generally limited to less than the transport mean free path, which is the average distance a photon can travel before being absorbed or scattered. Typical mean free paths in biological tissues range within the order of 100 microns [5].

For deeper tissue penetration on the order of millimeters up to centimeters, the information from highly scattered photons needs to be included in the imaging process. Early macroscopic optical imaging methods used flat illumination for probe excitation and acquired planar images of the fluorescence. However, while these planar methods are often used for preclinical studies involving optical imaging, they are not quantitative and may lead to inaccurate images as the signal recorded is modulated by depth and tissue optical properties in an unknown fashion [6]. For this reason, the urge to develop tomographic techniques evolved as it is crucial to quantify probe concentration and spatially resolve probe localization.

In this chapter, we discuss the progress made in the development of quantitative tomographic techniques to resolve fluorophore concentration in vivo, describe the theoretical foundations of the techniques, and show several application examples. Furthermore, we give an overview of currently investigated optimizations of the described methods that have just recently emerged. We also provide an introduction to photoacoustic tomography as a promising new technique that could help in the development of improved fluorescence tomography systems.

17.2 From Planar Imaging to Tomography

17.2.1 Prerequisites

Crucial to all fluorescence-based optical imaging techniques is the availability of suitable molecular probes. Among other criteria, these probes can be distinguished according to:

- *Target:* Most probes are either unspecific blood-pooling agents, or they target specific receptor molecules, the activity of specific proteases, protein-protein interactions, gene expression, or other cellular processes.
- *Tagging method:* Depending on the target, probes are either unspecific, targeted—meaning that they attach themselves to their target (e.g., by the use of an antibody) such that the specific signal becomes visible after blood clearance of unbound probes—or activatable, such that the probe only creates a signal after activation by the target.
- *Probe type*: Apart from the most often used organic fluorescent dyes—with indocyanine derivates being the most popular—there are also some anorganic dyes under development, such as quantum dots or gold nanoshells, that offer certain advantages, such as high quantum efficiency, tunable emission wavelengths, and low photobleaching. Furthermore, by transfecting genes for light-emitting proteins, such as luciferases or fluorescent proteins, cells can be forced to synthesize their own dyes. This can be used, for example, for cell tracking in metastasizing tumors [7, 8].
- *Method of excitation:* Light emission is stimulated chemically in the case of bioluminescence or by use of an external light source for fluorescence excitation.
- *Emission wavelength, excitation wavelength* (if applicable).

For the development of imaging hardware, only the latter two categories are of greater importance. The choice of wavelength for fluorescent probes, for example, can solve or create an abundance of further problems, either due to the fact that tissue is highly absorbing or due to autofluorescence [5, 9]. For bioluminescence imaging (BLI), both effects only play a minor role as background noise is very low because of the absence of autoluminescence in most organisms. However, bioluminescence requires delivery of a substrate such as luciferin to bioluminescent target cells through the organism and its chemical barriers, a complex biochemical process [10], while fluorescence only requires the propagation of photons to the molecule, a much simpler physical process.

17.2.2 Bioluminescence and Fluorescence Imaging

Planar imaging techniques for fluorescence and bioluminescence signals have been the working horses for biomedical research involving optical molecular probes. These techniques are easy to implement and offer high throughput. Due to the pronounced scattering features of tissue and their relatively high absorption, however, signals are detected only from very limited depths of a few millimeters inside tissue, and resulting images are not absolutely quantitative [5]. Sometimes it is argued that planar imaging can be quantitative, at least if used in the same animal within a longitudinal study. However, it has been shown that even within the same animal, the change of signal amplitude due to the scattering of light can be misleading when trying to compare signal sources in this animal [6].

Thus, it is important to develop quantitative tomographic imaging strategies for both bioluminescence and fluorescence. This chapter covers mostly fluorescent tomographic techniques. While it is possible to use a tomographic approach for BLI by including spectral information [11, 12], method development is still at an early stage. Furthermore, reconstructions require an even more detailed a priori knowledge than necessary for fluorescence tomography, such as tissue structure and emission spectra of the targeted luciferase.

17.2.3 Data-Collection Modes

Figure 17.1 shows a comparison of the different features exhibited by different data-collection modes. Here, simulated fluorescence and bioluminescence signals caused by two sources at different depths within a slab are presented for planar as well as tomographic techniques. In general, bioluminescence as well as fluorescence signals can be detected from any side of the object. For fluorescence-based methods, signal detection on the same side as the external source is called reflectance mode, while detection on the opposite side is called transmission mode. Bioluminescence does not require an external source but is stimulated through a chemical compound that is metabolized by a specific enzyme (a luciferase), emitting photons during that process.

As can be seen in Figure 17.1, bioluminescence signals are heavily surface weighted, just like fluorescence signals acquired in reflectance mode. The signal originating from the emitter closest to the surface dominates the detected photon intensities. In transmission mode, however, both sources appear in the detected signal. The source hidden deeper in the tissue as seen from the detector appears less bright, and the distribution of light appears wider as it is more affected by scattering due to the longer path length. Over all, however, the signal seems less surface weighted. The properties of detected reflectance and transmission signals are caused by the fact that the photon flux created by the exterior source is strongly attenuated by the scattering within the tissue, exciting more the emitter closer to the source. The detector, on the other hand, is also more sensitive to emitters located near to it. In reflectance mode, both effects increase the sensitivity toward the superficial emit-

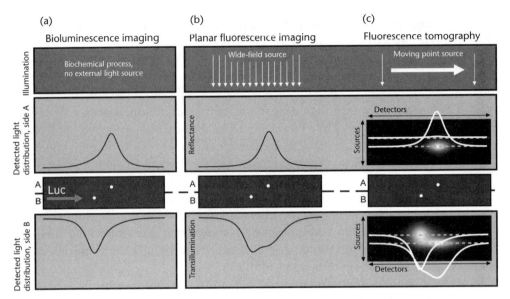

Figure 17.1 Differences between possible data-collection modes in optical imaging and the obtained information content. The shown curves and images present simulated signals of two point inclusions 6 mm distant to each other and hidden at a depth of 3 mm from either side of a 1 cm thick slab of tissuelike properties ($\mu_a = 0.3$ cm^{-1}, $\mu'_s = 10$ cm^{-1}). In all cases, emitted signals are shown for both sides of the slab. (a) For bioluminescence, a biochemical compound stimulates the emission of light. (b) Planar fluorescence imaging requires a homogeneous wide-field light source. The reflectance signal, obtained from the same side as the excitation, is similar to the bioluminescence signal in (a) but even more surface weighted. The intensity profile in transillumination mode, however, shows both emitters having comparable intensities. (c) For tomographic data acquisition, a point source is scanned over the object, and fluorescence distributions are recorded for each of these excitation points. These distributions are depicted as images, with the horizontal axis being the detector position, as before, and the vertical axis describing the different source positions, while gray values show the intensity. The intensity profiles from two exemplary sources are depicted in the images. Clearly, in tomographic mode, a lot more information is acquired regarding the position, depth, and intensity of the inclusions. Again, data obtained in transillumination mode provides better signal dynamics.

ter. In transmission mode, emitters close to the source are usually far from the detector, and vice versa, so both effects compensate for each other to some extent. This effect has lately been used for transillumination imaging of fluorescent proteins [13] as it is simple yet powerful, although it lacks the quantitative capabilities.

While planar fluorescence imaging employs a homogeneous wide-field source, tomographic acquisition is performed using a collimated point source that is moved to different positions, acquiring fluorescence intensities for all detectors at each. Obviously, a lot more data is obtained in this way, which allows for volumetric reconstruction (see Section 17.3.2). As Figure 17.1 shows, again in transillumination mode the signal from the superficial emitter dominates the detected profiles. However, the superficial emitter is not visible in all intensity profiles; if the dynamic range of the detector is adapted for each acquisition, those curves not containing a signal in Figure 17.1 will actually show some signal from the deeply hidden emitter, although it will be much weaker than in transillumination mode. Again, however, transillumination mode offers the highest information content at the best contrast. Both emitters are actually separable by looking at the two profiles depicted in the figure.

17.3 Fluorescence Molecular Tomography

To date, a significant number of novel imaging methods are emerging—among them fluorescence molecular tomography (FMT), which allows for quantitative volumetric reconstructions instead of providing only qualitative planar images of fluorescence. Fluorescence-based tomographic techniques were derived from the more general framework of diffuse optical tomography (DOT) in the mid-1990s. They aim to noninvasively estimate a spatial map of fluorescent probe concentration by illuminating the object under investigation with light at the excitation wavelength and subsequently measuring the generated fluorescence light distribution on the outer boundaries. By changing the position of the (usually collimated) light source, a number of measurements become available, allowing for tomographic reconstruction, just as in the case of DOT. One of the main differences from DOT, however, is the use of continuous excitation light; this becomes possible as the recovery of fluorescence is a linear process with only one unknown, the concentration (see Section 17.3.2).

17.3.1 Hardware Development

The first FMT systems included a number of continuous-wave sources and time-integrating detectors coupled to the object under investigation via light-guiding fibers [14]. The geometrical arrangement of sources and detectors was fixed such that the imaged object either had to be compressible enough to conform to that geometry or resulting gaps between object and source/detector fibers had to be filled with an optically matching liquid, usually a mixture of Intralipid, water, and ink to match the scattering and absorption coefficients of the object. Due to the fixed number of sources and detectors, resolution was limited; due to the use of a matching fluid, imaging procedures proved to be complex for small animals, which had to be embedded in the fluid, yet still able to breathe. However, the use of a fixed geometry minimizes the computational effort as it greatly simplifies solving the forward model.

A second-generation system restricted the angular coverage to approximately a mere 120° by placing the animal in a chamber with a slab geometry instead of a cylindrical geometry. One side of the chamber contained a fixed array of source fibers; the other side was made of glass and allowed a CCD camera to be used as a more flexible detection system, providing literally hundreds of detector measurements by using individual groups of binned pixels as one detector in a postprocessing step. In phantom experiments, submillimeter resolution was reported for this kind of system [15].

With these first- and second-generation systems (see Figure 17.2), it was difficult to correlate reconstructed fluorescent sources with the anatomical position

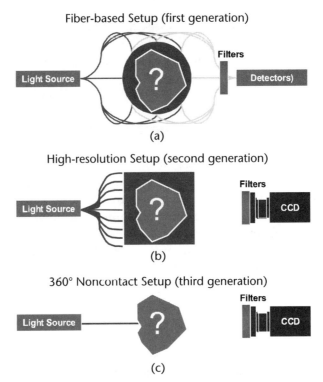

Figure 17.2 Different generations of fluorescence-mediated molecular tomography (FMT) systems. (a) Schematic drawing of a first-generation system, employing a fixed pattern of light-guiding fibers for detection and excitation from 360° of view around a cylindrical geometry. (b) Depiction of a second-generation system with planar geometry, using a CCD camera for detection. Experimental procedures required the mouse to be embedded in an optically matching fluid. Spatial resolution is on the order of 1 mm or better. (c) Third-generation systems do not require matching fluids or fibers, yielding high image performance together with a rendering of the animal's geometry.

inside the animal's body as no information on the shape or interior structure of the animal was obtained.

One of the most pronounced developments in recent years [16] is the implementation of noncontact imaging systems, which use a collimated free laser beam instead of light-guiding fibers as sources and a lens-coupled CCD camera as a multidetector array as employed in the second-generation systems (see [9] and references therein). By obtaining images from the outer surface of the animal, its shape can first be deduced and subsequently used to set up an adequate photon propagation model for that specific geometry. The latest generations of noncontact systems allow a full 360° view around the animal, and a large number of source-detector pairs yields high-resolution images, with a resolution of better than 1 mm in small animals. Figure 17.2 shows the development of different FMT generations from fixed-geometry, fiber-coupled systems to fully noncontact ones.

17.3.2 Image Reconstruction

Most often, FMT systems use a forward model based on the diffusion approximation to the radiative transport equation [17]:

$$[-\nabla D \nabla + \mu_a] U_m(\mathbf{r}) = n(\mathbf{r}) U_x(\mathbf{r}) \tag{17.1}$$

In (17.1), D and μ_a are the possibly spatially varying diffusion and absorption coefficients, $n \propto c$ is some function proportional to the concentration c of fluorochrome, and U_x/U_m describes the photon density at the excitation/emission wavelengths. For applications where absorption is low compared to the reduced scattering coefficient μ'_s, the diffusion coefficient is given by $D = \frac{1}{3}(\mu'_s)^{-1}$; if absorption is high, a better model results by using $D = \frac{1}{3}(\mu'_s + \alpha\mu_a)^{-1}$ with some adapted α [18]. If the optical coefficients are given, either by approximating them with constants or by obtaining them through some other imaging method (see the following sections), an explicit solution to (17.1) is expressed using the Green's functions of (17.1):

$$U_m(\mathbf{r}) = \int_{\mathbf{r}' \in V} G_m(\mathbf{r}, \mathbf{r}') n(\mathbf{r}') U_x(\mathbf{r}') d\mathbf{r}' \tag{17.2}$$

Equation (17.2) is a linear system that can be inverted using standard methods to yield n, a measure of concentration, for each voxel $\mathbf{r}'$ in volume V. For inversion, it is required to know the photon density U_x, which is usually modeled using the same Green's functions as U_m, thus assuming identical optical properties at both the excitation and emission wavelengths.

It is important to note that in order to calculate G, it is necessary to properly model boundary effects (i.e., the loss of light due to a tissue-air interface). Early FMT systems used a fixed geometry to simplify these calculations, but the development of proper analytical approximations and fast finite element solvers, in addition to increased computing power, have eliminated these limitations.

When applying (17.2) to real data, it must be considered that, apart from noise, individual detectors, even if pixels on a CCD, might have a different sensitivity for photon detection. Furthermore, the power of the source might depend on its position due to different tissue coupling efficiencies and, in the case of light-guiding fibers, to differing loss within the fibers. The photon density U_x is thus described as $U_x = \Theta_s U_x^0$, with source intensity Θ relative to the photon density created by a unit source U_x^0. This expression can be used in (17.2) such that $U_m = \Theta_s U_m^0$, with U_m^0 being the emitted photon density induced by unit source U_x^0. Detection occurs according to some detector sensitivity Θ, such that the detected photon densities $\hat{U}_x, \hat{U}_m$, become $\hat{U}_x = \Theta_d \Theta_s U_x^0$ and $\hat{U}_m = \Theta_d \Theta_s U_m^0$, respectively.

The effect of the different sensitivities and source intensities for different sources and detectors can be eliminated by reconstructing according to the normalized ratio $\hat{U}_m/\hat{U}_x = U_m^0/U_x^0$ instead of using (17.2) directly. It has been shown that this normalized approach also has advantages in the presence of heterogeneities of the optical coefficients [19].

17.3.3 Intrinsic Resolution Limits

The resolution of FMT techniques is limited by one or more of the following factors:

- *Number of sources and detectors:* The inverse problem of image reconstruction in FMT is highly ill-posed and ill-conditioned [17]. To reduce both effects, it is helpful to obtain data from as many source-detector pairs as possible. It has been shown that even for very small detector separations, the information content of the forward model (and thus the reconstruction quality) is ever increasing [20]. While for first-generation FMT systems the problem size (i.e., the number of measurements) was fixed due to the fixed number of light-guiding fibers, for CCD-based noncontact systems, the maximum number of data points is no longer restricted by imaging hardware but by available computer memory for reconstruction and the desired reconstruction time.

- *Accuracy of the theoretical model:* It is known that the diffusion equation, the most commonly used approximation to the radiative transport equation, is only valid for relatively large source-detector distances, high scattering, and low absorption [17]. For smaller objects, other models have been tried, including a Fokker-Planck approximation [21] for mesoscopic resolution or a modified Radon model for early photons at low scatter order [22]. However, even the radiative transport equation does not model all effects of light propagation as it considers photons to be individual particles, not interfering waves.

- *Accuracy of the assumed tissue properties:* While diffuse optical tomography (DOT) recovers tissue parameters during reconstruction, for the linear models of fluorescence excitation in continuous-wave mode, the spatially varying absorption and scattering coefficients need to be given prior to reconstruction. Usually, if nothing else is known, a homogeneous tissue having a mean absorption and scattering coefficient is assumed. This technique can be stabilized by normalization of emission with transillumination images [19], as described in Section 17.3.2.

- *Dynamic range of the detector:* Due to the scattering properties of tissues, obtained projection data exhibit a wide dynamic range. Furthermore, the more deeply the sources are localized inside the tissue, the smaller the differences between their signals become, and good dynamic resolution is required to separate them.

- *Size of investigated object:* As it gets more difficult to separate sources when hidden more deeply in an object, it follows that the thicker a specimen is, the lower the achievable resolution becomes for a given imaging setup.

- *Stability of source intensity and detector sensitivity:* Minute differences in the signal have significant influence on the reconstructed results as discussed above. Therefore, it is obvious that shifts in source intensity or detector sensitivity will disturb the reconstruction. If the shift is negligible between the acquisition of both the fluorescence images and the images at excitation wavelength, a normalization of the fluorescence with the excitation image will cure this defect (see Section 17.3.2).

17.4 FMT-Derived Imaging Modalities

Fluorescence-mediated molecular tomography (FMT) has developed from a highly experimental technique into a more established method. Advances in instrumentation and theoretical modeling enable the use of very large data sets consisting of many projections, allowing for whole-body small-animal imaging [9]. To date, the method has been validated in a number of preclinical application cases, such as measurement of tumor vascularization/blood volume [23], tumor progression under therapy [6], lymphatic function [24], protease activity [14, 25], and detection of fluorescent proteins [26–28]. Some of the recent developments and applications are detailed in the following.

17.4.1 Noncontact FMT

Noncontact FMT methods use a model for free-space transmission of the diffuse exitance from an object's surface to a detector, in addition to the diffusion modeling inside the object [9, 29]. Together with appropriate ways of treating the boundary conditions of the diffusion equation, the need for matching fluids and a fixed geometry is eliminated. These free-space systems additionally allow the acquisition of data arbitrarily at many projection angles, resulting in an arbitrary number of detector measurements. A single CCD camera is generally used in experiments to detect light emitted from the complexly shaped surface of the specimen, employing a noncontact forward model that correctly describes this geometry.

In addition to simplifying experimental procedures by eliminating fibers and matching fluids, a step necessary to increase applicability and acceptance of FMT, the method enabled the acquisition of a sufficient number of measurements for high-resolution reconstruction, which requires roughly 10^4 to 10^6 source-detector pairs [20]. Figure 17.3 depicts examples of noncontact imaging results [30].

17.4.2 Fluorescent Protein Tomography

Fluorescent proteins (FPs) offer a wide range of biological in vivo applications, ranging from the elucidation of gene activation and the functions of proteins within cells, to the biodistribution of immune, stem, and cancer cells, to the evaluation of drug candidates [9, 31]. While the first available proteins emitted in the green to yellow wavelength range, more and more synthetically created fluorescent proteins have been developed that emit farther in the red spectrum [32], nearly reaching the near-infrared region optimal for optical imaging in tissues. However, only very recently have these proteins reached a brightness and stability that is in any way comparable to the properties of green and yellow fluorescent proteins (GFP, YFP), and to date these new proteins have been applied in only a very few studies.

To image fluorescent protein expression in high resolution in vivo, confocal and multiphoton microscopy can be used, but they can only depict superficial locations down to a few hundred micrometers and in a very limited field of views [33]. Planar imaging methods are another alternative, but they suffer from the high level of autofluorescence present in the visible part of the spectrum and are thus often used in an invasive manner, removing the skin of the animal prior to imaging; other sys-

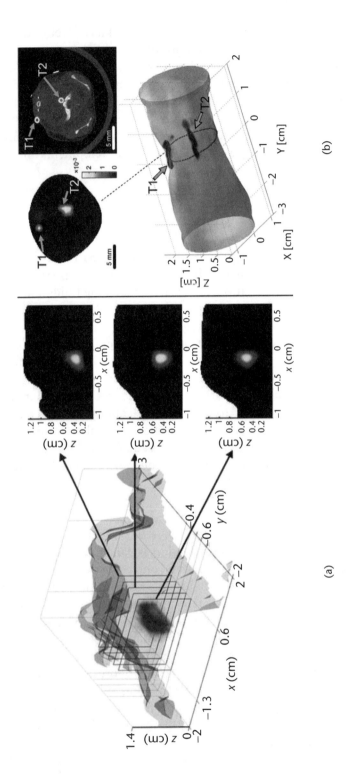

Figure 17.3 Results obtained using noncontact FMT. (a) A fluorescent tube was inserted into the esophagus of a euthanized nude mouse. On the left-hand side, the mouse shape is depicted as captured by a photogrammetric camera, containing a rendering of the tube. Small images on the right depict individual slices from the reconstructed volume. The system used an imaging chamber similar to a second-generation FMT system; thus, only one side of the outer boundaries was acquired. For details, refer to [29]. (b) Fully 360° noncontact results from a euthanized mouse containing two implantations. The outer boundaries were estimated using a volume carving technique based on white-light images acquired with the system's CCD. The images shown on top depict a slice of the reconstructed fluorescence concentration (left) as well as an X-ray CT slice (right) in which the two implanted tubes are marked. For details refer to [30].

tems try to improve the differentiation between fluorescence and autofluorescence by means of color separation [34].

Due to the high absorption and autofluorescence in the visible part of the spectrum, whole-body imaging of GFP- and YFP-labeled cells requires excellent optical filters and ultimate detection sensitivity—even more so if deeply located cells need to be detected as well, and quantification of protein concentration is required. To perform fluorescence tomography as described above, the forward model based on the diffusion approximation needs to be modified by using $D = \frac{1}{3}(\mu'_s + \alpha\mu_a)^{-1}$ for the diffusion coefficient (see Section 17.3.2). Figure 17.4 shows results from an in vivo imaging study. Fluorescence reflectance images are depicted as well and contain only autofluorescent signals, while tomographic reconstructions of FP emission are possible and deliver accurate results [18].

17.4.3 Mesoscopic Fluorescence Tomography

For the longitudinal imaging of small living entities such as developing insects, animal embryos, or the extremities of common small animals, neither microscopic nor macroscopic tomographic imaging approaches are suitable. For these applications, the former still do not offer sufficient penetration depths and fields of view, while the latter usually employ diffusion-based modeling, not accurate for small objects. A modified forward model in combination with an FMT setup suitable for microscopic imaging has been presented as what is called mesoscopic tomography [21].

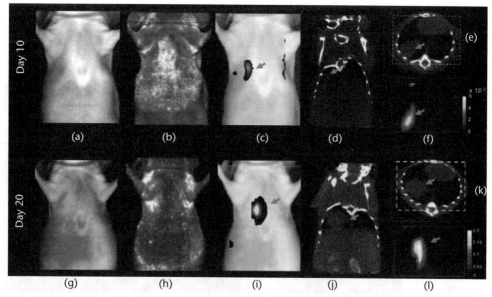

Figure 17.4 Fluorescent protein tomography (FPT) of GFP-labeled lung cancer cells. Depicted images were obtained after (a–f) 10 days and (g–l) 20 days of tumor growth. (a, g) White-light image of the mouse as positioned in the imaging system. (b, h) Reflectance images obtained using epi-illumination. Fluorescence signals originate from autofluorescence only; tumor-specific signals cannot be detected. (c, i) Coronal slice from the reconstructed FPT data set at a depth of approximately 7 mm below the skin, overlaid on the white-light image. (d, j) Coronal and (e, k) axial X-ray CT slices. Tumor sites are depicted with small arrows. (f, l) Axial slices from FPT data set. These slices correspond to the dashed rectangles shown in (e) and (k). For more details, see [18].

Previously, for the mentioned application cases, optical clearing methods were proposed; however, they can only be used ex vivo [35, 36]. These methods were demonstrated on mouse embryos and adult mouse brains, both objects having a thickness of up to 15 mm.

Optical clearing uses chemical compounds to level the refractive indices between tissue cells to reduce or eliminate scattering. Projection images of the treated specimen can then be tomographically reconstructed using approaches based on line integrals, as is known from X-ray CT.

Mesoscopic FMT, however, has recently proved its capability to noninvasively image insect development over time [21] (see also Figure 17.5). Pupae of *Drosophila melanogaster*, having a thickness of less than 1 mm, were imaged using a microscope-coupled 360° noncontact FMT setup. It was shown that even for those small objects, reconstruction methods based on line integrals do not yield sufficient resolution and accuracy. Instead, the Fokker-Planck approximation to the equation of radiative transfer was used, which can be used for high forward scattering, which is generally present in thin biological tissues. The imaging setup allowed visualization of GFP-labeled salivary glands as well as monitoring of wing-disc development over time.

17.4.4 Further Developments

Aside from the applications and methods described above, a number of other modifications to the general framework of FMT-based imaging modalities have been performed or are actively being researched. These changes include:

- *Using multiple wavelengths for excitation and detection:* A conventional FMT system uses one laser wavelength and a fixed set of emission filters. By using

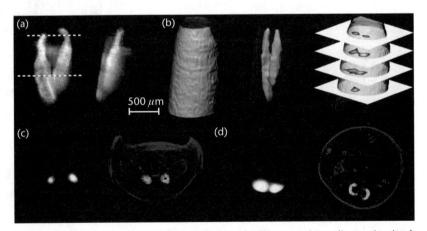

Figure 17.5 FMT at mesoscopic resolution: imaging of GFP-expressing salivary glands of *Drosophila melanogaster* imaged using a noncontact FMT setup coupled to a microscope. (a) Projection images of the salivary glands at 0° and 90° projection angles. The dashed lines mark the position of the two histological sections shown in (c, d). (b) Renderings of the reconstructed results, showing the outer surface of the pupae as established from bright-light images, a rendering of the reconstruction within that surface, and five exemplary slices. (c, d) The bottom row shows two exemplary slices together with histological results. For a detailed description of the experiments, refer to [21].

different excitation wavelengths, several different fluorochromes can be distinguished. This is particularly useful for applications, where the concentration of a specific probe needs to be related to the blood volume present; blood volume can be reliably estimated using FMT and appropriate blood-pooling agents [23].

On the detector side, the separation of many incoming wavelengths can help in eliminating autofluorescence in acquired images by correlating detected spectra with the probe's actual emission spectrum [37].

- *Adding time resolution:* As known from diffuse optical tomography, in addition to the use of a continuous-wave (CW) source, there are two operational modes for time-resolved operation, time-domain (TD) and frequency-domain (FD) operation. In TD mode, ultrafast light pulses probe the sample while detectors need to record incoming photons as a function of time. Recently, advances in the design of photomultipliers have lead to the development of gated CCD cameras with a time resolution on the order of 100 ps. These time-discrimination systems allow for the separation of detected photons according to arrival time and thus enable the rejection of highly diffuse photons. This might help increase resolution and sensitivity in diffuse optical tomography, but only proof-of-principle studies such as [22] have been published so far.

  Another possibility is FD mode. Here, a modulated light source at some frequency f is used for excitation. This induces a diffuse photon-density wave of the same frequency in the transilluminated medium. Detectors need to measure the light intensity and phase shift of the photon wavefront. These FD methods have been used to extract fluorescence lifetime in order to separate autofluorescence from desired probe emission, as well as for estimation of optical properties [38–40]. In general, FD methods are not as sensitive to ambient light as CW and TD methods, but they require very high modulation frequencies to achieve better results than CW mode.

- *Multimodality imaging:* The reconstruction according to (17.1) requires prior knowledge of the optical coefficients within the imaged specimen. While the normalized approach stabilizes the results with respect to absorptive heterogeneities [19], a better model description could potentially cover heterogeneities in the diffusion coefficient as well and thus further improve reconstruction quality. A special implementation of a combined imaging modality is described in Section 17.5.2.

17.5 Photoacoustic Tomography

Photoacoustic tomography (PAT) [9, 41] is an emerging technique capable of recovering the optical absorption coefficients in tissues by detecting ultrasonic waves originating from a photoacoustic interaction of a short laser pulse with tissue. The incident light pulse will be absorbed by tissue cells, instantaneously creating a small temperature elevation and thus a thermal expansion. The expansion in turn gives rise to an acoustic pressure wave, which will propagate through the sample and subsequently be detected on the sample's outside as an acoustic signal. While the effect can be observed with any radiation that will increase sample temperature, such as microwaves, the use of visible light is especially useful in the context of bioimaging.

Since PAT's first reported use for biological purposes [42], different systems have been developed for preclinical use [43], and even clinical applications for optical mammography have been proposed [44–46]. Compared to other optical whole-body techniques, PAT offers an excellent resolution of a few hundred microns, which can even be improved by coupling the technique to a microscope [47, 48]. By using several different wavelengths, it is possible to distinguish different chromophores and thus use the technique for fluorophore detection or blood-oxygenation measurements [48–51].

17.5.1 Photoacoustic Theory

Theoretically, the pressure wave p following the absorption of a very short light pulse of fluence U is modeled using the wave equation [41]:

$$\frac{1}{v_s^2} \frac{\partial^2 p(\mathbf{r},t)}{\partial t^2} - \nabla^2 p(\mathbf{r},t) = \frac{\beta \mu_a}{C} \frac{\partial U(\mathbf{r},t)}{\partial t} \tag{17.3}$$

In (17.3), further coefficients are the speed of sound (v_s) in the media, the mass density (β), the isobaric volume expansion coefficient (C), and the optical absorption coefficient for the incident wavelength (μ_a), all of which are possibly varying according to spatial coordinate or wavelength. One simplification included in this equation is the negligence of thermal conduction (i.e., the resolution is limited by the duration of the incident light pulse, which needs to be short enough to confine the thermal energy within one voxel of the reconstructed data set).

For reconstruction, it is first necessary to relate the acoustic signal measured on the outer surface of the imaged object, which is the integration of the pressure wave over all internal pressure sources, to the presence of pressure sources p_s within the tissue. Recently, a general back-projection algorithm was proposed [52], which is based on the surface integral over the outer surface S' of the investigated object:

$$p_s(\mathbf{r}) = \frac{1}{2\pi} \oiint_{\mathbf{r}' \in S'} \frac{\bar{t} \partial p(\mathbf{r}', \bar{t})/\partial t - p(\mathbf{r}', \bar{t})}{|\mathbf{r} - \mathbf{r}'|^3} n_{\mathbf{r}'} \cdot (\mathbf{r} - \mathbf{r}') d\mathbf{r}' \bigg|_{\bar{t} = (\mathbf{r} - \mathbf{r}')/v_s} \tag{17.4}$$

Equation (17.4) is a linear system on the time-based measurements of sound pressure on the surface of the investigated object, theoretically requiring full surface coverage. To relate sound pressure p_s to optical absorption μ_a, it is necessary to assume that the pressure relaxation during the laser pulse is insignificant [53], yielding:

$$\mu_a(\mathbf{r}) = \frac{C^2}{\beta v_s} \frac{p_s(\mathbf{r})}{U(\mathbf{r})} \tag{17.5}$$

In (17.5), U is the local magnitude of laser fluence during the laser pulse. Regarding the approximation validity, laser pulses of less than 100 ns duration fulfill both requirements, heat confinement as well as insignificant pressure relaxation in biological tissues [53].

In order to solve (17.5) it is obviously necessary to obtain an estimate of photon density U, which in turn requires a model of light propagation and prior knowledge about the optical tissue coefficients. During reconstruction, the forward model used to calculate U and the resulting absorption μ_a can be iteratively refined if necessary.

17.5.2 Combined FMT-PAT Imaging

As PAT targets the intrinsic absorption of tissue, it is not per se a molecular or functional imaging modality, but rather a morphological one. By using different wavelengths at the same time, it can, however, be used to target contrasts of different biological chromophores, such as the difference in absorption spectra between oxy- and deoxyhemoglobin to determine tissue oxygenation [50]. Furthermore, fluorescent dyes could act as contrast agents, specifically increasing the absorption of targeted biostructures; again, by using multiple wavelengths, absorption spectra of the fluorophore can more easily be distinguished from intrinsic tissue absorption, yielding a sensitivity in the femtomolar range and resolution on the order of a few hundred microns [49].

Another interesting approach is the emerging combination of PAT and FMT [53] (see Figure 17.6). For optimal performance, FMT requires proper knowledge about the tissue structure (i.e., the spatially varying scattering and absorption coefficients). While it has been shown that the normalization of emission images with transillumination images stabilizes reconstruction outcome [19], for large heterogeneities, deviations will still be observed. As PAT can spatially resolve the tissue absorption coefficients for any given wavelength, it is straightforward to feed these results into the forward model used for FMT reconstruction. An initial study reported that this approach improved the quality of reconstructions in terms of localization accuracy as well as spatial resolution [53].

17.6 Summary

The emerging fluorescence-based imaging techniques described herein present an important advancement in the field of optical small-animal imaging. The advantages of optically active molecular probes—high specificity, no radiation safety issues for synthesis and application, high stability, the ability to create optical switches via molecular beacons, and the possibility of using different emission wavelengths simultaneously—can only develop their full potential for biomedical research if used in conjunction with accurate, noninvasive, quantitative in vivo tomographic techniques that are able to make use of the aforementioned properties.

Fluorescence tomography is currently transforming into a reliable, validated imaging technique of constantly improving spatial resolution. Although the method will never reach resolutions common to microscopy, it offers very high sensitivity in the femtomolar range. Furthermore, the probes used for fluorescence microscopy or other ex vivo techniques are the same as those used for FMT. Thus, a longitudinal

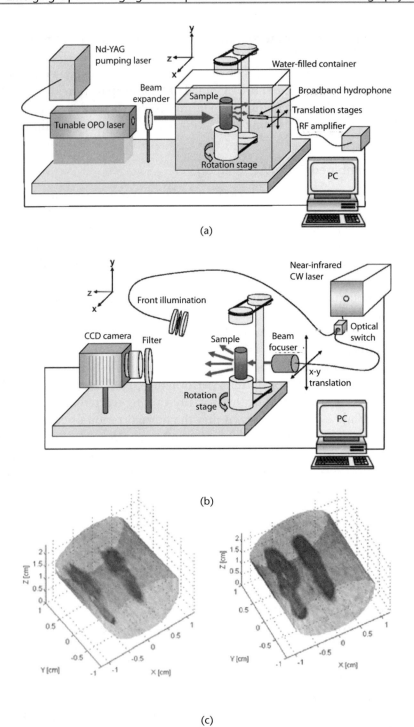

Figure 17.6 Results from combined fluorescence and photoacoustic tomography (see [53]). (a) Photoacoustic setup. The expanded beam of a pulsed, tunable laser is directed onto the sample, which is mounted on a rotation stage. Induced photoacoustic signals are recorded by an acoustic hydrophone, which can be translated along the vertical axis. Total acquisition time for each experiment is approximately 30 minutes. (b) Setup of a 360° noncontact FMT scanner using a continuous-wave laser diode at 748 nm and a cooled CCD camera. (c) Rendering of FMT results obtained with an optically inhomogeneous, cylindrical phantom containing two fluorescent inclusions. Left: Reconstructions using optical properties as established by PAT. Right: Reconstructions using a homogeneous model. The reconstructed inclusions are larger in size and shifted in position compared to the combined PAT/FMT images and the actual situation.

FMT study can always be validated in the end using microscopy on tissue sections of study animals.

We are furthermore convinced that the immanent combination of optical with morphological imaging systems such as PAT or X-ray CT will create a new generation of FMT systems showing unprecedented resolution, sensitivity, and reliability. This will further increase the acceptance and usability of FMT-derived methods.

References

[1] Rudin, M., and R. Weissleder, "Molecular imaging in drug discovery and development," *Nat. Rev. Drug Disc.* 2(2) (2003): 123–131.

[2] Helmchen, F., and W. Denk, "Deep tissue two-photon microscopy," *Nat. Methods* 2(12) (2005): 932–940.

[3] Yuste, R., "Fluorescence microscopy today," *Nat. Methods* 2(12) (2005): 902–904.

[4] Low, A. F., et al., "Technology insight: Optical coherence tomography—current status and future development," *Nat. Clin. Prac. Cardiovasc. Med.* 3(3) (2006): 154–162.

[5] Weissleder, R., and V. Ntziachristos, "Shedding light onto live molecular targets," *Nat. Med.* 9(1) (2003): 123–128.

[6] Ntziachristos, V., et al., "Visualization of antitumor treatment by means of fluorescence molecular tomography with an annexin V-Cy5.5 conjugate," *Proc. Natl. Acad. Sci. USA* 101(33) (2004): 12294–12299.

[7] Hoffman, R. M., "Recent advances on in vivo imaging with fluorescent proteins," in Kevin F. Sullivan (ed.), *Fluorescent proteins, second edition*, Methods in Cell Biology 85, London: Academic Press, 2008, 485–495.

[8] Ikeda, N., et al., "Comprehensive diagnostic bronchoscopy of central-type early-stage lung cancer," *Lung Canc.* 56(3) (2007): 295–302.

[9] Ntziachristos, V., et al., "Looking and listening to light: The evolution of whole-body photonic imaging," *Nat. Biotechnol.* 23(3) (2005): 313–320.

[10] Massoud, T. F., and S. S. Gambhir, "Molecular imaging in living subjects: Seeing fundamental biological processes in a new light," *Genes Develop.* 17(5) (2003): 545–580.

[11] Wang, G., et al., "Recent development in bioluminescence tomography," *Curr. Med. Imag. Rev.* 2(4) (2006): 453–457.

[12] Dehghani, H., et al., "Spectrally resolved bioluminescence optical tomography," *Opt. Lett.* 31(3) (2006): 365–367.

[13] Zacharakis, G., et al., "Normalized transillumination of fluorescent proteins in small animals," *Mol. Imag.* 5(3) (2006): 153–159.

[14] Ntziachristos, V., et al., "Fluorescence molecular tomography resolves protease activity in vivo," *Nat. Med.* 8(7) (2002): 757–760.

[15] Graves, E. E., et al., "A submillimeter resolution fluorescence molecular imaging system for small animal imaging," *Med. Phys.* 30(5) (2003): 901–911.

[16] Hielscher, A. H., "Optical tomographic imaging of small animals," *Curr. Opin. Biotechnol.* 16(1) (2005): 79–88.

[17] Arridge, S. R., "Optical tomography in medical imaging," *Inverse Problems* 15(2) (1999): R41–R93.

[18] Zacharakis, G., et al., "Volumetric tomography of fluorescent proteins through small animals in vivo," *Proc. Natl. Acad. Sci. USA* 102(51) (2005): 18252–18257.

[19] Soubret, A., J. Ripoll, and V. Ntziachristos, "Accuracy of fluorescent tomography in the presence of heterogeneities: Study of the normalized born ratio," *IEEE Trans. Med. Imag.* 24(10) (2005): 1377–1386.

[20] Graves, E. E., et al., "Singular-value analysis and optimization of experimental parameters in fluorescence molecular tomography," *J. Opt. Soc. Am. A—Opt. Image Sci. Vision* 21(2) (2004): 231–241.

[21] Vinegoni, C., et al., "In vivo imaging of *Drosophila melanogaster* pupae with mesoscopic fluorescence tomography," *Nat. Methods* 5 (2008): 45–47.

[22] Turner, G. M., et al., "Complete-angle projection diffuse optical tomography by use of early photons," *Opt. Lett.* 30(4) (2005): 409–411.

[23] Montet, X., et al., "Tomographic fluorescence imaging of tumor vascular volume in mice," *Radiology* 242(3) (2007): 751–758.

[24] Sharma, R., et al., "Quantitative imaging of lymph function," *Am. J. Physiol.—Heart Circ. Physiol.* 292(6) (2007): H3109–H3118.

[25] Nahrendorf, M., et al., "Dual channel optical tomographic imaging of leukocyte recruitment and protease activity in the healing myocardial infarct," *Circ. Res.* 100(8) (2007): 1218–1225.

[26] Garofalakis, A., et al., "Three-dimensional in vivo imaging of green fluorescent protein-expressing T cells in mice with noncontact fluorescence molecular tomography," *Mol. Imag.* 6(2) (2007): 96–107.

[27] Tam, J. M., et al., "Improved in vivo whole-animal detection limits of green fluorescent protein-expressing tumor lines by spectral fluorescence imaging," *Mol. Imag.* 6(4) (2007): 269–276.

[28] Zacharakis, G., et al., "Fluorescent protein tomography scanner for small animal imaging," *IEEE Trans. Med. Imag.* 24(7) (2005): 878–885.

[29] Schulz, R. B., J. Ripoll, and V. Ntziachristos, "Experimental fluorescence tomography of tissues with noncontact measurements," *IEEE Trans. Med. Imag.* 23(4) (2004): 492–500.

[30] Deliolanis, N., et al., "Free-space fluorescence molecular tomography utilizing 360 degrees geometry projections," *Opt. Lett.* 32(4) (2007): 382–384.

[31] Hoffman, R. M., "The multiple uses of fluorescent proteins to visualize cancer in vivo," *Nat. Rev. Canc.* 5(10) (2005): 796–806.

[32] Shaner, N. C., P. A. Steinbach, and R. Y. Tsien, "A guide to choosing fluorescent proteins," *Nat. Methods* 2(12) (2005): 905–909.

[33] Harisinghani, M. G., et al., "Splenic imaging with ultrasmall superparamagnetic iron oxide ferumoxtran-10 (AMI-7227): Preliminary observations," *J. Comput. Assist. Tomog.* 25(5) (2001): 770–776.

[34] Hoffman, R. M., and M. Yang, "Whole-body imaging with fluorescent proteins," *Nat. Protoc.* 1 (2006): 1429–1438.

[35] Sharpe, J., "Optical projection tomography," *Annu. Rev. Biomed. Eng.* 6 (2004): 209–228.

[36] Dodt, H. U., U. Leischner, A. Schierloh, N. Jährling, C. P. Mauch, K. Deininger, J. M. Deussing, M. Eder, W. Zieglgänsberger, and K. Becker, "Ultramicroscopy: Three-dimensional visualization of neuronal networks in the whole mouse brain," *Nat. Methods* 4(4) (2007): 307–308.

[37] Zavattini, G., et al., "A hyperspectral fluorescence system for 3D in vivo optical imaging," *Phys. Med. Biol.* 51(8) (2006): 2029–2043.

[38] Keren, S., et al., "A comparison between a time domain and continuous wave small animal optical imaging system," *IEEE Trans. Med. Imag.* 27 (2008): 58–63.

[39] Roy, R., A. Godavarty, and E. M. Sevick-Muraca, "Fluorescence-enhanced three-dimensional lifetime imaging: A phantom study," *Phys. Med. Biol.* 52(14) (2007): 4155–4170.

[40] Kumar, A. T. N., et al., "Time resolved fluorescence tomography of turbid media based on lifetime contrast," *Opt. Exp.* 14(25) (2006): 12255–12270.

[41] Wang, L. H. V., "Ultrasound-mediated biophotonic imaging: A review of acousto-optical tomography and photo-acoustic tomography," *Dis. Mark.* 19(2–3) (2003): 123–138.

[42] Wang, X. D., et al., "Photoacoustic tomography of biological tissues with high cross-section resolution: Reconstruction and experiment," *Med. Phys.* 29(12) (2002): 2799–2805.

[43] Xu, M. H., and L. H. V. Wang, "Photoacoustic imaging in biomedicine," *Rev. Sci. Instr.* 77(4) (2006): 041101.

[44] Manohar, S., et al., "Photoacoustic mammography laboratory prototype: Imaging of breast tissue phantoms," *J. Biomed. Opt.* 9(6) (2004): 1172–1181.

[45] Gu, H. M., S. H. Yang, and L. Z. Xiang, "Photoacoustic tomography and applications in the medical clinic diagnosis," *Prog. Biochem. Biophys.* 33(5) (2006): 431–437.

[46] Ku, G., et al., "Thermoacoustic and photoacoustic tomography of thick biological tissues toward breast imaging," *Technol. Canc. Res. Treat.* 4(5) (2005): 559–565.

[47] Zhang, H. F., K. Maslov, and L. V. Wang, "In vivo imaging of subcutaneous structures using functional photoacoustic microscopy," *Nat. Protoc.* 2(4) (2007): 797–804.

[48] Zhang, H. F., et al., "Functional photoacoustic microscopy for high-resolution and noninvasive in vivo imaging," *Nat. Biotechnol.* 24(7) (2006): 848–851.

[49] Razansky, D., C. Vinegoni, and V. Ntziachristos, "Multispectral photoacoustic imaging of fluorochromes in small animals," *Opt. Lett.* 32 (2007): 2891–2893.

[50] Wang, X. D., et al., "Noninvasive imaging of hemoglobin concentration and oxygenation in the rat brain using high-resolution photoacoustic tomography," *J. Biomed. Opt.* 11(2) (2006): 024015.

[51] Zhang, H. F., et al., "Imaging of hemoglobin oxygen saturation variations in single vessels in vivo using photoacoustic microscopy," *Appl. Phys. Lett.* 90(5) (2007): 053901.

[52] Xu, M. H., and L. H. V. Wang, "Universal back-projection algorithm for photoacoustic computed tomography," *Physic. Rev. E* 71(1) (2005): 016706.

[53] Razansky, D., and V. Ntziachristos, "Hybrid photoacoustic fluorescence molecular tomography using finite-element-based inversion," *Med. Phys.* 34 (2007): 4293–4301.

CHAPTER 18
From Benchtop to Boardroom: Staying Market Focused*

David A. Benaron

Sitting in a pitch-black room at Stanford, Chris Contag and I stared at a Petri dish streaked with the genetically transformed bacteria that his wife, Pam, had engineered. Slowly, our eyes adapted to the darkness, and we began to see the faint colonies of glowing green bacteria. At that instant, I knew we could change biomedical imaging by noninvasively sensing small populations of these genetically labeled cells in the bodies of living animals. Later, as the full implications of this event became clear, I remained awake well into the night.

Shortly thereafter, the Contags suggested we had something that could really pull in grants. "No," I countered. "What we have is a really good company." And with that, Xenogen was born, eventually reaching a $112 million valuation at public offering in 2004, followed by acquisition by Caliper in 2006. Xenogen, with its proprietary ability to noninvasively track infection, cancer, and stem cells down to just a few hundred cells (when millions of cells were required before), remains the standout leader in optical molecular imaging a decade later.

So, what made this a biophotonics company and not just a series of grants?

18.1 Identify the Market

The first step to a successful entrepreneurial business is to identify your product-specific market. This determines who the customers are, how to build a sales team, and how large the return on investment may ultimately be. You can't just say, "We address cancer," as such top-down methods grossly overestimate how your product will be used. Rather, you say, "We address the diagnosis of prostate cancer, for which there are x tests per year, costing y." If you address a new market, you need to consider how you will induce demand when demand is currently zero. Consider whether your idea is a one-trick pony or can serve as a platform for a series of products, services, or licenses that would support a growing company.

---

*This chapter is based on "Seeing the Light Through the Eyes of an Entrepreneur," an article that originally appeared in *SPIE Professional Magazine* in April 2008 (http://spie.org/x24276.xml) and was modified with permission as a derivative work thereof.

Failing to reach clarity on this issue is the single most common error in business plans from inventors, especially when they try to value their own invention. The specific market is the key and defines the potential business value—and it creates the story line for investment in your business. For Xenogen, our discovery was directed to a large and growing market, lead selection in drug discovery, which allowed Xenogen to attract the multiple financing rounds required to launch the product. For FirstScan, we started with the market. We first looked only where billion-dollar markets and significant market growth we expected: oncology, women's health, and age-related illnesses. We next identified an unmet need for the early detection and screening of breast cancer, a product-specific market we estimated at $10 billion per year. Last, we estimated the cost to bring a device to market: $5 million to develop, $20 million to clinically test, and $75 million to launch, leaving a reasonable risk-adjusted return and clear milestones for reducing risk and increasing value at each stage.

Only then did we look for the right technology. We selected optical spectroscopy with tissue-component characterization (fat, water, heme, wavelength shift, and other markers) as being the most robust and closest to clinical use. We identified who had existing technology rights and in-licensed these rights from the University of California, MIT, the University of Pennsylvania, and others, collecting over 70 patents directed toward this device and market. Then, through the creation of an affiliate, FirstScan (an alliance between Spectros, the University of California at Irvine, MIT, the University of Pennsylvania, and other partners), we set out to develop a molecular-sensing clinical device for the early and specific detection of breast cancer and other metabolic diseases, a market estimated at $10 billion per year. Only when these structures were in place, including a path to exit, did we raise the first $5 million privately to build the first commercial prototype and take this to trial.

18.2 Technology Alone Has Little Value

From the viewpoint of any strategic partner or investor you approach, there are many reasons why technology alone has little initial business value. Companies see a stream of inventors pass through, and the story is always the same: please give me a few million dollars to prove my technology, and for this opportunity to invest, I will offer certain limited rights.

The flaw with this approach is that there are nearly always a half-dozen similar inventions, and each inventor claims his or her invention works best. Companies worry that with too early an investment, they will bet on the wrong horse or that the problem will turn out to be better served using an unrelated technology. In fact, corporations receive strong financial disincentives for such R&D investments from Wall Street, which rewards them only for sales in the prior fiscal quarter, not for R&D.

From a small-business viewpoint, this is a critical aspect. I assume that all the technologies on the benchtop will work, and the key becomes understanding if there is a market there once they do. This is not to say that technology always has little or no business value. Indeed, proprietary technology that addresses a need more effectively or cheaply than others has a very high commercial value. Controlling a gateway technology protects your company's market and raises your value during acquisition or public offering.

18.3   Find a Business Mentor

Finding a good business leader and mentor is a first step in distinguishing your business from the background noise.

When you decide to develop your new product as a business, your new company will no longer be about you and your amazing idea. Rather, it changes to focuses on a reasonably maximized return on the capital received from investors to begin and run the company, which is a market-driven story, not a technology- or inventor-driven story. Managing a company at this new stage requires very different skills than inventing, such as a dispassionate objectivity that inventors often lack. It also requires fluency in financial terms and deal structures that will make or break the success as well as comfort with the objective metrics that will evaluate your start-up effort. You also must be able to manage investor expectations.

Those varied skills can and do exist at times in one inventor entrepreneur. But, if you don't have sufficient knowledge or the experience to take a company from funding through exit, you will most likely fail to attract the right people and the smart capital you need to start the business. Remember, marketing costs dwarf technology development costs, and you will need someone who can raise and manage all aspects of the growing business.

The time to start looking for a business-trained partner is before you begin to raise money. Preferably, find a partner who has business experience in your market and someone who will mentor you. We followed this approach at Xenogen. I was already a physician and inventor and had trained in optical biophysics with Britton Chance at the University of Pennsylvania by the time we glimpsed that glowing bacteria. Similarly, Pamela Contag was a microbiologist with experience in market and opportunity valuations, and she had independently conceived of the same idea. However, we needed someone who better understood business and would show the venture capital community that an investment with us would be properly managed.

18.4   Tell a Story Using the Right Terms

In many respects, building a business (raising capital, closing deals, talking to strategic partners, and executing public offerings) is really all about telling a good story using the right terms.

The bottom line for entrepreneurs is that it is not about how smart you are or how well you can describe the technology. Rather, it is about having the right skill set and the right vocabulary to convince the right investors as well as to lead the company. Entrepreneurs think projects and knowledge are exciting, while management eschews distractions and seeks simple, sound-bite clarity. If you don't think you could tell the same, unchanging story, day after day, with the same excitement or look investment bankers in the eye and tell them enthusiastically, "We expect the company to continue to outperform the sector for the foreseeable future," and mean it, then you need a good business person at the top.

In contrast, at Spectros, I had been through the process several times. In this case, we recruited several trial CEOs, but none had the enthusiasm or insight of the founding team. We focused the company on advanced molecular sensing and imaging devices that shed light on life-threatening diseases, including cancer and ischemia, a condition in which tissues receive insufficient blood flow. Spectros's flagship T-Stat product was the first device labeled by the U.S. FDA as "sensitive to ischemia." Red Herring recently evaluated Spectros and the ischemia market and estimated annual sales could reach $3 billion in monitors and up to $10 billion in sensors and probes, which dwarfs the mature pulse oximetry market.

18.5 Focus Is the Key

With the right technology, people, and market understanding in hand, you can focus on exactly what your product or business will be, with focus being key. When you are adequately focused, you usually can describe your specific market in a sentence. Here are some examples: "FirstScan is a women's health company focused on early molecular screening for breast cancer, allowing for improved survival and reduced treatment toxicity." Or, "Spectros is a molecular detection company focused on the real-time detection of ischemia, the final common pathway for nearly all organ failure and death in the hospital."

Use your core mission as a sword (or mantra) to cut through anything that is off topic or tangential. For many entrepreneurs, the hardest thing to do is to remain focused and say no to interesting tangents and distractions. Listen carefully to what comes your way, but turn down vastly more opportunities than you accept.

It's important to show you can be, at least in theory, successful with your first product. If you can do this, you have differentiated yourself from academic efforts in a second way. Still, pick good, flexible people and have a backup plan. Few successful medical device companies find success with Plan A. Genentech is a classic example. The first drugs on Genentech's list were industrial chemicals and food-processing additives; none of its first real successes were even on that list (in this regard, I recommend Cynthia Robbins-Roth's *From Alchemy to IPO: The Business of Biotechnology* [1]).

Focus should not be confused with a narrow skill set. Don't hire people just because they do exactly what you *think* your company is going to need, unless they serve at the lowest levels. Things change, as noted above. Rather, hire people who are great to work with, flexible, and insightful. If you hire your team just for their unique skills, when the company evolves, these talented but specialized people will be like fish out of water. Instead, if you just hire good people, then when the seas change, your team members can ride the changes out and capitalize on their knowledge to become excellent in whatever area the company chooses. Again, for more reading on this, try Jim Collins's *Good to Great* [2].

18.6 Build Value

If you have a focused plan, proper business involvement, and a clear path to market, it is finally time to raise some funds. Timing is everything. Green businesses are hotly fundable in 2008, just as biotech was in the 1980s and the Internet was in the 1990s. The same goes for exit strategies.

The best you can do is create value for your company at each step. If you weigh every decision along the way by how it serves the core mission and builds value, you will be in the best position for all contingencies, whether this means raising more funds, keeping investors happy, doing a deal, or selling the company.

Of course, raising value at each step is not always possible; here, building value minimizes the depth of the crashes. Xenogen was hours away from going public in January 2001 when investor appetite for initial public offerings (IPOs) vanished, values fell, and significant additional investment was required. Spectros found that its first market dried up when a surgical procedure changed, but it didn't have a second product ready yet. Having an experienced board and mature, flexible investors with the patience to weather such changes is essential to keep the team going through such trying times.

One way to build early value is to provide services while your product is in development. Both Spectros and Xenogen provided subcontract services as a way to ensure early income and hone target-market skills. Another route is outlicensing. If this is done outside of your product focus, both the licensee and licensor can profit. For example, Spectros was the first to demonstrate and patent multiwavelength pulse oximetry spectroscopy use to noninvasively measure the concentration of substances in the bloodstream, such as total hemoglobin, the most common laboratory test in the United States, and carboxyhemoglobin. Spectros held very early core intellectual property on an array of biophotonic medical devices, including optical contrast-guided surgery, automated tissue classification and identification, multiwavelength oximetry and CO-oximetry, and tissue-guided surgical tools, as well as implantable and other optical physiology monitors. Here, Spectros proposed licensing to target firms (such as to Masimo, a biophotonics company that completed its IPO in 2007 and achieved a valuation of more than $2 billion for introducing multispectral pulse oximetry to the market). With this model in hand, Spectros began to seek licensing more aggressively. Such an approach worked well at Xenogen and allowed for licenses that generated significant income for the company from users of the technology.

18.7 Conclusions

In the end, entrepreneurship is not for everyone. There are real risks to personal income and career when you leave a secure academic or middle-management life. Begin by understanding yourself. What do you want and expect from a start-up? Are you comfortable with rapid change? What will you do if you fail?

When I was still in academics in the 1990s, the founder of the glucose-monitoring company LifeScan (still a billion-dollar division of J&J) told me that if I didn't leave medicine, I would always wonder what might have been. He was right.

Xenogen went public in 2004, and Spectros was profitable by 2007, with a revenue growth of 38% in 2006, while FirstScan is just making its transition from benchtop to business. Picking your stock symbol and watching it trade, seeing what you helped invent being used in universities and operating rooms everywhere, and knowing that lives have been saved or improved by what you helped create are experiences that are hard to beat.

References

[1] Robbins-Roth, C., *From Alchemy to IPO: The Business of Biotechnology*, Cambridge, MA: Perseus Publishing, 2000.

[2] Collins, J., *Good to Great: Why Some Companies Make the Leap . . . and Others Don't*, New York: HarperCollins Publishers, 2001.

About the Editors

Fred S. Azar is the external projects lead and a scientific investigator in the Department of Imaging and Visualization at Siemens Corporate Research Inc. (Princeton, New Jersey), where he is currently developing multimodal and optical imaging technologies for tracking and predicting cancer. Dr. Azar led the team that developed the first software prototype platform capable of integrating multimodal optical imaging data with X-ray mammography and magnetic resonance images of the breast and organized the first international conference dedicated to multimodal biomedical optical imaging. Dr. Azar served as a reviewer for several journals including *Academic Radiology, Theoretical Medicine, IEEE Transactions on Biomedical Engineering,* and *Medical Image Analysis.* He holds more than 15 provisional patents/patents, has given over 40 publications/invited talks, and has worked in the past for several leading institutions such as Sarnoff Corporation, the Montreal Neurological Institute, and GE Medical Systems. Dr. Azar earned a Ph.D. in bioengineering at the University of Pennsylvania and an M.S. in bioengineering at the Ecole Centrale Paris. He is currently pursuing an executive M.B.A. degree at the Wharton School.

Xavier Intes is an assistant professor in the Department of Biomedical Engineering at the Rensselaer Polytechnic Institute (RPI), Troy, New York. Prior to joining RPI, Dr. Intes was the chief scientist of Advanced Research Technologies Inc., Canada, a leader in optical molecular imaging. He has cowritten more than 80 published peer-reviewed papers in the field and serves as a reviewer for several science and engineering journals, including *Applied Optics, Optics Express, Medical Physics, JOSA A, Journal of Biomedical Optics, Technology in Cancer Research and Treatment, Optics Letters, IEEE Transactions in Medical Imaging, Neuroimage,* and the *Proceedings of the National Academy of Sciences.* He received a Ph.D. in physics from the Université de Bretagne Occidentale, France.

List of Contributors

Desmond C. Adler
50 Vassar Street
Room 36-345
Research Laboratory of Electronics
Massachusetts Institute of Technology
Cambridge, MA 02139
United States
e-mail: dadler@mit.edu

Aaron D. Aguirre
50 Vassar Street
Room 36-345
Research Laboratory of Electronics
Massachusetts Institute of Technology
Cambridge, MA 02139
United States
e-mail: aaguirre@mit.edu

Margarete K. Akens
Sunnybrook Health Sciences Centre
Room UB-19
2075 Bayview Avenue
Toronto, Ontario
M4N 3M5
Canada
e-mail: makens@uhnres.utoronto.ca

Simon Arridge
Department of Computer Science
University College London (UCL)
Room No. 5.04
Malet Street Engineering Building
London WC1E 6BT
United Kingdom
e-mail: S.Arridge@cs.ucl.ac.uk

Fred S. Azar
Department of Imaging and Visualization
Siemens Corporate Research Inc.
755 College Road East
Princeton, NJ 08540
United States
e-mail: FredAzar@alumni.upenn.edu

David A. Benaron
Spectros Corporation
Suites 100-109
4370 Alpine Road
Portola Valley, CA 94028
United States
e-mail: dbenaron@spectros.com

David Boas
Martinos Center for Biomedical Imaging
Massachusetts General Hospital
Harvard Medical School
Bldg. 149, 13th Street
Charlestown, MA 02129
United States
e-mail: dboas@nmr.mgh.harvard.edu

Stefan Carp
Martinos Center for Biomedical Imaging
Massachusetts General Hospital
Harvard Medical School
Bldg. 149, 13th Street
Charlestown, MA 02129
United States
e-mail: carp@nmr.mgh.harvard.edu

Colin M. Carpenter
Thayer School of Engineering
Dartmouth College
8000 Cummings Hall
Hanover, NH 03755
United States
e-mail: Colin.M.Carpenter@dartmouth.edu

Albert E. Cerussi
Beckman Laser Institute and Medical Clinic
University of California, Irvine
1002 Health Sciences Road East
Irvine, CA 92612
United States
e-mail: acerussi@uci.edu

Yu Chen
2330A Jeong H. Kim Engineering Building
Fischell Department of Bioengineering
University of Maryland
College Park, MD 20742
United States
e-mail: yuchen@umd.edu

Bruce A. Drum
Food and Drug Administration
9200 Corporate Boulevard
Rockville, MD 20850
United States
e-mail: bad@cdrh.fda.gov

Qianqian Fang
Martinos Center for Biomedical Imaging
Massachusetts General Hospital
Harvard Medical School
Bldg. 149, 13th Street
Charlestown, MA 02129
United States
e-mail: fangq@nmr.mgh.harvard.edu

James G. Fujimoto
Dept. of Electrical Engineering and
Computer Science
Research Laboratory of Electronics
Massachusetts Institute of Technology
77 Massachusetts Avenue
Cambridge, MA 02139
United States
e-mail: jgfuji@mit.edu

Pavel A. Fomitchov
GE Healthcare—Life Sciences
800 Centennial Avenue
Bldg. 3
Piscataway, NJ 08855
United States
e-mail: pavel.fomitchov@ge.com

Andrew J. Healey
GE Healthcare—Bio-Sciences
Nycoveien 2
P.O. Box 4220 Nydalen
NO-0401 Oslo
Norway
e-mail: andrew.healey@ge.com

Gavin Henry
Mivenion GmbH
Robert-Koch-Platz 4-8
10115 Berlin
Germany
e-mail: gavin.henry@bayerhealthcare.com

Nola M. Hylton
Magnetic Resonance Science Center
Helen Diller Family Comprehensive Cancer Center
University of California, San Francisco
1 Irving Street
Room A-C109
San Francisco, CA 94143
United States
e-mail: Nola.Hylton@radiology.ucsf.edu

Xavier Intes
Biomedical Engineering Department
Rensselaer Polytechnic Institute
110 8th Street
Troy, NY 12180-3590
United States
e-mail: intesx@rpi.edu

Shudong Jiang
Thayer School of Engineering
Dartmouth College
8000 Cummings Hall
Hanover, NH 03755-8000
United States
e-mail: Shudong.Jiang@Dartmouth.edu

Mario Khayat
ART Advanced Research Technologies
2300 Alfred Nobel, Technoparc Saint-Laurent
Montreal QC H4S 2A4
Canada
e-mail: mkhayat@art.ca

Catherine Klifa
Magnetic Resonance Science Center
Helen Diller Family Comprehensive Cancer Center
University of California, San Francisco
1 Irving Street
Room A-C109
San Francisco, CA 94143
United States
e-mail: klifa@mrsc.ucsf.edu

Ville Kolehmainen
Department of Physics
University of Kuopio
P.O. Box 1627
FIN-70211 Kuopio
Finland
e-mail: ville.kolehmainen@uku.fi

Soren D. Konecky
Department of Physics and Astronomy
University of Pennsylvania
209 South 33rd Street
Philadelphia, PA 19104-6396
United States
e-mail: skonecky@student.physics.upenn.edu

Ang Li
Beckman Laser Institute and Medical Clinic
University of California, Irvine
1002 Health Sciences Road East
Irvine, CA 92612
United States
e-mail: lia@uci.edu

Kai Licha
Mivenion GmbH
Robert-Koch-Platz 4-8
10115 Berlin
Germany
e-mail: kai.licha@chemie.fu-berlin.de

D. Lothar Lilge
Ontario Cancer Institute
Princess Margaret Hospital
610 University Avenue, Room 7-416
Toronto, Ontario M5G2M9
Canada
e-mail: lilge@uhnres.utoronto.ca

Stephen J. Lomnes
Sunstone Biosciences, Inc.
3701 Market Street
4th Floor
Philadelphia, PA 19104
United States
e-mail: steve.lomnes@sunstones.com

Hiroshi Mashimo
VA Boston Medical Center
VAMC Research 151
1400 VFW Parkway
West Roxbury, MA 02132
United States
e-mail: hiroshi.mashimo@med.va.gov

Vasilis Ntziachristos
Institute for Biological and Medical Imaging (IBMI)
Technical University of Munich
Helmholtz Center Munich
Ingolstädter Landstraße 1
85764 Neuherberg
Germany
e-mail: v.ntziachristos@tum.de

List of Contributors

Christos Panagiotou
Department of Computer Science
University College London (UCL)
Room No. 5.08
Malet Street Engineering Building
London WC1E 6BT
United Kingdom
e-mail: c.panagiotou@cs.ucl.ac.uk

T. Joshua Pfefer
Food and Drug Administration
10903 New Hampshire Avenue
Bldg. 62
Rm. 1222
Silver Spring, MD 20993-0002
United States
e-mail: Joshua.pfefer@fda.hhs.gov

Daqing Piao
School of Electrical and Computer Engineering
Oklahoma State University
202 Engineering South
Stillwater, OK 74078-5032
United States
e-mail: daqing.piao@okstate.edu

Brian W. Pogue
Thayer School of Engineering
Dartmouth College
8000 Cummings Hall
Hanover, NH 03755
United States
e-mail: Brian.W.Pogue@dartmouth.edu

Michael Schirner
Mivenion GmbH
Robert-Koch-Platz 4-8
10115 Berlin
Germany
e-mail: schirner@mivenion.com

Ralf B. Schulz
Institute for Biological and Medical Imaging (IBMI)
Technical University of Munich
Helmholtz Center Munich
Ingolstädter Landstraße 1
85764 Neuherberg
Germany
e-mail: r.schulz@dkfz.de

Martin Schweiger
Department of Computer Science
University College London (UCL)
Room No. 5.07
Malet Street Engineering Building
London WC1E 6BT
United Kingdom
e-mail: martins@medphys.ucl.ac.uk

Juliette Selb
Martinos Center for Biomedical Imaging
Massachusetts General Hospital
Harvard Medical School
Bldg. 149
13th Street
Charlestown, MA 02129
United States
e-mail: juliette@nmr.mgh.harvard.edu

Natasha Shah
Beckman Laser Institute and Medical Clinic
University of California, Irvine
1002 Health Sciences Road East
Irvine, CA 92612
United States
e-mail: nshah@uci.edu

Bruce J. Tromberg
Beckman Laser Institute and Medical Clinic
University of California, Irvine
1002 Health Sciences Road East
Irvine, CA 92612
United States
e-mail: bjtrombe@uci.edu

Thomas D. Wang
Division of Gastroenterology
Department of Biomedical Engineering
University of Michigan
109 Zina Pitcher Pl. BSRB 1522
Ann Arbor, MI 48109-2200
United States
e-mail: Thomaswa@umich.edu

Arjun G. Yodh
Department of Physics and Astronomy
University of Pennsylvania
209 South 33rd Street
Philadelphia, PA 19104-6396
United States
e-mail: yodh@dept.physics.upenn.edu

Index

3D-DOT/3D-MRI image-registration, 144–51
2D-signatures flowchart, 150
    challenges, 144
    global flowchart, 150
    intensity-based, 145
    nonrigid algorithm, 146–48
    parameter space, 148
    projection geometries, 146
    projection images, 146
    similarities measure, 146–48
3D forward modeling, 190
5-ALA, 227, 228, 230, 231

A

Ablation mechanisms, 320–21
Absorbers, optical tissue phantoms, 243
Absorption, 3–4
    coefficient spectra, 4
    decoupling, 65–70
    near-infrared (NIR), 59
    scatter phantom composition, 242–45
Absorptive stains, 42
Ac/dc attenuation rate, 68
Acquisition system, 283–84
Adjoint Fréchet derivative, 104–5
Aim and scope, this book, *xix–xx*
    From Alchemy to IPO: The Business of Biotechnology (Robbins-Roth), 366
Anatomical imaging, 126–28
Applicator array, 93
Aqueous suspension phantoms, 251–53
    advantages, 251
    container choice, 252–53
    example, 252
    See also Optical phantoms
Arterial-spin-labeling (ASL), 130
Autofluorescence, 265
    endoscopy, 39
    imaging (AFI), 41
    tissue type and, 265
Avalanche photodiode (APD), 69

B

Bayesian framework, 102, 103
Best linear unbiased estimator (BLUE), 192
Bioluminescence imaging (BLI), 344, 345
Blood-oxygen-level-dependent (BOLD)
    gradient-echo, 128
    MRI imaging, 128, 233
    spin-echo, 128
Body cavities, PDT in, 231–32
Breast cancer, 276–77
    DOS in, 163–82
    screening and diagnosis, 185–86
    statistics, 276
Breast cancer imaging
    DOT advances, 187–88
    dynamic, under mechanical compression, 194–98
    modalities, 276
    optical technology, 277
    sensitivity, 186
    specificity, 186
    TOBI/DBT, 193–94
    tomographic system, 188–90
Breast-contour imaging (BCI), 284
Breast MRI image segmentation, 151–52
    illustrated, 151
    workflow, 152
Breast-only PET (BPET), 209–10, 216
Business mentors, 365

C

Calibration coefficient estimation, 190–91
Canadian Medical Devices Regulations (CMDR), 281
Center for Devices and Radiological Health (CDRH), 305
    approvals, 313
    Product Classification Database, 307
    See also FDA regulation
Center for Drug Evaluation and Research (CDER), 305, 313
Cerebral blood flow (CBF), 129

Cerebral blood volume (CBV), 129
Cerebral plasma volume (CPV), 129, 210
Charge-coupled device (CCD)
　camera, 210, 348
　detector, 20
　exposure, 213, 214
　intensified (ICCD), 39
Chemotherapy
　ctTHb decrease during, 180
　neoadjuvant, monitoring/predicting, 163, 176–81
　treatment sequence, 177
Chromoendoscopy, 42–43
　chemical straining, 42
　with dyes, 42
　results, 43
Cimmino algorithm, 234
Clinical indication, 279–80
Clinical plan, 286
Clinical trials, 286–94
　clinical plan, 286
　pilot studies, 286–87
　tissue-characterization, 287–94
　See also Medical device commercialization
cMRI, 171–74, 176
　high-resolution, 181
　measurements, 176
Collection optics, 267–68
Complete lymph node biopsy (CLNB), 260
Complications
　in coronary artery bypass graft (CABG), 262
　rate, reducing, 261–62
Compression force recordings, 197
Computed tomography (CT)
　contrast, 254
　DOT (CT-DOT), 101
Confocal microscopy, 19–30
　defined, 20
　dual-axes, 20, 25–27
　EC-3870K, 21, 22
　endoscope-compatible, 20–22
　fluorescence sensitivity, 27
　illustrated, 21
　introduction to, 19–20
　MKT Cellvizio-GI, 23–25
　Optiscan, 21, 22
　peptide binding on, 29
Contact pressure map, 197–98
Continuous-wave (CW) ablation, 321
Continuous-wave detection, 70
Contrast agents, 327–37
　clinically approved, 329
　fluorescent nanoparticles, 331–32
　fluorophore conjugates, 330–31
　fluorophores as, 328–30
　introduction, 327–28
　MRI/optical imaging, 332–35
　multimodality probes, 332–37
　optical probes, 328–32
　SPECT/PET, 335–36
　summary and conclusions, 337
　therapy/optical imaging, 336–37
　See also Probes
Contrast-enhanced MRI, 185
Contrast media, 262–63
Contrast stains, 42
Coregistration with MRI, 163, 164–76
　case studies, 169–74
　cMRI, 171–74
　discussion, 175–76
　DOS instrumentation and measurements, 164–66
　fibroadenoma, 170–71
　invasive ductal carcinoma, 170
　materials and methods, 164–67
　MRI measurements, 166–67
　normal volunteers, 168–69
　results, 167–74
　subjects, 164
　See also Magnetic resonance imaging (MRI)
Coronary artery bypass graft (CABG) procedures, 262
Cross-sectional imaging, 44–51
　multimodality, 47–51
　OCT, 44–45
　three-dimensional OCT, 46–47
　ultrahigh-resolution OCT, 45–46

D

Data-collection modes, 345–47
Deexcitation, 228
Deoxyhemoglobin (Hb), 277
Detectors, 268
Development process, 277–86
　clinical indication, 279–80
　design control, 285–86
　effective, 277–78
　feedback, 278
　general device description, 282–85
　product definition, 278–79
　regulatory risk classification, 282
　synchronization, 278
　target markets, 280–82
　See also Medical device commercialization

Index

Diffuse optical imaging (DOI), 210–12
    clinical studies, 275–94
    fluorescence (FDOI), 205, 207, 212–14
    image reconstruction, 211–12
    initial research phase, 206
    instrumentation, 210
    with MRI, 163–82
    with PET imaging, 205–20
    with X-ray imaging, 185–99
Diffuse optical spectroscopy (DOS)
    anatomical imaging, 126–28
    in breast cancer, 163–82
    image-based guidance workflow, 152–53
    lipid content, 174
    measurements, 164–66
    with MRI, 125–36
    MRI-guided, 109
    as noninvasive bedside technique, 143
    predictive value, 179
    sensitivity, 177–80
    software platform, 142–43
    THC, 174
    tissue oxygen saturation, 174
    validation by high-resolution cMRI, 181
    water content, 174
Diffuse optical techniques, 59
Diffuse optical tomography (DOT), 59–94, 102–8, 347
    for breast cancer imaging, 187–88
    computed tomography (CT-DOT), 101
    continuous-wave, 70
    data of human subjects, 155–57
    defined, 59, 102
    detector decoding, 62–65
    forward model, 103
    forward problem, 103–6
    frequency-domain, 68–69
    imager, 73–76
    instrumentation, 60
    integrated with MRI, 75–76
    integrated with ultrasound, 74–75
    inverse problem, 106–8
    measurement instrumentation, 93
    MRI (MRI-DOT), 101
    NIR, 60, 141
    novel instrumentation approaches, 76–93
    photon origin differentiation, 60–65
    reconstruction, 70–73, 142
    software platform, 141–42
    source encoding methods, 62–65
    source-encoding requirement, 61–62
    source spectral encoding, 76–85

    spatial resolution, 108
    time-domain, 66–67
    transrectal applicator, 85–93
    ultrasound (US-DOT), 101
Diffuse reflectance spectroscopy (DRS), 34
Diffusion approximation (DA), 103
Diffusion equation, 8–9
Diffusion-weighted MR imaging (DWI), 133
Diffusivity, 112
Digital breast tomosynthesis (DBT), 185
Direct Fréchet derivative, 104
Discrete spectral encoding, 76–78
Doppler ultrasonography, 185
Dual axes confocal microscope, 25–27
    actuation, 25
    defined, 25
    fluorescence detection, 26–27
    illustrated, 26
    imaging parameter comparison, 28
    MEMS mirror, 25
    See also Confocal microscopy
Dynamic breast imaging, 194–98
    contact pressure map under compression, 197–98
    experimental setup, 194–95
    tissue dynamics, 195–97
    See also Breast cancer imaging
Dynamic contrast-enhanced MRI (DCE-MRI), 127
Dynamic F-FDG PET imaging, 235

E

Edge prior information, 111
Elastic scattering spectroscopy (ESS), 34, 35
Emission filtering, 267–68
Endoscope-compatible confocal microscopy, 20–22
Endoscopy, 33–51
    autofluorescence, 39
    cross-sectional imaging, 44–51
    introduction to, 33
    light-induced fluorescence (LIFE), 39–40
    point-probe spectroscopy techniques, 33–39
    wide-field imaging, 39–44
Entropy
    information, 115
    joint, 116–18
    as measure of randomness, 116
Excitation
    deexcitation and, 228
    power density, 267
    sources, 267

F

Failure-mode effects and criticality analysis (FMECA), 285
FDA
  authorizing legislation, 304
  history, 304
  mission, 304
  organizational chart, 306
  organizational structure, 305
FDA regulations, 305–15
  Class I, 308–9
  Class II, 309
  Class III, 309
  classification, 307–9
  combination products and contrast agents, 313
  early premarket interactions, 310–11
  good practices, 314–15
  guidance documents, 313–14
  institutional review boards, 310
  investigational device exemption, 310–11
  postmarket issues, 312–13
  Premarket Approval, 312
  Premarket Notification, 311
  premarket submissions, 311–12
  presubmission meeting, 310
  regulatory submission aids, 313–14
  See also Medical device regulation
Finite element mesh (FEM), 109
Finite element method (FEM), 106, 190
Fluorescein, 262–63
Fluorescence, 4–6
  compounds, 5–6
  confocal microscopy sensitivity, 27
  defined, 4–5
  FMN, 5
  ICG, 216–19
  NAD+, 5
  OCT and, 48–51
  properties, 5
  reflectance-based, 265–67
Fluorescence DOI (FDOI), 205, 207, 212–14
  fluorophore concentration, 213
  reconstruction, 213
  scan protocol, 212
  success, 214
  in vivo, 219
Fluorescence imaging, 39–41, 345
  AFI system, 41
  dysplasia identification, 40
  LIFE, 39–40
  planar, 346
Fluorescence molecular tomography (FMT), 347–50
  developments, 354–55
  fluorescent protein tomography, 351–53
  generations, 348
  hardware development, 347–48
  image reconstruction, 349
  intrinsic resolution limits, 350
  mesoscopic fluorescence tomography, 353–54
  modalities, 351–55
  multimodality imaging and, 355
  multiple wavelengths and, 354–55
  noncontact, 351
  PAT imaging combination, 357
  time resolution and, 355
Fluorescence spectroscopy, 36–37
  defined, 36
  with exogenous contrast agents, 37
  for HGD, 36–37
  for LGD, 37
  probe depths, 36
Fluorescent-labeled peptides, 28
Fluorescent nanoparticles, 331–32
Fluorescent protein tomography, 351–53
Fluorophores, 328–30
  conjugates, 330–31
  dissolved in aqueous solution, 244
  optical tissue phantoms, 243
Focus, 366
Forward problem, 103–6
  adjoint Fréchet derivative, 104–5
  direct Fréchet derivative, 104
  forward operator, 104
  See also Diffuse optical tomography (DOT)
Fourier-domain OCT, 47
Frequency-based multiplexing, 63–64
  advantage, 64
  defined, 63
  operator, 63
  See also Source encoding
Frequency-domain detection, 68–69
  defined, 68
  instrumentation, 69
  technique illustration, 68
Frequency-domain photon-migration (FDPM), 164–65
Functional MRI (fMRI), 129
  in EEG/MEG inverse problem, 108
  optical imaging and, 129
  See also Magnetic resonance imaging (MRI)
Fusing function, 186–87

Index

G

Gamma rays, 9
Gauss-Newton method, 107, 113
Gd-DTPA, 135
Gelatin phantoms
  defined, 245
  disadvantage, 248–49
  mixing procedure, 248
  recipe, 248
  See also Optical phantoms
Generalized Gaussian Markov random field (GGMRF) functionals, 111
Global accuracy, 153–54
Global Harmonization Task Force (GHTF), 303
Good Clinical Practice (GCP), 314, 315
Good Laboratory Practice (GLP), 314–15
Good Manufacturing Practice (GMP), 314, 315
Good to Great (Collins), 366
G-protein-coupled receptors (GPCRs), 330
Gradient-echo BOLD, 128
Guidance documents, 313–14

H

HANDHELD, 142, 143
  current session, 152–53
  defined, 152
  reference session, 152
  sensors, 153
  workflow, 152–53
Hemodynamic imaging
  MRI and Optical imaging, 128–31
  quantification, 131
  by spread spectral encoding, 84–85
  tumor vascular, 130
High-grad dysplasia (HGD)
  fluorescence spectroscopy and, 36
  PDT for, 232
  scattering spectroscopy and, 34, 35
Hydrogel-based phantoms, 245–49
  disadvantage, 248–49
  gelatin, 245
  mixing procedure, 248
  recipe, 248
  water encapsulation, 245
  See also Optical phantoms

I

ICG fluorescence, 216–19
  absorption contrast, 219
  fDOI in humans with, 219
  use of, 216
India ink, 243
Indocyanine green, 262
Inelastic scattering, 38
Intensified CCD (ICCD), 39
Intensity-based registration, 145
International harmonization, 303–4
Intracranial PDT, 232
Intraoperative NIR fluorescence imaging, 259–69
  autofluorescence, 265
  collection optics, 267–68
  complication rate reduction, 261–62
  considerations, 262–68
  contrast media, 262–63
  detectors, 268
  emission filtering, 267–68
  excitation, 267
  future, 268–69
  long-term efficiency of primary treatment, 260–61
  medical needs addressed by, 259–62
  optical design considerations, 265–67
  tissue penetration depth, 263–65
Inverse problem, 106–8
  discretization of unknowns, 107
  finite element method (FEM), 106
In vivo microscopy, 19–30
Iron oxide nanoparticles, 336
Iterative closest point (ICP)-based algorithm, 153

J

Jablonski diagram, 229
Joint entropy, 116–18
  defined, 116
  illustrated, 117
  interpretation, 117
  low, 118

L

Labeling, 302
Laser-assisted in situ keratomileusis (LASIK), 320
Laser diodes (LDs), 76–78
  multiple, for spectral encoding, 83
  spectral-encoding technique, 81
Light-emitting diode (LED), 81
  idealized, 82
  output, 82
  superluminescent (SLED), 81
Light-induced fluorescence endoscopy (LIFE), 39–40

Light propagation, 6–9
  diffusion equation, 8–9
  forward model, 7–9
  fundamentals, 6–7
  Monte Carlo (MC) method, 8
  radiation transport equation (RTE), 7, 8
Light-scattering spectroscopy (LSS), 34, 35, 36
Lipid microparticles, 244
Low-coherence interferometry (LCI), 44
Low-grade dysplasia (LGD)
  fluorescence spectroscopy for, 37
  scattering spectroscopy for, 34, 35
Lymphatic staging, 260

M

Magnetic resonance imaging (MRI), 9
  BOLD imaging, 128
  breast image segmentation, 151–52
  contrast-enhanced, 185
  coregistration with, 163, 164–76
  DOS with, 125–36
  DOT (MRI-DOT), 75–76, 101
  dynamic contrast-enhanced (DCE-MRI), 127
  functional (fMRI), 108, 129
  hemodynamic measures, combining, 128–31
  kinetic contrast parameter changes, 174
  nonconcurrent, application to, 155–57
Magnetic resonance (MR)
  BOLD signal, 128
  breast tumor characterization, 127
  coil size, 134
  contrast, 133–34
  diffusion-weighted imaging, 133
  Gd-DTPA, 135
  optical imaging, 127
  structural data, 126
  weighted images, 127
Market identification, 363–64
Maximum randomness, 117
Mechanical tissue relaxation, 196
Medical device commercialization
  clinical indication, 279–809
  clinical plan, 286
  clinical trials, 286–94
  conclusions, 294
  design control, 285–86
  development process, 277–86
  general device description, 282–85
  introduction, 275–76
  pilot studies, 286–87
  product definition, 278–79
  regulatory risk classification, 282
  target markets, 280–82
  tissue-characterization trials, 287–94
Medical device regulation, 299–322
  classification, 307–9
  combination products and contrast agents, 313
  conclusions, 322
  early premarket interactions, 310–11
  effectiveness, 301
  FDA, 305–15
  fundamental concepts, 300–302
  good practices, 314–15
  international harmonization, 303–4
  introduction, 299–300
  labeling, 302
  optical safety hazards, 315–22
  postmarket, 301, 312–13
  premarket, 301
  premarket submissions, 311–12
  regulatory submission aids, 313–14
  risk evaluation, 301–2
  safety, 301
  standards, 302
  throughout the world, 302–4
Medical device reporting (MDR), 312
Medical Devices Directive (MDD), 281
Mesoscopic fluorescence tomography, 353–54
Metronomic PDT (mPDT), 236
Micro-electro-mechanical systems (MEMS), 20, 30
MKT Cellvizio-GI, 23–25
  beam scanning, 23–24
  defined, 23
  illustrated, 23
  images, 24
  imaging parameter comparison, 28
  key features, 25
  for lung, 25
  See also Confocal microscopy
Molecular imaging, 27–30, 41–42
  miniaturized endoscope devices, 42
  promises of, 41
Monomolecular multimodal imaging agents (MOMIAs), 336
Monte Carlo (MC) method, 8
Motion tracking, 154–55
MRI-guided DOS, 109
MRI-guided optical imaging reconstruction, 131–33
MRI-inferred prior information, 110

MRI/optical imaging probes, 332–35
    design illustration, 334
    light scattering, 333
Multimodal DOT, 101–19
    conclusions, 119
    introduction to, 101–2
    priors and regularization, 111–19
    reconstruction, 108–11
Multimodality
    optical/MR instruments, 134
    priors, 111–13
    reconstruction, 108–11
    regularization, 113–19
Multimodality imaging, 9–13
    history, 9–10
    with OCT, 47–51
    optical, 10–13
    optical phantoms, 241–54
    tissue phantoms, 245–53
    wide-field, 43–44
Multimodality probes, 332–37
    optical imaging and MRI, 332–35
    optical imaging and SPECT/PET, 335–36
    optical imaging and therapy, 336–37
Multimodality spectroscopy, 38–39
Mutual information
    in medical imaging, 114
    reconstruction with, 118
    regularization with, 113–19

N

Nanoparticle structures, 332
Narrowband imaging (NBI), 43
Near-infrared (NIR)
    absorption, 59, 178
    diffuse propagation, 59
    DOT, 60, 141
    image reconstructions, 72–73, 74
    intraoperative fluorescence imaging, 259–69
    light, 59
    reduced-scattering spectra, 178
    video-rate imaging, 78
Negative predictive value (NPV), 29
Neoadjuvant chemotherapy monitoring/
        predicting, 163, 176–81
    binary classification, 177–79
    chemotherapy treatment sequence, 177
    discussion, 180–81
    DOS predictive value, 179
    DOS sensitivity, 177–80
    materials/methods, 176–77
    measurement sequence, 177
    patient characteristics, 177
    results, 177–80
    tertiary classification, 179–80
Noncontact FMT, 351
Nonlinear image reconstruction, 190

O

Optical and Multimodal Imaging Platform for
        Research Assessment and Diagnosis
        (OMIRAD), 142
    analysis, 144
    input, 143
    registration, 144
    segmentation, 144
    visualization, 143–44
    workflow, 143–44
Optical coherence tomography (OCT), 44–51
    applying to noninvasive imaging, 93
    defined, 44
    EUS and, 47–48
    fluorescence and, 48–51
    integration, 45
    LCI basis, 44
    LIF combined with, 49
    multimodal, 101–19
    multimodality imaging with, 47–51
    speckle variance, 235
    spectral-domain, 47
    swept-source, 47
    three-dimensional, 46–47
    ultrahigh-resolution (UHR), 45–46
    uses, 45
    wide-field fluorescence combined with, 50–51
Optical frequency-domain imaging (OFDI), 47
Optical imaging
    case example, xviii–xix
    dynamic, 188
    introduction to, 1–13
    MRI hemodynamic measures combined
        with, 128–31
    multimodality, 10–13
    multimodality probes for, 332–37
    photon scatter sensitivity, 133
    software platforms, 141–58
    technologies, xvii–xviii
Optical/MR
    combination, 128–31
    contrast agents, 135–36
    hardware challenges, 134–35
    multimodality instruments, 134
    outlook, 136

Optical/MR (continued)
  reconstruction techniques, 131–33
Optical phantoms, 241–54
  absorption, 242–45
  aqueous suspension, 251–53
  classes, 247
  conclusions, 253–54
  fluorophores, 243
  hydrogel-based, 245–49
  introduction to, 241–42
  for multimodal imaging, 245–53
  polyester resin, 249–51
  RTV silicon, 249–51
  scattering agents, 246
  scatter phantom composition, 242–45
  short-term usage, 244
  spectrum, 244
  See also Multimodality imaging
Optical probes, 328–32
  fluorescent nanoparticles, 331–32
  fluorophore conjugates, 330–31
  fluorophores, 328–30
Optical properties, 70–76
  diffuse optical tomography, 73–76
  tomographic image reconstruction, 70–73
Optical safety hazards, 315–22
  photochemical damage, 316–17
  photomechanical damage, 320–22
  photosensitivity, 318
  photothermal effects, 318–20
  See also Medical device regulation
Optiscan confocal imaging system, 21, 22
Oxyhemoglobin (HbO_2), 277

P

Penetration depth, 263–65
  in diffuse optics regime, 263
  as function of light wavelength, 264
Pentax EC-3870K confocal microscopy, 21, 22
  images, 22
  imaging parameter comparison, 28
  system elements, 21
  See also Confocal microscopy
Peptides
  fluorescent-labeled, 28
  as molecular probes, 28
PET/CT, 186
PET/DOI, 214–20
  breast-only, 216
  clinical observations, 214–19
  ICG fluorescence, 216–19
  summary, 219–20
  whole-body, 214–16
Phase delay, 68
Photoacoustic tomography (PAT), 355–57
  combined FMT imaging, 357
  defined, 355
  system development, 356
  theory, 356–57
Photochemical damage, 316–17
Photodynamic therapy (PDT), 48, 225–36
  adjuvant intracranial, 232
  basics, 227–30
  in body cavities, 231–32
  cosmetic tissue healing, 231
  current indications, 225
  defined, 225
  delivery, 235
  efficacy, 229
  enabling/improving, 225
  future of, 236
  HGD and, 232
  light activation, 235
  limitations, 233
  long-term treatments, 236
  metronomic (mPDT), 236
  model therapy, 225
  monitoring, 235–36
  mutagenic effects, 229
  oncological applications, 226
  optical imaging techniques, 226
  orders of magnitude, 229
  Photofrin-mediated, 232
  photosensitizers for, 336
  probes for, 336–37
  for solid tumors, 233–35
  superficial applications, 230–31
  tissue-response models, 230
  use of, 236
  vascular damage magnitude, 235
  whole-bladder, 232
Photofrin, 227
Photomechanical damage, 320–22
Photomultiplier tube (PMT), 74
  detectors, 76
  sensitivity and gain, 69
Photosensitivity, 318
Photosensitizers, 228
Photothermal effects, 318–20
Phototoxicity, 316
Pilot studies, 286–87
Planar fluorescence imaging, 346
Plasma-mediated ablation, 322

Point-probe spectroscopy, 33–39
Polyester resin phantoms, 249–51
Polymer microparticles, 244
Positive predictive value (PPV), 29
Positron emission tomography (PET), 9, 10, 207–10
   breast-only (BPET), 209
   defined, 205, 207
   DOI and, 205–20
   F-FDG, 209
   fundamentals, 207–8
   image reconstruction, 208–9
   instrumentation, 209–10
   probes, 336
   system matrix, 208
   tomographs, 207
   whole-body tomographs, 209
   See also PET/CT; PET/DOI
Premarket
   approval (PMA), 282, 312
   interactions, 310–11
   notification, 311
   submissions, 311–12
   See also Medical device regulation
Pressure distribution, 198
Priors
   spatial, 192
   spectral, 191–92
   structural, 111–13
Probability density function, 115, 149
Probes
   fluorescent nanoparticles, 331–32
   fluorophore conjugates, 330–31
   fluorophores, 328–30
   multimodality, 332–37
   optical, 328–32
   for optical imaging and MRI, 332–35
   for optical imaging and SPECT/PET, 335–36
   for optical imaging and therapy, 336–37
Product definition, 278–79
Prostate imaging, 85

Q
Quantum dots (QDs), 331

R
Radiation transport equation (RTE), 7, 8
   defined, 8
   diffusion approximation (DA) to, 103
   independent variables, 9

Raman scattering, 3
Raman spectroscopy, 38
Rayleigh scattering, 3
Receiver-operating-characteristic (ROC) curves, 291, 292
Reconstruction
   DOT, 70–73, 142, 211–12
   MRI-guided optical imaging, 131–33
   multimodality, 108–11
   with mutual information, 118
   nonlinear image, 190
   PET image, 208–9
   simultaneous image, 190–91
   spread spectral encoding, 83–84
   tomographic image, 70–73
Reflectance-based fluorescence, 265–67
Region-of-interest (ROI)
   analysis, 194
   tissue-characterization trials, 290
Registration
   2D-2D, 246
   3D-DOT/3D-MRI, 144–51
   intensity-based, 145
   OMIRAD, 144
   of volumetric data sets, 146
Regularization
   examples, 118–19
   with mutual information, 113–19
   structural prior, 111–13
   term, 111
Regulation. *See* Medical device regulation
Regulatory risk classification, 282
Regulatory submission aids, 313–14
Resin-based phantoms, 249–51
   CT images, 249
   defined, 249
   procedure, 250
   recipe, 250
   RTV, 250–51
   See also Optical phantoms
Resonance Raman scattering, 3
Risk evaluation, medical device regulation, 301–2
RTV silicone phantoms, 249–51

S
Safety
   in medical device regulation, 301
   optical, hazards, 315–22
   tissue-characterization trials, 293–94
Sagittal transrectal DOT applicator, 88–93
   experimental results, 91–93

Sagittal transrectal DOT applicator (continued)
    probe illustration, 89
    simulation for, 88–90
    See also Transrectal applicator
Scattering, 2–3
    agents, 244, 246
    defined, 2
    inelastic, 38
    Raman, 3
    Rayleigh, 3
Scattering spectroscopy, 34–36
    DRS, 34
    ESS, 34, 35
    LSS, 34, 35, 36
Scatter phantom composition, 242–45
Segmentation
    breast MRI image, 151–52
    OMIRAD, 144
Sentinel lymph node biopsy (SLNB), 260
Short-term usage phantoms, 244
Silicone phantoms, 250, 251
Simultaneous image reconstruction, 190–91
Single photon emission computed tomography (SPECT), 9, 10
Singlet oxygen luminescence, 230
SoftScan optical breast-imaging device, 280
    acquisition system, 283–84, 286
    defined, 282
    evolution, 287
    review workstation, 284–85
    See also Medical device commercialization
Software platforms, 141–58
    3D-DOT/3D-MRI, 144–51
    DOS, 142–43
    DOT, 141–42
    OMIRAD, 142, 143–44
    technologies, 143–53
Solid tumors, PDT for, 233–35
Source encoding
    in DOT, 61–62
    frequency-based multiplexing, 63–64
    methods, 62–65
    time-based multiplexing, 62–63
    wavelength-based multiplexing, 64–65
Spatial prior, 71, 192
Specific update ratio (SUR), 228
Speckle variance OCT, 235
SPECT/PET/optical imaging probes, 335–36
Spectral-domain OCT, 47
Spectral encoding, 64–65, 76–85
    discrete, 76–78

LD-based, 81
    rapid NIR tomography, 78–81
    spread, 80–85
Spectral prior, 191–92
Spectroscopy
    diffuse reflectance (DRS), 34
    elastic scattering (ESS), 34, 35
    fluorescence, 36–37
    light-scattering (LSS), 34, 35, 36
    multimodality, 38–39
    point-probe techniques, 33–39
    Raman, 38
    scattering, 34–36
Spin-echo BOLD, 128
Spread spectral encoding, 80–85
    characteristics, 82–84
    hemodynamic imaging by, 84–85
    light sources, 81–82
    linear fiber bundle, 82–83
    low-coherence source, 80
    reconstruction uncertainty, 83–84
    shift-free configuration, 80–81, 83–84
    by single wideband light source, 80–81
    See also Spectral encoding
Structural priors, 111–13
    diffusivity, 112
    examples, 113
    TV, with partial edges weighting, 116
    TV, with sum edges weighting, 115
Superluminescent diode (SLD), 81, 82
    defined, 81
    output, 82
    sources, 81
Superluminescent LED (SLED), 81
Swept-source OCT, 47

T

Target markets, 280–82
Target registration error (TRE), 156
Temporal point spread function (TPSF), 67
Three-dimensional OCT, 46–47
Tikhonov total variation, 111
Time-based multiplexing, 62–63
    advantage, 63
    defined, 62
    operator, 62–63
    See also Source encoding
Time-domain detection, 66–67
Time-of-flight detection, 67
Time-resolved Optical Absorption and Scattering Tomography (TOAST), 211

Tissue-characterization trials, 287–94
  descriptive statistics, 293
  effectiveness, 293–94
  lesion types, 290
  mean and standard deviation, 291
  objectives, 288
  optical properties, 289
  population demographics, 288–89
  preliminary sensitivity/specificity analysis, 289–93
  primary/secondary efficacy variables, 288
  ROC curve, 292
  ROI selection, 290
  safety, 293–94
  See also Medical device commercialization
Tissue optics, 2–6
  absorption, 3–4
  fluorescence, 4–6
  Raman scattering, 3
  scattering, 2–3
Tissue penetration depth, 263–65
Tissue phantoms, 241–54
  absorption, 242–45
  aqueous suspension, 251–53
  classes, 247
  conclusions, 253–54
  fluorophores, 243
  hydrogel-based, 245–49
  introduction to, 241–42
  for multimodal imaging, 245–53
  polyester resin, 249–51
  RTV silicon, 249–51
  scattering agents, 246
  scatter phantom composition, 242–45
  short-term usage, 244
  spectrum, 244
  See also multimodality imaging
Titanium-dioxide, 244
TOBI/DBT imaging
  clinical trial, 192–94
  defined, 192
  imaging (breasts with tumors/benign lesions), 193–94
  imaging (healthy breasts), 193
  ROI analysis, 194
  See also Tomographic optical breast-imaging (TOBI) system
Tomographic image reconstruction, 70–73
  illustrated, 71
  model-based NIR, 72–73

Tomographic optical breast-imaging (TOBI) system, 188–90
  defined, 188
  optical probes, 189
  photos, 189
  See also TOBI/DBT imaging
Tomosynthesis, 188–90
  spatial prior from, 192
  unit, 190
TOOKAD, 234, 235
Total hemoglobin concentration (THC), 155–57
  average values, 156
  distribution, 156
Transrectal applicator, 85–93
  for sagittal DOT imaging, 88–93
  for transverse DOT imaging, 86–88
  See also Diffuse optical tomography (DOT)
Transverse transrectal DOT applicator, 86–88
  internal-application images, 87, 88
  probe illustration, 87
  probe size, 86
  See also Transrectal applicator
Tumor response, 280
Tumor-to-background ratio (TBR), 216

U

Ultrahigh-resolution (UHR) OCT, 45–46
Ultrasound
  DOT integration with, 74–75
  DOT (US-DOT), 101

V

Value, building, 367
Vascular-space occupancy (VASO), 131
Visualization, OMIRAD, 143–44

W

Wavelength-based multiplexing, 64–65
  advantage, 65
  defined, 64
  operator, 64–65
  See also Source encoding
White metal-oxide powders, 244
Whole-bladder PDT, 232
Whole-body PET and DOI, 214–16
Wide-field imaging, 39–44
  chromoendoscopy, 42–43
  fluorescence imaging, 39–41
  molecular imaging, 41–42
  multimodality wide-field imaging, 43–44

narrowband imaging (NBI), 43
See also Multimodality imaging
Workflow
   breast MRI image, 152
   HANDHELD, 152–53
   image-based guidance, 152–53
   OMIRAD, 143–44

X

X-ray imaging, 9
   DOI with, 185–99
   mammography, 187